Imaging Complications of Gastrointestinal and Biliopancreatic Endoscopy Procedures

Massimo Tonolini
Editor

Imaging Complications of Gastrointestinal and Biliopancreatic Endoscopy Procedures

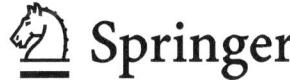

Editor
Massimo Tonolini
Department of Radiology
Luigi Sacco University Hospital
Milan
Italy

ISBN 978-3-319-31209-5   ISBN 978-3-319-31211-8   (eBook)
DOI 10.1007/978-3-319-31211-8

Library of Congress Control Number: 2016941181

Printed on acid-free paper

This Springer imprint is published by Springer Nature
The registered company is Springer International Publishing AG Switzerland

To Kumsa
who made me a father

During the last decades, digestive endoscopy significantly developed not only as a diagnostic technique but also in its operative-therapeutic applications.

Endoscopy increasingly has replaced surgery and previous radiological approaches in a variety of conditions, which up to some years ago required a surgical approach, such as endoscopic submucosal dissection of intramucosal tumors or endoscopic drainage of pseudocysts. In the diagnostic field, for instance, fine needle aspiration (FNA) of pancreatic masses is currently performed under echoendoscopy (EUS), whereas until a few years ago it required CT or ultrasound guide.

Over time some endoscopic methods, such as endoscopic retrograde cholangiopancreatography (ERCP), acquired an almost exclusive therapeutic role since the diagnosis increasingly relied on other modalities including CT, magnetic resonance imaging (MRI), and EUS.

This evolution has surely contributed to increase the risks related to endoscopic procedures.

In this scenario, the relationship between endoscopists and radiologists has become increasingly close in the past 20 years. Indeed, the accurate knowledge of the potential risks of operative endoscopic techniques requires collaboration between endoscopists and radiologists for two main reasons. First, advanced endoscopy increases the potential risk of perforation: when iatrogenic perforation is suspected, the contribution of the radiologist becomes essential both to make the diagnosis and to guide the treatment strategy. Second, with operative endoscopic procedures, the risk is not limited to perforation but encompasses other complications such as post-ERCP pancreatitis (where contrast-enhanced CT is crucial to assess the severity) and dislocation of metallic or plastic gastrointestinal or biliopancreatic stents. For instance, in my personal experience, a plastic stent placed in the common bile duct may dislodge, ulcerate, and penetrate the contralateral wall to the papilla of Vater, an occurrence which requires dedicated attention by the radiologist to reach a comprehensive diagnosis.

Therefore, when a complication occurs, a radiologist with appropriate knowledge on possible endoscopy-related injuries and with experience in interventional radiology is indispensable in treatment decision-making and sometimes in treating the complication itself, such as to drain intra-abdominal abscesses.

The therapeutic choice certainly requires not only support from the radiologist but also consultation with the surgeon, which allows to solve some challenging occurrences; this means that an interdisciplinary consultation before any complicated procedure is indispensable.

Besides the technical expertise, the endoscopist should possess a thorough clinical knowledge in order to better accomplish the procedure, to prevent risks related to it, and also to face them appropriately when they occur. The skilled endoscopist is always ready to approach any occasional and unforeseeable situation, even when they are not so simple. Thorough preparation and experience allow the endoscopist both to take the necessary precautions to reduce and prevent iatrogenic injuries and to adequately face the complications; as a result, the related morbidity and mortality will diminish over time.

With this in mind, not only is the the endoscopist manually performing a procedure, but also his/her work relies on accurate experience and knowledge in many areas: medical, oncological, surgical, and radiological. This expanded knowledge in multiple fields allows the endoscopist to face possible adverse outcomes and to plan an effective therapy.

In the future, digestive endoscopy will continue to be performed in the operative-therapeutic field, and emerging methods such as EUS will allow further applications of endoscopic procedures in different fields.

This could possibly lead to an increase of complications related to digestive endoscopy. The role of the endoscopist will be to prevent and reduce the related risks and that of the radiologist to recognize them and guide the endoscopist in his/her work so that the procedures can find wide application in clinical practice.

This book has clear radiological images and provides a comprehensive coverage of possible complications of endoscopy, which can help the operator in his/her "delicate" work.

Milan, Italy   Pietro Gambitta, MD

Contents

Massimo Tonolini

1.1 Background

Nowadays, gastrointestinal (GI) endoscopy is extensively used worldwide for diagnosis, screening, treatment and surveillance of a wide spectrum of alimentary tract symptoms and disorders. An estimate of 15–20 million endoscopies are performed annually in the United States. Although generally considered safe techniques with limited contraindications, digestive endoscopic procedures are associated with a non-negligible morbidity and occasional mortality. However, the true range and incidence of post-GI endoscopy adverse events are much greater than typically appreciated. In the past decade, hospitalisation rates of 1.1 % and 0.5 % were reported after upper GI endoscopy and colonoscopy, respectively [1, 2].

By reviewing more than 18,000 outpatient digestive endoscopies, a recent study disclosed that one out of 127 patients sought medical attention at emergency department (ED) within 2 weeks from the procedure. Hospital visit rates reached 0.79 % (95 % confidence interval 0.63–0.88 %), 1.07 % (CI 0.84–1.35 %), 0.84 % (CI 0.69–1.03 %) and 0.95 % (CI 0.75–1.19 %) for all endoscopies, upper GI, colonoscopies and screening colonoscopies, respectively, without statistically significant difference between these groups. The mean time of ED presentation after the procedure was 6 days (median 5.5 days) after upper GI endoscopy and 5.2 days (median 3.5 days) for colonoscopy. The commonest complaints were abdominal pain (47 %), digestive tract bleeding (12 %) and chest pain (11 %), followed by pneumonia and fever. The impressive range of reported adverse events included fall, exacerbation of congestive heart failure, dehydration, bowel perforation, syncope, atrial fibrillation, vomiting, back or neck pain, diarrhoea, transient ischaemic attack or cerebrovascular stroke, acute appendicitis, urinary retention, myocardial infarction, asthma, hepatic encephalopathy, hypoglycaemia, small bowel obstruction, cardiac arrest, deep venous thrombosis, acute pancreatitis and adynamic ileus. Approximately one-third of all ED visits were considered related to the recent endoscopic procedure, and more than half (56.7 %) of these resulted in hospitalisation. Interestingly, only one death was considered procedure related [3].

Firstly, the range, risk and severity of post-GI endoscopy complications significantly widened with the expansion of minimally invasive therapeutic interventions such as foreign body retrieval, stricture or anastomotic dilatation, positioning of gastroesophageal, duodenal or colonic stents, endoluminal haemostasis and variceal sclerotherapy, ablation of mucosal lesions, polypectomy, endoscopic mucosal resection and submucosal dissection [4–6].

M. Tonolini
Radiology Department, "Luigi Sacco" University Hospital, Via G.B. Grassi 74, Milan 20157, Italy
e-mail: mtonolini@sirm.org

© Springer International Publishing Switzerland 2016
M. Tonolini (ed.), *Imaging Complications of Gastrointestinal and Biliopancreatic Endoscopy Procedures*, DOI 10.1007/978-3-319-31211-8_1

Secondly, percutaneous endoscopic gastrostomy (PEG) has become established as the preferred minimally invasive technique to provide long-term nutrition support and prevent lung aspiration in patients with dysphagia or impaired swallowing and to palliate inoperable upper aerodigestive tumours. Despite the growing operators' experience, due to the steady increase in referrals, PEG-related complications are commonly encountered in most general hospitals and may occur during or shortly after insertion or result from devices left in place for a long time. The overall post-PEG complication rate approaches 21 %. Major occurrences are reported in approximately 3–4 % of patients but often need urgent surgery and are associated with a significant (17 %) mortality [7, 8].

Thirdly, due to the widespread availability of non-invasive imaging techniques such as magnetic resonance cholangiopancreatography (MRCP) and multidetector computed tomography (CT), during the last decade, endoscopic retrograde cholangiopancreatography (ERCP) transitioned from a diagnostic tool towards a primarily therapeutic procedure. Currently indispensable in surgical practice, ERCP is widely used to treat several biliopancreatic (BP) diseases and often allows obviating surgery. However, despite improvements in periprocedural care, ERCP has a non-negligible post-procedural morbidity (estimated in the range 4–10 % overall) and mortality (0.5–1.4 %). The incidence of ERCP-specific complications largely varies according to the underlying disease, patients' age and comorbidities, complexity of the procedure and operator's experience. In particular, the risk is significantly increased by operative techniques such as use of balloons and dilating catheters, tissue sampling, mechanical lithotripsy and wire baskets for stone extraction and positioning of plastic and metallic biliary stents [9–14].

1.2   Approach to Post-endoscopy Complications

Due to the large number of diagnostic and therapeutic GI and BP endoscopic procedures currently performed, clinicians and radiologists are increasingly faced with suspected iatrogenic complications, which represent a major cause of concern and often have unspecific clinical and laboratory manifestations [1–6, 9, 15]. Among post-endoscopy complications, medication-related cardiorespiratory and systemic events include oversedation, flushing, respiratory depression, aspiration, arrhythmias, hypertension, hypotension and vasovagal fainting, angina, myocardial infarction and stroke in descending order or frequency. With the increased use of operative techniques, PEG-related, specific GI endoscopy and post-ERCP complications such as perforation, bleeding, luminal obstruction and infections are increasingly encountered, particularly in elderly patients or with comorbidities [4–6, 9, 14, 15].

According to the guidelines issued by the American and European Societies for Gastrointestinal Endoscopy and by the World Society of Emergency Surgery (WSES), diagnosis and management of post-endoscopy complications should rely upon a combination of physical, laboratory and imaging data. Early diagnosis is essential in optimising management and outcome of post-endoscopy complications, particularly to triage those occurrences that require prolonged hospitalisation and to choose the most appropriate therapeutic approach between conservative treatment, surgery and endoscopic, percutaneous or endovascular interventions [6, 16].

Aimed at gastroenterologists, general surgeons and radiologists, this practical volume discusses the incidence, mechanisms, patient- and procedure-related risk factors, clinical features and treatment options (including endoscopic haemostasis, perforation closure, transarterial embolisation, percutaneous drainage and surgery) of post-endoscopy complications. The radiologic chapters review and illustrate with several case examples the imaging appearances of the commonest and unusual occurrences after upper GI endoscopy, ERCP (including sphincterotomy and positioning of biliary endoprosthesis), PEG positioning, colonoscopy, stricture dilatation and anorectal procedures. Since clinical assessment of severely ill patients is usually difficult, emphasis is placed on the pivotal role of CT to allow prompt efficient triage of endoscopy-specific complications. According to published guidelines and to our experience, multidetector CT represents the ideal imaging modality to identify intraluminal or extravisceral haemorrhage; signs of mediastinal, peritoneal or retroperitoneal perforation; acute pancreatitis; and infections [14, 16–19].

Specific attention is devoted to complications related to oesophageal, gastroduodenal and colorectal stents, to the issue of video capsule retention during small bowel capsule endoscopy and to iatrogenic colonoscopy perforations in patients with Crohn's disease and ulcerative colitis. Finally, a dedicated chapter discusses the role and possibilities of interventional radiology in the treatment of complications after digestive and biliopancreatic endoscopy.

By providing an increased familiarity with clinical and imaging manifestations of endoscopy-related complications, this book aims to enable radiologists and clinicians to diagnose and treat them in a timely fashion. The widespread use of CT will increasingly allow early diagnosis of post-endoscopy complications, thus preventing harmful delays and ultimately decreasing the iatrogenic morbidity and costs [6, 16].

References

1. Zubarik R, Fleischer DE, Mastropietro C et al (1999) Prospective analysis of complications 30 days after outpatient colonoscopy. Gastrointest Endosc 50:322–328
2. Zubarik R, Eisen G, Mastropietro C et al (1999) Prospective analysis of complications 30 days after outpatient upper endoscopy. Am J Gastroenterol 94:1539–1545
3. Leffler DA, Kheraj R, Garud S et al (2010) The incidence and cost of unexpected hospital use after scheduled outpatient endoscopy. Arch Intern Med 170:1752–1757
4. Ben-Menachem T, Decker GA, Early DS et al (2012) Adverse events of upper GI endoscopy. Gastrointest Endosc 76:707–718
5. Green J (2006) Complications of gastrointestinal endoscopy. British Society of Gastroenterology, London. Available at: http://www.bsg.org.uk/pdf_word_docs/complications.pdf. Accessed July 4th, 2015
6. Paspatis GA, Dumonceau JM, Barthet M et al (2014) Diagnosis and management of iatrogenic endoscopic perforations: European Society of Gastrointestinal Endoscopy (ESGE) position statement. Endoscopy 46:693–711
7. Gomes CA Jr, Lustosa SA, Matos D et al (2012) Percutaneous endoscopic gastrostomy versus nasogastric tube feeding for adults with swallowing disturbances. Cochrane Database Syst Rev (3):CD008096
8. Jain R, Maple JT, Anderson MA et al (2011) The role of endoscopy in enteral feeding. Gastrointest Endosc 74:7–12
9. Anderson MA, Fisher L, Jain R et al (2012) Complications of ERCP. Gastrointest Endosc 75:467–473
10. Kapral C, Duller C, Wewalka F et al (2008) Case volume and outcome of endoscopic retrograde cholangiopancreatography: results of a nationwide Austrian benchmarking project. Endoscopy 40:625–630
11. Silviera ML, Seamon MJ, Porshinsky B et al (2009) Complications related to endoscopic retrograde chol angiopancreatography: a comprehensive clinical review. J Gastrointest Liver Dis 18:73–82
12. Stapfer M, Selby RR, Stain SC et al (2000) Management of duodenal perforation after endoscopic retrograde cholangiopancreatography and sphincterotomy. Ann Surg 232:191–198
13. Glomsaker T, Hoff G, Kvaloy JT et al (2013) Patterns and predictive factors of complications after endoscopic retrograde cholangiopancreatography. Br J Surg 100:373–380
14. Tonolini M, Pagani A, Bianco R (2015) Cross-sectional imaging of common and unusual complications after endoscopic retrograde cholangiopancreatography. Insights Imag 6:323–338
15. Cotton PB (2006) Analysis of 59 ERCP lawsuits; mainly about indications. Gastrointest Endosc 63:378–382; quiz 464
16. Sartelli M, Viale P, Catena F et al (2013) 2013 WSES guidelines for management of intra-abdominal infections. World J Emerg Surg 8:3
17. Catalano O, De Bellis M, Sandomenico F et al (2012) Complications of biliary and gastrointestinal stents: MDCT of the cancer patient. AJR Am J Roentgenol 199:W187–W196
18. Pannu HK, Fishman EK (2001) Complications of endoscopic retrograde cholangiopancreatography: spectrum of abnormalities demonstrated with CT. Radiographics 21:1441–1453
19. Wax BN, Katz DS, Badler RL et al (2006) Complications of abdominal and pelvic procedures: computed tomographic diagnosis. Curr Probl Diagn Radiol 35:171–187

Complications of Upper Digestive Endoscopy

2

Alessandra Dell'Era

2.1 Upper Gastrointestinal Endoscopy: An Overview

Upper gastrointestinal endoscopy (UGIE) is a very common procedure performed to diagnose and treat a wide range of disorders. UGIE allows to investigate the upper digestive tract in case of anaemia and symptoms such as dyspepsia, dysphagia, vomiting and heartburn and diagnose (and eventually treat) the cause of haematemesis or melaena [1]. It is also used to follow up Barrett oesophagus and gastric ulcers.

2.1.1 The Procedure

UGIE, also known as oesophago-gastroduodenoscopy (EGDS), is an endoscopic procedure by which a scope (a flexible tube with a camera on the tips) is used to examine the upper GI tract. During UGIE the scope is inserted through the mouth and passed through the oesophagus, the stomach and the duodenum. During the withdrawal of the endoscope, while in the stomach, a

A. Dell'Era
Gastroenterology Unit, "Luigi Sacco" University Hospital, Via G.B. Grassi 74, Milan 20157, Italy

Department of Clinical and Medical Sciences, Università degli Studi di Milano, Via G.B. Grassi 74, Milan 20157, Italy
e-mail: alessandra.dellera@unimi.it

J-manoeuvre is performed to retroflex and accurately visualise the fundus and the gastro-esophageal junction. During the procedure air is inflated, water is injected and fluids aspirated to achieve a better visualisation. It can be used only to visualise the upper GI tract, but, usually, biopsies are taken.

By means of UGIE, interventional procedures can be performed (e.g. stents can be placed to treat stenosis, substances can be injected to treat haemorrhages and fine needle biopsies can be taken if an ultrasound-equipped endoscope is available).

2.1.2 Patient- and Procedure-Related Risk Factors and Contraindications

Contraindications to all medical procedures are all the situations in which the risks overweigh the benefits [1]. *Absolute contraindications* of UGIE are shock, acute myocardial infarction and perforation. *Relative contraindications* are cardiac arrhythmias, recent myocardial infarction, poor patient cooperation and neoplasms of the oropharyngeal tract (which may impede the passage of the endoscope).

In case of diagnostic and, more so, interventional endoscopy, the endoscopist should operate in the appropriate setting and should be trained in the endoscopic technique and management of all the possible complications.

M. Tonolini (ed.), *Imaging Complications of Gastrointestinal and Biliopancreatic Endoscopy Procedures*, DOI 10.1007/978-3-319-31211-8_2

2.2 Complications of Diagnostic Endoscopy

Complications of UGIE can be divided into those related to sedation (not treated in this chapter), diagnostic endoscopy and interventional endoscopy. Many of them are preventable and all should be recognised as soon as possible to institute the appropriate treatment. The imaging appearances of iatrogenic perforation and intraluminal bleeding are discussed in the following chapters.

Complications related to diagnostic evaluations are rare, with a rate of 0.13 % and an associated mortality of 0.004 % [2, 3].

2.2.1 Aspiration

UGIE is associated to a significant risk of *aspiration* (0.3–1.0 %) [4] that may cause pneumonia and eventually death. *Risk factors* for aspiration include elderly age, chronic illness, gastrointestinal bleeding, gastric outlet obstruction, depressed mental status, supine positioning and oversedation:

Clinical manifestations: severe coughing during/soon after endoscopy, onset of cyanosis and severe desaturation

Prevention: the endoscopist can reduce this risk by avoiding excessive sedation and gastric air insufflation, aspirating gastric contents before and after endoscopy.

Diagnosis: a chest X-ray should be performed.

Treatment options: in case of suspicion of aspiration, the patient should be stimulated to cough, secretions should be aspired from the mouth/throat and increased O2 should be given. In case of a confirmed aspiration, antibiotics should be started.

2.2.2 Bleeding

Severe *haemorrhage* occurs in 0.02–0.06 % of upper endoscopies [3]. *Risk factors* include antiplatelet therapy and anticoagulation [2]. Current guidelines state that biopsies can be performed in patients on anticoagulants within a therapeutic range and in those on NSAIDS and standard-dose aspirin [5].

Clinical and laboratory manifestations: immediate diagnosis can be made during endoscopy if bleeding (e.g. after a biopsy) does not stop. Late bleeding can be observed as melaena/haematemesis or a drop in haemoglobin levels.

Prevention: careful examination of the upper GI tract during withdrawal of the endoscope to identify potential bleeding sites and clip placement of the bleeding source to prevent further bleeding

Diagnosis: is usually made by repeated endoscopy

Treatment options: operative UGIE to treat the bleeding source is warranted; surgical intervention may be needed if endoscopy is not effective.

2.2.3 Perforation

Perforation in diagnostic upper GI endoscopy is a rare complication with an incidence of 0.008–0.04 % and a mortality rate of 0.001 % [2, 3]. *Risk factors* in patients with normal anatomy include all the sites where natural narrowing of the oesophagus occur (cricopharyngeus, aortic knob, diaphragmatic hiatus); anatomic anomalies (e.g. Zenker's or epiphrenic oesophageal diverticula, benign or malignant oesophageal strictures and mass lesions) contribute to perforation in up to 50 % of cases [6–8]. Endoscopist-dependent risk factors are blind or forced intubation and poor skill.

Clinical and laboratory manifestations: patients typically present with pain, tachycardia, fever, dysphagia, odynophagia, respiratory distress or sepsis [6–9]. Leucocytosis and pleural effusion may also be present. Recognition within 24 h provides a mortality benefit (<10 % versus >50 %).

Diagnosis: perforations may be diagnosed by plain radiograph of the neck and/or chest that shows air outside the lumen. Contrast media may help localise the perforation; however, a negative study does not rule out a perforation [10].

Treatment options: the approach depends on the size and site of the perforation, the clinical conditions of the patient and the overall prognosis. Treatment consists of clip placement on the perforation if it is recognised during endoscopy. Broad-spectrum antibiotics and, eventually, surgical repair may be needed. In selected patients without evidence of sepsis, with small perforations or significant comorbidities, nonsurgical management may be appropriate.

2.3 Complications of Therapeutic Endoscopy

Therapeutic endoscopy is associated with a tenfold increased risk of complications compared with diagnostic endoscopic. The reasons, besides those specifically related to the therapeutic technique performed, are longer procedures and need for a prolonged and sometimes deeper sedation [2].

2.3.1 Upper Gastrointestinal Dilation

Upper GI dilation is performed to widen a part of the upper GI tract, in order to allow the passage of food, using different techniques, such as wire-guided polyvinyl dilators (e.g. Savary–Gilliard) or balloon dilators. The most common complications are perforation, pain, haemorrhage and bacteraemia/sepsis. The overall *perforation* rate is 2–3 % with a mortality rate of 1 % and depends on the indication for the dilation. In the setting of benign peptic strictures, perforation is less common than in malignant strictures (1–2 % with a mortality of 0.5 % versus 4–6 % with a mortality of 2–3 %) [11–13]. The risk of perforation in dilations for achalasia is lower, being 0–7 % with a 1 % mortality, provided a graded dilation technique with low-compliance balloons is used [14].

Risks factors for perforation following oesophageal dilatation are inexperienced endoscopist, angulated or complex strictures and blind passage of weighted bougies.

Prevention: wire-guided or endoscopically controlled techniques should be used, performing radiographic screening when the stricture is complex/tortuous, associated to a large hiatus hernia

or diverticula or when the guidewire passage is difficult [15].

For *clinical and laboratory manifestations*, *diagnosis* and *treatment options*, refer to the paragraph on perforation in diagnostic endoscopy.

2.3.2 Oesophageal Stents

Oesophageal stents are used to establish oesophageal patency in neoplastic or peptic stenosis, relieving obstructive symptoms.

Self-expanding metal stents (SEMS) or self-expanding plastic stents (SEPS) are the most commonly used stents placed during UGIE for the treatment of malignant or benign oesophageal strictures [16, 17].

Post-placement complications occur in up to 20–40 % of cases with a mortality rate about 3 % [18]. The most common complication is *pain* (20 % of cases), followed by *stent migration* (5–15 %), *tumour ingrowth* (with the use of covered stents, 10–20 %) and food *impaction* (5–15 %). *Perforation* is a rare complication with the use of SEMS which have minimal dilation (1–2 %). *Haemorrhage* rate is difficult to evaluate, especially for stents placed for neoplasms, because often it cannot be distinguished from bleeding from the neoplasm.

Clinical and laboratory manifestations: stent migration, food impaction and tumour ingrowth can be suspected because of the recurrence of obstructive symptoms. Perforation can be often recognised during stent placement; sometimes symptoms as described above can lead to suspect perforation.

Prevention: blind dilation of malignant strictures should be avoided [11]. Expandable stents are preferable to non-expandable plastic stents [18, 19]. Covered stents may help preventing stent occlusion caused by tumour ingrowth.

Diagnosis: imaging appearances of specific stent-related complications are discussed in Chap. 4.

Treatment options: tumour ingrowth can be treated with thermal ablative techniques or insertion of another stent [20]. In case of stent migration, the stent should be removed and another stent placed. For treatment of *perforation* and *haemorrhage*, see the above paragraphs in diagnostic endoscopy.

2.3.3 Polypectomy and Endoscopic Mucosal Resection

Polyps of the upper gastrointestinal tract are a less common finding than in the lower gastrointestinal tract. They can be removed by biopsy forceps in case of diminutive size or by snare, in case of larger size. *Endoscopic mucosal resection* (*EMR*) and *endoscopic submucosal dissection* (*ESD*) are used to remove flat/depressed/sessile lesions of the superficial layers of the gastrointestinal tract by lifting the mucosal lesion injecting fluid into the submucosal layer and removing the lesion by snare (sometimes using a cap) or dedicated devices according to the technique.

Complications of *gastric polypectomy* are not frequent and include haemorrhage and perforation [21]. In case of *EMR/ESD*, complications are more frequent. *Bleeding* occurs in up to 1–45 % of the procedures, particularly in larger lesions and in the periprocedural period [22]. *Perforation* occurs in 4–10 % of ESD procedures and in 0.3–0.5 % of EMR [23]; it can be due to deeper muscle layer resection or to excessive cautery that causes transmural burn and delayed perforation.

Prevention: injection of adequate volume of fluid and identification of possible scarring in case of previous EMR

For *clinical and laboratory manifestations*, *diagnosis* and *treatment options*, see above.

2.3.4 Gastric Variceal Tissue Adhesive Injection

Gastric variceal bleeding should be treated, according to current recommendations, with intravariceal tissue adhesive injection [24]. The tissue adhesive, once in contact with the blood, polymerises forming a cast that occludes the varix; the glue can be mixed with lipid-soluble contrast agent Lipiodol to enhance radiopacity (even though this can cause slightly longer polymerisation times). The risks of the procedure are potentially fatal since the embolisation of the glue (2–5 %) may occur to the lungs, spleen, portal vein, inferior vena cava and brain, and extrusion of the glue plug may occur leading to massive bleeding [25].

Clinical manifestations depend on the site of the embolisation, ranging from neurologic impairment, dyspnoea and abdominal pain. Massive bleeding may present with haematemesis and/or melaena.

Diagnosis of the embolisation site can be done with X-ray or CT scan.

Treatment: no specific treatment is available for glue emboli, but symptomatic therapy.

References

1. ASGE Standards of Practice Committee, Early DS, Ben-Menachem T et al (2012) Appropriate use of GI endoscopy. Gastrointest Endosc 75:1127–1131
2. Silvis SE, Nebel O, Rogers G et al (1976) Endoscopic complications. Results of the 1974 American Society for Gastrointestinal Endoscopy Survey. JAMA 235:928
3. Froelich F, Gonvers J, Vader J et al (1999) Appropriateness of gastrointestinal endoscopy: risk of complications. Endoscopy 31:684–686
4. Eisen GM, Baron TH, Dominitz JA et al (2002) Complications of upper GI endoscopy. Gastrointest Endosc 55:784–793
5. Eisen GM, Baron TH, Dominitz JA et al (2002) Guideline on the management of anticoagulation and antiplatelet therapy for endoscopic procedures. Gastrointest Endosc 55:775–779
6. Pettersson G, Larsson S, Gatzinsky P et al (1981) Differentiated treatment of intrathoracic oesophageal perforations. Scand J Thorac Cardiovasc Surg 15:321–324
7. Schulze S, Pedersen VM, Hoier-Madsen K (1982) Iatrogenic perforation of the esophagus. Acta Chir Scand 148:679–682
8. Wychulis AR, Fontana RS, Payne WS (1969) Instrumental perforation of the esophagus. Dis Chest 55:184–189
9. Larsen K, Jensen B, Axelsen F (1983) Perforation and rupture of the esophagus. Scand J Thorac Cardiovasc Surg 17:311–316
10. Sawyer R, Phillips C, Vakil N (1995) Short- and long-term outcome of esophageal perforation. Gastrointest Endosc 41:130–134
11. Hernandez LV, Jacobson JW, Harris MS (2000) Comparison among the perforation rates of Maloney, balloon and Savary dilation of esophageal strictures. Gastrointest Endosc 51:460–462

12. Clouse RE (1996) Complications of endoscopic gastrointestinal dilation techniques. Gastroenterol Clin N Am 6:323–341

13. Newcomer MK, Brazer SR (1994) Complications of upper gastrointestinal endoscopy and their management. Gastroenterol Clin N Am 4:551–570

14. Nair LA, Reynolds JC, Parkman HP et al (1993) Complications during pneumatic dilation for achalasia or diffuse esophageal spasm: analysis of risk factors, early clinical characteristics, and outcome. Dig Dis Sci 38:1893–1904

15. Riley SA, Attwood SE (2004) Guidelines on the use of oesophageal dilatation in clinical practice. Gut 53(Suppl 1):i1–i6

16. Hindy P, Hong J, Lam-Tsai Y et al (2012) A comprehensive review of esophageal stents. Gastroenterol Hepatol 8:526–534

17. Sharma P, Kozarek R, Practice Parameters Committee of American College of Gastroenterology (2010) Role of esophageal stents in benign and malignant diseases. Am J Gastroenterol 105:258–273

18. Mangiavillano B, Pagano N, Arena M et al (2015) Role of stenting in gastrointestinal benign and malignant diseases. World J Gastrointest Endosc 7: 460–480

19. Knyrim K, Wagner HJ, Bethge N, Keymling M, Vakil N et al (1993) A controlled trial of an expansile metal stent for palliation of esophageal obstruction due to inoperable cancer. N Engl J Med 329:1302–1307

20. Jacobson BC, Hirota W, Baron TH et al (2003) The role of endoscopy in the assessment and treatment of esophageal cancer. Gastrointest Endosc 57:817–822

21. ASGE Standards of Practice Committee, Ben-Menachem T, Decker GA et al (2012) Adverse events of upper GI endoscopy. Gastrointest Endosc 76: 707–718

22. Okano A, Hajiro K, Takakuwa H et al (2003) Predictors of bleeding after endoscopic mucosal resection of gastric tumours. Gastrointest Endosc 57:687–690

23. ASGE Technology Committee, Kantsevoy SV, Adler DG et al (2008) Endoscopic mucosal resection and endoscopic submucosal dissection. Gastrointest Endosc 1:11–18

24. de Franchis R, On behalf of the Baveno V Faculty (2010) Revising consensus in portal hypertension: report of the Baveno V consensus workshop on methodology of diagnosis and therapy in portal hypertension. J Hepatol 53:762–768

25. Binmoeller K (2000) Glue for gastric varix: some sticky issues. Gastrointest Endosc 52:298–301

Imaging Techniques, Normal Post-procedural Findings and Complications After Upper Gastrointestinal Endoscopy

3

Massimo Tonolini

3.1 Introduction

Upper gastrointestinal endoscopy (UGIE) is commonly performed to investigate a wide range of symptoms and treat several digestive tract disorders, even in elderly patients and in those with significant comorbidities. The largest series reported a very low (0.14–0.2%) complication rate. However, despite the general impression of safety, diagnostic and therapeutic oesophago-gastroduodenoscopy (EGDS) remains an invasive procedure which carries a potential for life-threatening complications and occasional mortality [1–3].

Since a few years ago, the majority (almost 60%) of adverse events were cardiopulmonary problems (hypoxia, arrhythmia, aspiration pneumonia, myocardial infarction, shock) related to sedation and analgesia. According to the European Society for Gastrointestinal Endoscopy (ESGE), post-UGIE complications will be increasingly encountered due to the growing number and complexity of endoscopies. Furthermore, the spectrum of complications widened since the use of advanced interventional procedures, including foreign body removal, stricture dilatation, haemostasis, ablative techniques using a variety of devices, endoscopic

mucosal resection (EMR) and endoscopic submucosal dissection (ESD). Occasionally, similar complications may occur after other types of instrumentation such as nasogastric tube placement, trans-oesophageal echocardiography and atrial radiofrequency ablation for cardiac diseases [1–3].

Unfortunately, iatrogenic complications are often unrecognised during UGIE. Symptoms of oesophageal or gastric injury include chest or abdominal pain, dysphagia and odynophagia, dyspnoea, haemodynamic instability, haematemesis or melaena, followed by clinical and laboratory signs of systemic inflammation at a later stage. Since early diagnosis substantially impacts the outcome, prompt investigation is warranted in patients with unusual complaints after UGIE [1, 3].

3.2 Oesophageal and Gastric Perforation

3.2.1 Incidence and Risk Factors

The commonest and most-feared complication of UGIE is intrathoracic or intra-abdominal perforation. Almost invariably associated with therapeutic EGDS, iatrogenic perforation (IP) after UGIE is very rare (estimated incidence 1/2,500–1/11,000) with exceptional mortality (0.001%) [4, 5]. Whereas the absolute number of IPs is

M. Tonolini
Radiology Department, "Luigi Sacco" University Hospital, Via G.B. Grassi 74, Milan 20157, Italy
e-mail: mtonolini@sirm.org

likely to increase because of the growing indications for therapeutic endoscopy, improvements in the endoscopic and surgical management of IPs might substantially reduce the associated morbidity and mortality [1–3].

IP may occur at the pharynx or oesophagus during blind passage of the endoscope (particularly with predisposing factors such as cervical osteophytes, oesophageal strictures and Zenker's diverticulum) or at the site of strictures. Although the incidence of damage during endoscopy is low (<0.04 %), due to its prevalence, endoscopy represents the commonest cause of oesophageal IPs. According to the ESGE, high-risk procedures include endoscopic dilatation of lower oesophageal sphincter in achalasia; dilatation of caustic, complex (angulated, multiple or long), malignant or radiation-induced strictures; foreign bowel removal; EMR for Barrett's oesophagus and ESD, the latter reaching a 5–10 % risk [1–3, 6].

In the stomach, IP may occur after snare polypectomy, argon plasma coagulation, cryotherapy and EMR. However, the highest-risk procedure is by far ESD that reaches a 6–10 % incidence of perforation particularly in larger lesions or located in the upper stomach and during prolonged procedures [3, 7, 8].

The ESGE recommends that symptoms or signs suggestive of IP following any endoscopic procedure should be carefully evaluated and documented with CT, to avoid diagnostic delay. The general principle of these guidelines is that diagnosis of post-UGIE complications and therapeutic choice between conservative and surgical requires integration of CT data with clinical features including timing of detection respect to procedure and oral alimentation, symptoms and signs of sepsis and shock [3].

3.2.2 Imaging Techniques and Findings

Traditionally, conventional radiographs are often acquired as the initial diagnostic procedure. Extraluminal air may be detected in upright lateral neck, chest and abdominal radiographs. Radiographic signs suggesting gastroesophageal injury include pneumomediastinum, mediastinal widening, hydropneumothorax and sudden appearance or increase of pleural effusion. The "Naclerio V" sign represents pneumomediastinum outlining the medial left hemidiaphragm and left lower lateral mediastinum. However, technically inadequate views in uncooperative patients and subtle or unspecific radiographic findings may result in critical diagnostic delays [9].

In the setting of suspected IP, fluoroscopic-contrast oesophagography (F-CE) is still largely employed as it typically confirms oesophageal perforation through the direct demonstration of extraluminal contrast medium (CM) extravasation. Its specificity approaches 100 %, but sensitivity for the detection of perforation is moderate (approximately 75 %). F-CE should be initially performed using ingestion of water-soluble iodine-based CM. Conversely, when perforation is a concern, barium sulphate preparations should be avoided, since extravasation will result in inflammatory reactions and fibrosing mediastinitis. The classic enteral water-soluble CMs such as diatrizoate meglumine are rapidly absorbed but are hyperosmolar; therefore, caution is necessary to avoid aspiration which may precipitate pulmonary oedema. Therefore, nonionic CMs such as iopromide or iomeprol are increasingly administered orally. Unfortunately, severely ill, bedridden patients may not be able to stand up and drink or may not tolerate oral CM or because of nausea, vomiting or pain [9–11].

Currently, plain radiographs are considered suboptimal (50–70 % sensitivity for pneumoperitoneum) compared to multidetector CT, which reliably detects minimal amounts of air, free or loculated fluid in the mediastinum and pleural or peritoneal cavity even before CM administration. Furthermore, compared to F-CE CT is much less cumbersome in critically ill and uncooperative patients and undoubtedly represents the imaging modality of choice for diagnosing deep infections. Intravenous CM administration is recommended unless contraindicated, since it improves the detection of secondary signs of perforation. To facilitate the identification of free intra- or extra-peritoneal air, scans should also be viewed at the lung or bone window settings. Multiplanar image review and appropriate sagittal or coronal reconstructions allow confident interpretation and

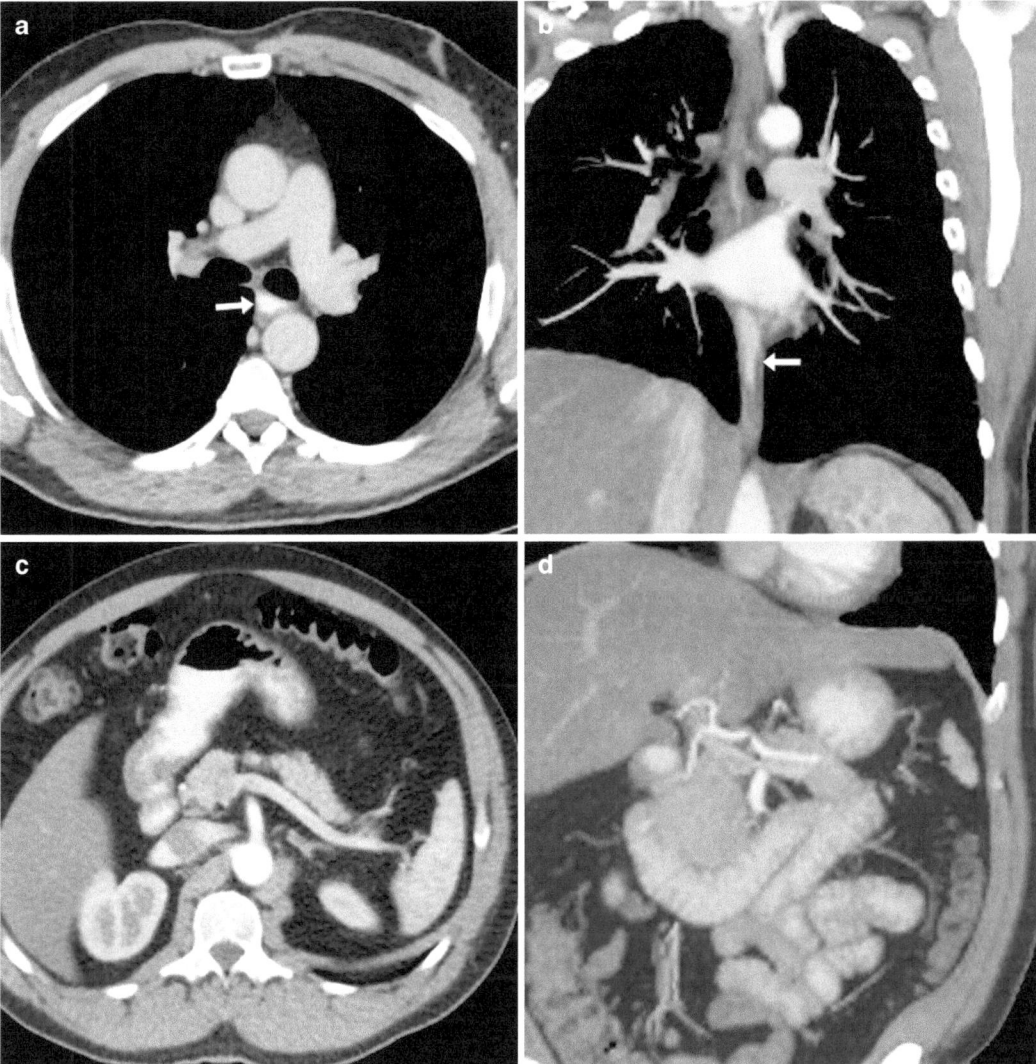

Fig. 3.1 Multiplanar images from multidetector CT-oesophagography acquired after oral ingestion of water-soluble contrast medium (CM) to rule out oesophageal perforation in a 35-year-old male complaining of odynophagia and severe dysphagia after oesophago-gastroduodenoscopy (EGDS). The non-dilated oesophageal lumen is filled by diluted CM (*arrows*) without appreciable extraluminal leak and pneumomediastinum. The ingested CM normally opacified the stomach, duodenum and jejunal loops (**c, d**)

visualisation of the entire extent of digestive tract injuries. However, in children and young adults, exposure to ionising radiation is of particular concern and must be taken into consideration before requesting and performing CT studies [11–16].

The estimated sensitivity and negative predictive value of CT versus F-CE are 100 % versus 66.7 % and 100 % versus 87.9 %, respectively; therefore, performing F-CE is unnecessary after negative CT findings for oesophageal perforation [17].

Furthermore, CT may be complemented with oral administration of 10 % diluted water-soluble iodine CM such as diatrizoate meglumine, iopromide or iomeprol. CT-oesophagography (Figs. 3.1 and 3.2) may represent the ideal "one-stop shop" technique to allow a rapid, comprehensive diagnosis of IP including identification of suggestive perioesophageal abnormalities, direct visualisation of oesophageal perforation and quantification of pleural and

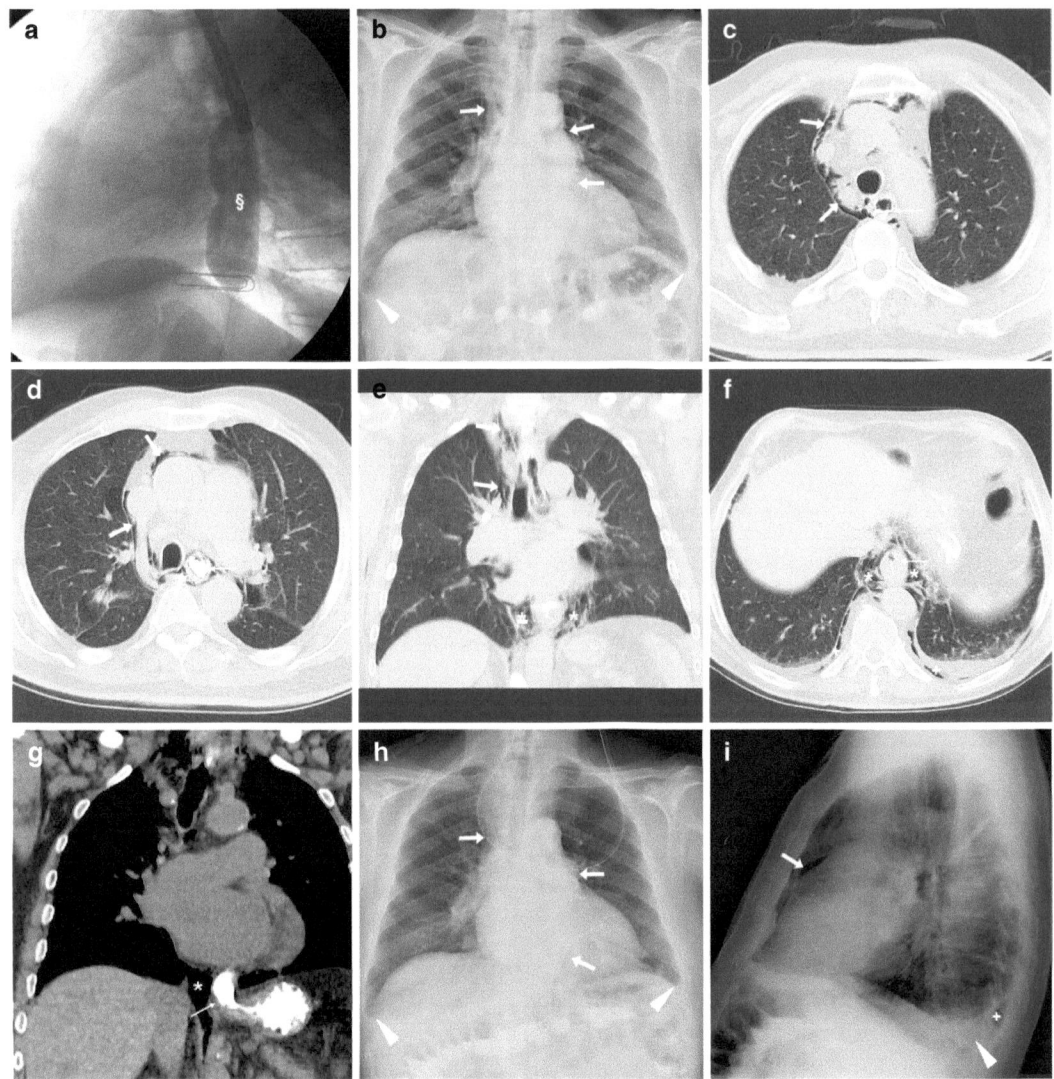

Fig. 3.2 An 82-year-old elderly male underwent balloon (§) dilatation of the distal oesophageal sphincter (**a**) to treat achalasia. Postoperative radiograph (**b**) obtained in a semisupine position detected appearance of pneumomediastinum (*arrows*) and of minimal pleural effusions (*arrowheads*). Multidetector CT-oesophagography (**c–g**) with ingestion of water-soluble CM confirmed moderate, diffuse pneumomediastinum (*arrows*), predominantly collected around the distal thoracic oesophagus (*). Note minimal atelectasis and pleural fluid, extrapleural air (+), opacified oesophageal lumen (*thin arrows*) and patent gastroesophageal junction (in **g**), absent extraluminal CM leakage in the mediastinum or pleural cavities. The patient remained stable under conservative treatment including positioning of nasogastric tube for oesophageal suction and feeding. Follow-up radiographs before discharge (**h**, **i**) showed mild decrease of pneumomediastinum, persistent pleural effusions (*arrowheads*) and extrapleural air (+ in **i**) (Partially reproduced from Open Access Ref. [22])

mediastinal contamination, without transferring the patient to or from the fluoroscopic suite [9–11].

Oesophageal IP after therapeutic endoscopic procedures may be categorised as superficial (mucosal laceration), intramural dissection and transmural (full-thickness) perforation. Representing an intermediate form of oesophageal injury, the rare intramural dissection is heralded by mural thickening with submucosal

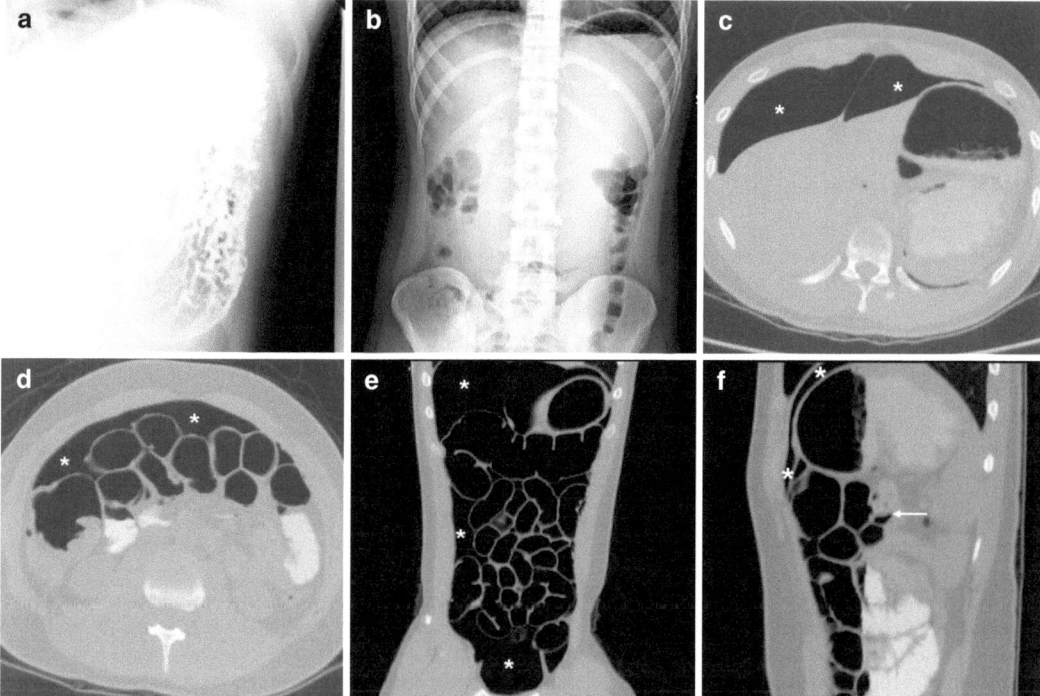

Fig. 3.3 A 16-year-old Chinese boy suffering from persistent vomiting and weight loss had endoscopic diagnosis of peptic ulcer of the pylorus with positive *Helicobacter pylori* microscopy. Double-contrast upper gastrointestinal study (**a**) depicted pyloric distortion with slow progression of barium CM. He failed to improve during prolonged medical treatment and subsequently experienced acute obstruction with radiographic confirmation of severe gastric dilatation (* in **b**). He was then hospitalised to undergo endoscopic dilatation. Immediately after the procedure, he suffered from severe abdominal pain. Urgent unenhanced CT (**c–f**) showed appearance of predominantly supramesocolic pneumoperitoneum (*), residual ingested CM and gaseous distension from endoscopic insufflation of most small and large bowel. The probable site of perforation was identified by careful scrutiny as a focal mural discontinuity (*thin arrow* in **f**). Laparotomy confirmed biliary peritonitis from prepyloric perforation in the site of known peptic stricture, which was repaired with suture and omentoplasty

distribution of gas, hyperattenuating blood or ingested CM. The CT signs of oesophageal injury include:

- Mural thickening (>5 mm or asymmetric)
- Mural discontinuity
- Oedematous infiltration ("fat stranding") of perioesophageal structures
- Focal perioesophageal air or fluid collection abutting the oesophagus
- Left-sided pleural effusion or hydropneumothorax
- Pneumomediastinum (Fig. 3.2)
- CM leakage into the mediastinum or pleural space, which is by far the most specific sign of transmural perforation [6, 9–11, 17]

Whereas oesophageal perforation typically results in pneumomediastinum, injuries to the distal thoracic oesophagus and oesophago-gastric junction may cause dissection of air inferiorly into the abdomen, either in an intra- or extraperitoneal location, thus mimicking a gastric perforation. Pneumoperitoneum (Figs. 3.3 and 3.4) is highly predictive indicator of perforation involving an intraperitoneal segment of the gastrointestinal tract (namely, the entire stomach and the first portion of the duodenum) but allows limited identification of the perforation site. Conversely, focal mural discontinuity (Fig. 3.3), CM leakage and localised extraluminal air or fluid collections (Figs. 3.4 and 3.5) are direct and highly predictive signs indicating the site of perforation. Borrowing

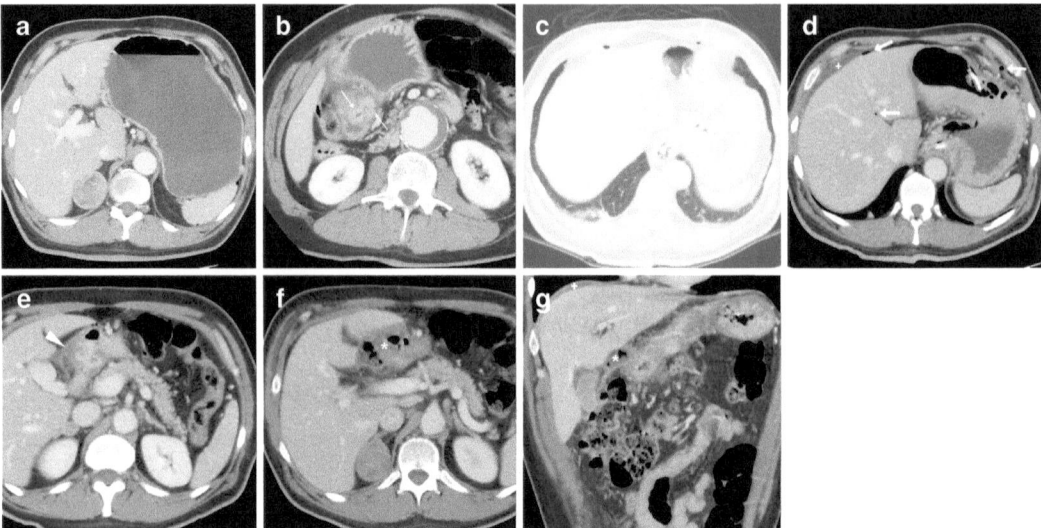

Fig. 3.4 A 56-year-old male suffering from severe vomiting and abdominal distension suggesting upper digestive tract obstruction was treated medically with nasogastric tube placement. Urgent CT revealed marked distension of the stomach with abundant endoluminal fluid (**a**), contracted pylorus and proximal duodenum with thickened wall and enhancing mucosa (*thin arrows* in **b**). The stricture was endoscopically confirmed and biopsied. A few days after endoscopic biopsy (which excluded neoplastic changes), repeated CT showed minimal pneumoperitoneum (*arrows* in **c**, **d**) and oedematous fat infiltration abutting the known stricture (*arrowhead* in **e**). A few days later repeated CT showed appearance of a mixed air–fluid collection (* in **f**, **g**) consistent with contained perforation. He ultimately recovered with conservative treatment

from experience with spontaneous perforations, the specificity of CT for identification of the perforation site probably falls in the range 75–90 %. Finally, IP involving the extraperitoneal second through fourth portions of the duodenum will result in retroperitoneal air or fluid [12, 18].

Notably, following ESD, extraluminal bubbles resulting from transmural air leak are commonly observed in up to half of patients and are not associated with increased hospital stay and unfavourable outcome. Therefore, the imaging finding of pneumomediastinum or pneumoperitoneum without endoscopic evidence of IP after gastroesophageal ESD should be interpreted together with clinical data before claiming that a perforation occurred [3, 19, 20].

3.3   Haemorrhage

Significant bleeding is rare (below 1 % of procedures) after diagnostic UGIE and mucosal biopsy and rarely requires intervention in the absence of coagulopathy, thrombocytopaenia or portal hypertension. Most cases are related therapeutic manoeuvres: haemorrhage may occur at the site of biopsy, polypectomy, EMR and especially ESD [1–3].

Urgent multidetector CT studies may reveal intraluminal hyperattenuating blood and intravenous CM extravasation indicating active gastrointestinal bleeding (see case 3.5.1). In the setting of acute abdomen, CT angiography had 85.2 % sensitivity and 92.1 % specificity for the detection of active bleeding [13, 14].

3.4   Treatment of Gastroesophageal Injuries

Management of iatrogenic UGIE complications should be tailored on the patient's conditions and prognosis, site and entity of perforation or haemorrhage. The ESGE guidelines recommend first-line endoscopic treatment within 12 h from injury using clips or other devices for sealing oesophageal and gastric perforations, especially those not exceeding 1 cm, and haemostasis with

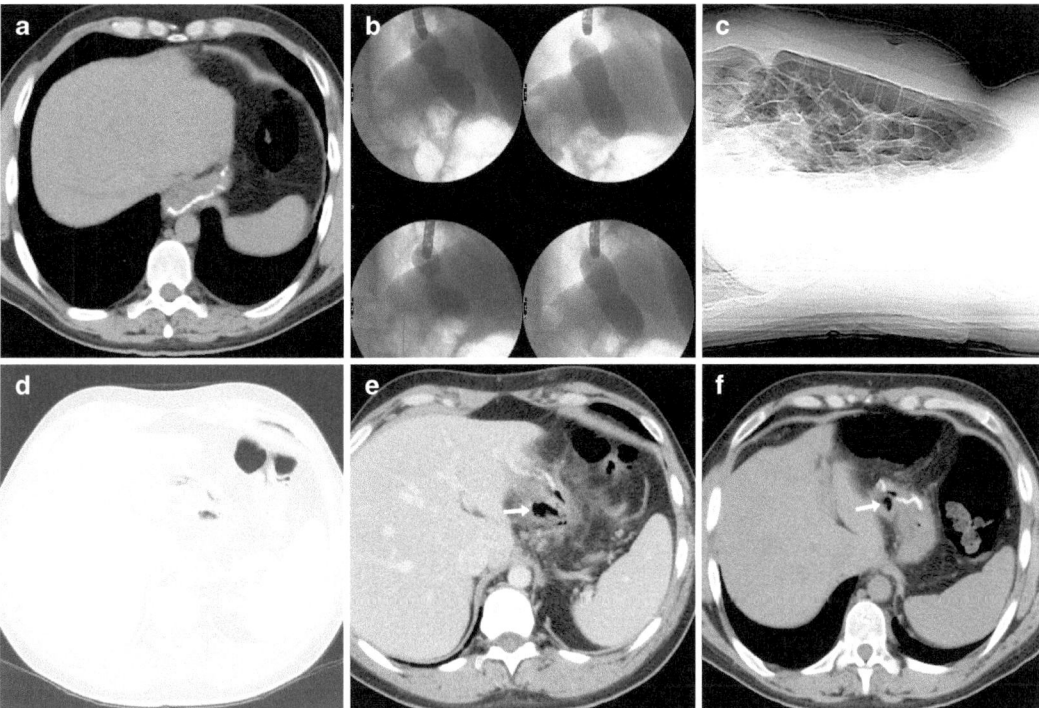

Fig. 3.5 A 33-year-old male with history of obesity and failed gastric fundoplication corrected with sleeve gastrectomy (SG) suffered from epigastric pain after endoscopic dilatation of a postsurgical gastric stricture; preprocedural unenhanced CT (**a**) showed hyperattenuating linear band consistent with SG surgical suture. During balloon dilatation (**b**) the patient did not experience adverse symptoms. A day later, tangential radiograph (**c**) did not show pneumoperitoneum. With worsening symptoms the patient underwent CT which showed localised extraluminal air (*arrows*) medially to the stomach (**d**, **e**). Follow-up unenhanced CT during conservative treatment 3 days later showed decreasing air collection (*arrow* in **f**), and the patient finally recovered

adrenaline, clips or thermal coagulation for bleeding. After a complicated UGIE, CT may be helpful to assess the efficacy of endoscopic perforation closure as it allows easy recognition of metallic clips (Fig. 3.6), which range within 8–16 mm in width [21].

With delayed diagnosis of IP, conservative management may be attempted provided that clinical and laboratory signs of sepsis and peritonitis are absent, and CT excludes luminal obstruction, abnormal collections, effusion or CM extravasation in the mediastinum, pleural or peritoneal cavity. Two CT findings, namely, free fluid and oral CM extravasation, are significantly associated with failure of nonoperative treatment. Asymptomatic IPs may be treated conservatively with hospitalisation, nil-by-mouth regimen, nasogastric suction, parenteral nutrition and intravenous administration of proton pump inhibitors, broad-spectrum antibiotics,

fluids and on-demand pain medication. Surgery is warranted in patients with large perforations, generalised peritonitis, sepsis or worsening clinical conditions, when CT reveals heavily contaminated mediastinal, pleural or peritoneal cavity and when nonoperative management fails. Primary closure may be attempted in non-diseased viscera; alternatively, surgical treatment requires resection or diversion [1–3].

3.5 Case Presentations

3.5.1 Intraluminal Bleeding and Mural Perforation After Diagnostic Upper Digestive Endoscopy

A 76-year-old woman had several comorbidities including chronic congestive heart failure, pulmonary hypertension, large gastric hiatal hernia

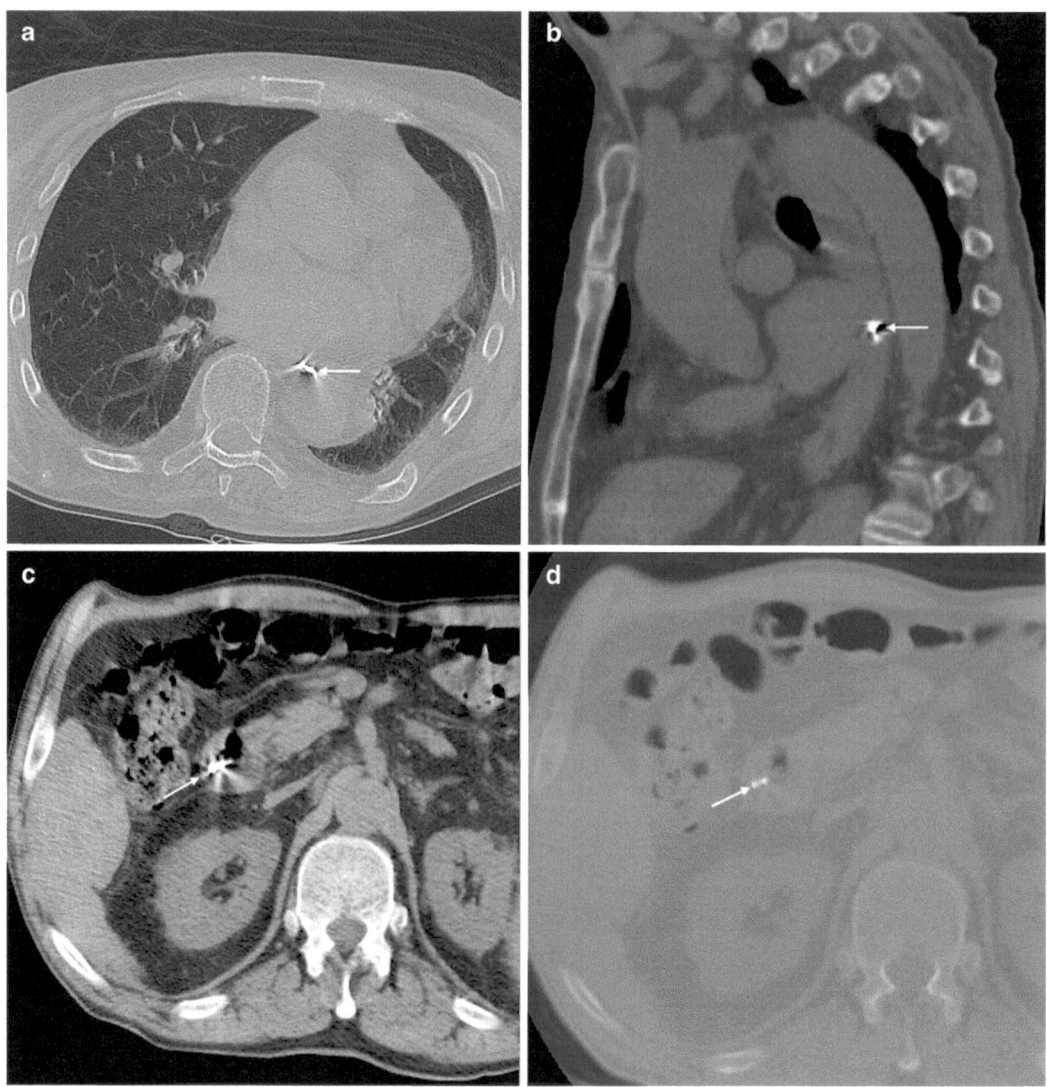

Fig. 3.6 Viewed at bone window settings, unenhanced axial (**a**) and sagittal (**b**) multidetector CT images following endoscopic sealing of iatrogenic perforation of the distal intrathoracic oesophagus confirmed the presence of metallic endoscopic clips (*thin arrows*) and excluded abnormal air or fluid collections in the mediastinum and pleural space. In a different patient, after endoscopic clipping of iatrogenic duodenal perforation, unenhanced CT showed clips (*thin arrows*) in the second duodenal portion and excluded air, fluid or abscess collections in the periduodenal retroperitoneum. The significant streaky artefacts during viewing at standard soft tissue settings (**c**) are reduced by rewindowing at bone settings (**d**)

and gallstones with previous episodes of acute cholecystitis treated medically. Upon emergency department admission for crampy abdominal pain, the attending surgeon requested UGIE. Endoscopy was interrupted for suspected complications soon after the endoscope impacted the gastric fundus wall, and the patient was immediately transferred to the CT suite. CT detected pneumoperitoneum and posterior pneumomediastinum surrounding a large hiatal hernia (Fig. 3.7a, b). In the herniated gastric fundus, hyperattenuating material suggesting fresh intraluminal blood (Fig. 3.7c) was noted on unenhanced images, and linear extravasation consistent with active bleeding was identifiable after intravenous CM injection (Fig. 3.7d, f).

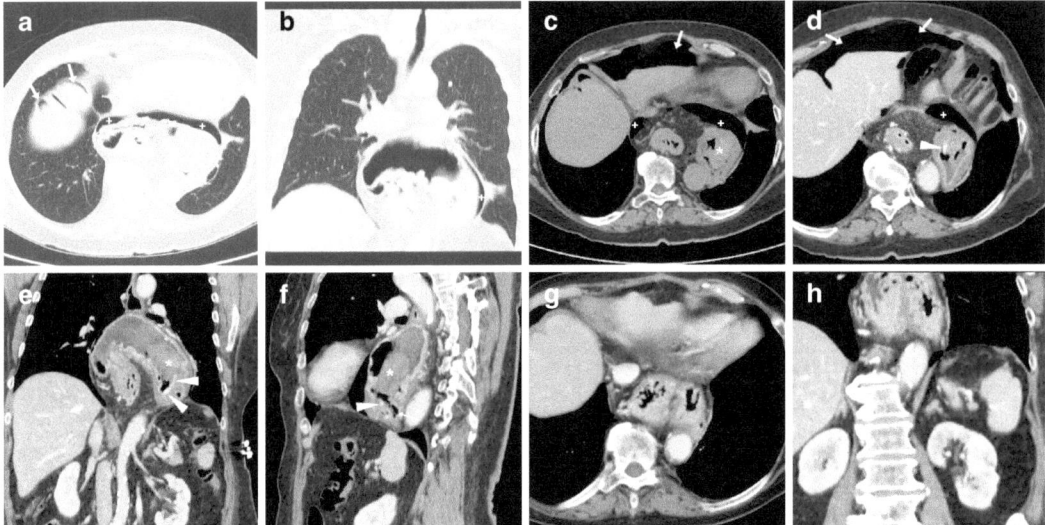

Fig. 3.7 Axial (**a**) and coronal (**b**) CT images viewed at lung window settings showed pneumoperitoneum (*arrowheads*) and large hiatal hernia containing rotated stomach consistent with chronic organoaxial volvulus surrounded by posterior pneumomediastinum (+). On unenhanced images (**c**) hyperattenuating material (***) was seen in the herniated gastric fundus suggesting fresh intraluminal blood. Multiplanar contrast-enhanced images (**d**, **f**) depicted linear CM extravasation (*arrows*) consistent with active intraluminal bleeding and a focal discontinuity of the gastric wall (*thin arrow*). One month after surgery, repeated CT (**g**, **h**) showed disappearance of extraluminal air and absent fluid collections, consistent with normal postoperative appearance (Partially reproduced with permission from Ref. [23])

Careful multiplanar study review allowed to detect a focal mural discontinuity consistent with iatrogenic perforation (Fig. 3.7f).

Considering the patient's worsening clinical conditions and comorbidities, urgent laparotomic surgery was required to repair a full-thickness gastric wall laceration with suture and omentopexy. After a prolonged postoperative course, follow-up CT 1 month after surgery (Fig. 3.7g, h) revealed normal postoperative appearances [23].

3.5.2 Pedunculated Liver Haemangioma: A Challenging Imaging Diagnosis with Potential Danger

An elderly male was referred to radiology to investigate suspected pyelonephritis. Physical examination and routine laboratory assays were unremarkable. His medical history included radical prostatectomy, previous myocardial infarction treated by percutaneous coronary stenting, severe carotid artery stenosis, nephrolithiasis and tubercular nephritis and hepatitis C virus-related chronic liver disease.

Incidentally, CT (Fig. 3.8a–d) detected a sizeable ovoid left-sided upper abdominal mass, extrinsic to the pancreas and spleen. Unknown from previous ultrasound reports, the lesion was mildly heterogeneous with peripheral calcifications and eccentric progressive foci of contrast enhancement. Additional unenhanced MRI (Fig. 3.8e, f) confirmed well-demarcated mass, extrinsically compressing the stomach without infiltration, with intermediate T1 and moderately high T2 signal.

Since the lesion's origin and nature were unclear, the patient underwent transgastric endoscopic ultrasound (EUS)-guided fine-needle aspiration biopsy (FNAB). Despite withdrawal of antiaggregation, immediately after EUS-FNAB, the patient suffered from severe hypotension and anaemisation. Immediate CT (Fig. 3.9) showed appearance of intralesional bleeding and massive haemoperitoneum. Emergency laparotomy was

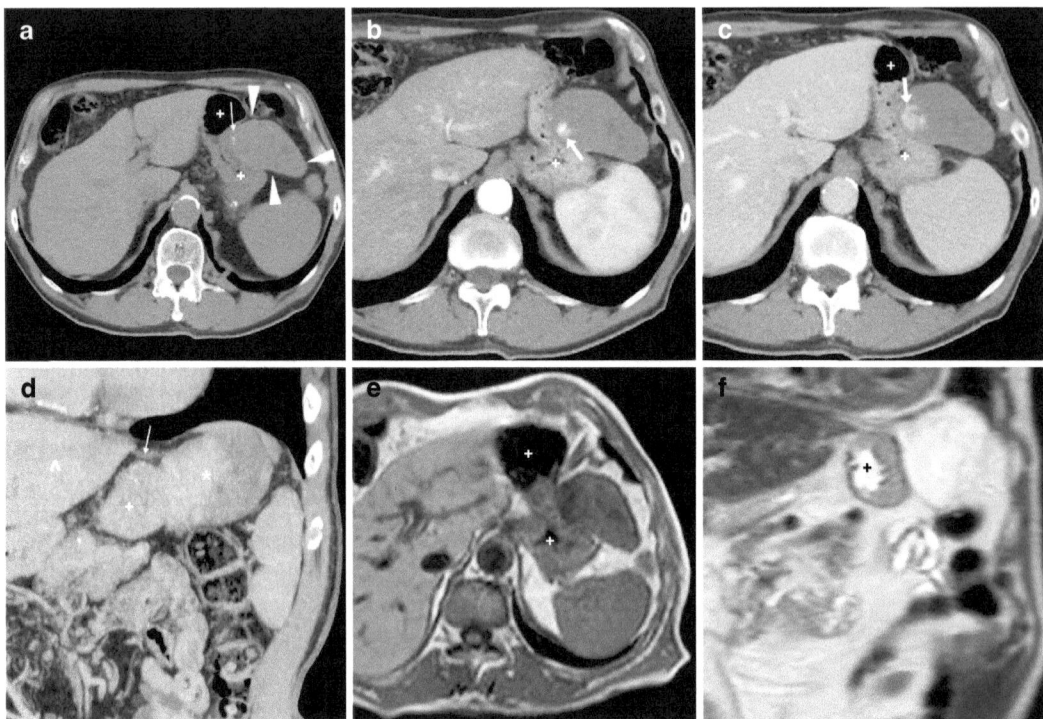

Fig. 3.8 A multidetector CT study performed for unrelated reasons revealed a 7×3.5 cm well-demarcated ovoid mass (*arrowheads*), moderately inhomogeneous with a few linear calcifications (*thin arrows*) on unenhanced scans (**a**), located ventrally to the spleen and compressing the stomach (+) medially. After intravenous contrast, arterial- (**b**) and venous-phase (**c**) acquisitions showed localised, eccentrically located foci of progressive enhancement (*arrows*). Conversely, most of the mass did not enhance. Delayed phase acquisition (**d**) showed persistent, more extensive enhancement of the medial portion of the mass (*arrows*). Retrospectively, focused reconstruction identified a very thin stalk (*thin arrows*) connecting the left-sided mass (*) abutting the stomach (+) to the left liver lobe (^), consistent with pedunculated liver haemangioma. Additionally, axial T1- (**e**) and coronal T2-(**f**) weighted MRI images confirmed a well-demarcated mass ventral to the spleen, extrinsically compressing the stomach (+) without signs of infiltration, with intermediate T1 and moderately high T2 signal intensity with a few strongly hyperintense internal foci (*thin arrows*) (Partially reproduced with permission from Ref. [24])

required to relieve haemoperitoneum and resect a bleeding brownish "spongy" mass attached to the liver margin, pathologically diagnosed as pedunculated cavernous haemangioma (PLH) [24].

Liver haemangiomas usually represent a straightforward imaging diagnosis unless atypical morphological or structural features are present. Whereas exophytic forms are uncommon, PLHs centred outside the liver margin are exceptional, and a recent literature review included only 24 cases. Predominantly found in females, PLHs are commonly asymptomatic despite large size (4–15 cm) and therefore incidentally discovered. Alternatively epigastric discomfort and symptoms from mass effect or complications such as spontaneous torsion and haemorrhage have been reported. Palpable, symptomatic or growing masses require surgical treatment, and laparoscopic resection may prevent potential traumatic rupture, torsion or intraperitoneal bleeding [25–29].

Despite similar CT attenuation, MRI signal intensity features and characteristic enhancement pattern compared to usual typical intraparenchymal haemangiomas, a correct preoperative diagnosis of PLH is reached in approximately 50 % of patients, since the thin stalk connecting the lesion to the liver is very difficult to identify. PLHs are commonly misinterpreted as other extrahepatic abnormalities such as exophytic gastric submucosal tumours, colon or adrenal masses,

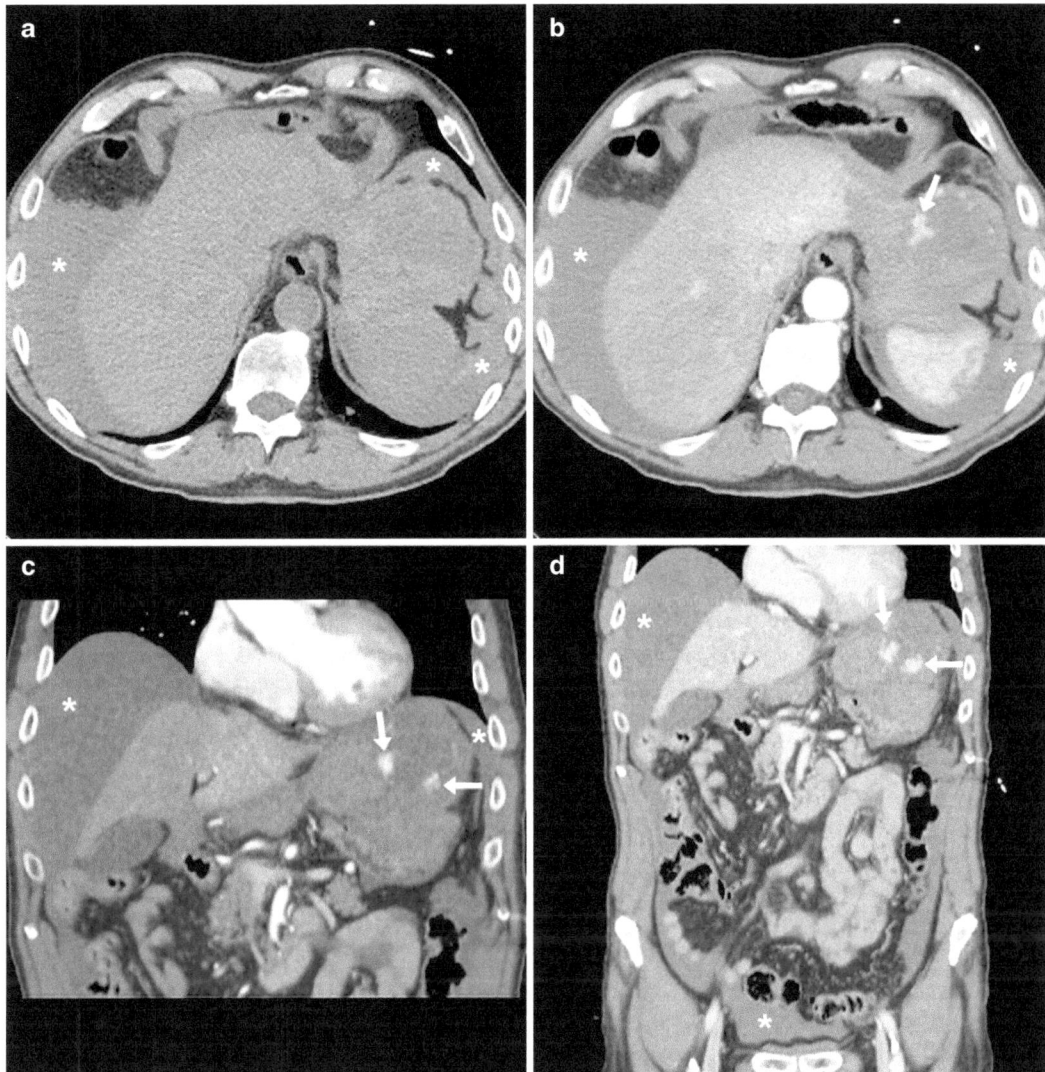

Fig. 3.9 One hour after endoscopic ultrasound-guided fine-needle aspiration biopsy, emergency CT showed appearance of massive hyperattenuating effusion (*) on unenhanced scans (**a**) consistent with hemoperitoneum. Arterial- (**b**, **c**) and venous (**d**) phase acquisitions con-firmed massive hemoperitoneum (*), and showed increasing size of the left-sided mass in Fig. 3.7 with perfusion foci (*arrows*) consistent with active bleeding (Partially reproduced with permission from Ref. [24])

sometimes as other benign and malignant liver lesions with exophytic growth [25–29].

Percutaneous puncture of a haemangioma was traditionally considered hazardous and requires interposition of liver tissue between the capsule and the lesion along the needle path. As this case exemplifies, misinterpretation of a PLH may result in potential danger from inappropriate procedures such as biopsy [25–27, 30].

EUS provides excellent visualisation of the sub-mucosal layers of the gastrointestinal tract as well as the adjacent organs and structures, but has limited ability to differentiate between inflammatory masses and tumour tissue. EUS-guided FNAB consistently provides accurate tissue diagnosis in a variety of intramural lesions of the oesophagus, stomach, duodenum and rectum/sigmoid and of extraintestinal abnormalities such as pancreatic and selected hepatobiliary lesions, lung neoplasms abutting the oesophagus, mediastinal and abdominal lymph nodes, perirectal and perigastric masses, adrenal and splenic lesions and idiopathic abdominal masses. Therefore, EUS-FNAB is increasingly used for lesions not amenable to or after unsuccessful percutaneous biopsy and in patients at increased risk of bleeding [31–35].

Generally considered safe, EUS-FNAB is associated with uncommon (1.6–6.3 % of cases), mostly minor, complications similar to those of UGIE and/or EUS alone, including fever, self-limiting local bleeding, with 1–2 % major occurrences requiring hospitalisation, and occasional severe or fatal occurrences. Whereas asymptomatic hyperamylasaemia is common in the first day after puncture, acute pancreatitis is rare (less than 2 %) but well known although rare complication of EUS-FNAB of pancreatic lesions, defined by upper abdominal pain plus elevation of serum amylase or lipase at least twice baseline levels [31–34, 36–42].

References

1. Ben-Menachem T, Decker GA, Early DS et al (2012) Adverse events of upper GI endoscopy. Gastrointest Endosc 76:707–718
2. Green J (2006) Guidelines on complications of gastrointestinal endoscopy. British Society of Gastroenterology, London. Available at: http://www.bsg.org.uk/pdf_word_docs/complications.pdf. Accessed July 4th, 2015
3. Paspatis GA, Dumonceau JM, Barthet M et al (2014) Diagnosis and management of iatrogenic endoscopic perforations: European Society of Gastrointestinal Endoscopy (ESGE) Position Statement. Endoscopy 46:693–711
4. Thill V, Simoens C, Mendes da Costa P (2010) Management of iatrogenic perforation after gastrointestinal endoscopy. Hepatogastroenterology 57:1465–1468
5. Misra T, Lalor E, Fedorak RN (2004) Endoscopic perforation rates at a Canadian university teaching hospital. Can J Gastroenterol 18:221–226
6. Zhou WZ, Song HY, Park JH et al (2015) Full-thickness esophageal perforation after fluoroscopic balloon dilation: incidence and management in 820 adult patients. AJR Am J Roentgenol 204:1115–1119
7. Kim M, Jeon SW, Cho KB et al (2013) Predictive risk factors of perforation in gastric endoscopic submucosal dissection for early gastric cancer: a large, multicenter study. Surg Endosc 27:1372–1378
8. Yoo JH, Shin SJ, Lee KM et al (2012) Risk factors for perforations associated with endoscopic submucosal dissection in gastric lesions: emphasis on perforation type. Surg Endosc 26:2456–2464
9. Madan R, Bair RJ, Chick JF (2015) Complex iatrogenic esophageal injuries: an imaging spectrum. AJR Am J Roentgenol 204:W116–W125
10. Suarez-Poveda T, Morales-Uribe CH, Sanabria A et al (2014) Diagnostic performance of CT esophagography in patients with suspected esophageal rupture. Emerg Radiol 21:505–510
11. Young CA, Menias CO, Bhalla S et al (2008) CT features of esophageal emergencies. Radiographics 28:1541–1553
12. Maniatis V, Chryssikopoulos H, Roussakis A et al (2000) Perforation of the alimentary tract: evaluation with computed tomography. Abdom Imaging 25:373–379
13. Artigas JM, Marti M, Soto JA et al (2013) Multidetector CT angiography for acute gastrointestinal bleeding: technique and findings. Radiographics 33:1453–1470
14. Garcia-Blazquez V, Vicente-Bartulos A, Olavarria-Delgado A et al (2013) Accuracy of CT angiography in the diagnosis of acute gastrointestinal bleeding: systematic review and meta-analysis. Eur Radiol 23:1181–1190
15. Wax BN, Katz DS, Badler RL et al (2006) Complications of abdominal and pelvic procedures: computed tomographic diagnosis. Curr Probl Diagn Radiol 35:171–187
16. Sartelli M, Viale P, Catena F et al (2013) 2013 WSES guidelines for management of intra-abdominal infections. World J Emerg Surg 8:3
17. Wu CH, Chen CM, Chen CC et al (2013) Esophagography after pneumomediastinum without CT findings of esophageal perforation: is it necessary? AJR Am J Roentgenol 201:977–984
18. Borofsky S, Taffel M, Khati N et al (2015) The emergency room diagnosis of gastrointestinal tract perforation: the role of CT. Emerg Radiol 22:315–327
19. Coriat R, Leblanc S, Pommaret E et al (2010) Transmural air leak following endoscopic submucosal dissection: a non-useful computed tomography finding. Endoscopy 42:1117; author reply 1118
20. Onogi F, Araki H, Ibuka T et al (2010) "Transmural air leak": a computed tomographic finding following endoscopic submucosal dissection of gastric tumors. Endoscopy 42:441–447
21. Shaish H, Gilet A, Gerard P (2015) "It's all foreign to me": how to decipher gastrointestinal intraluminal foreign bodies. Abdom Imag. In press
22. Tonolini M, Villa C (2015) EuroRAD Case 13193. Iatrogenic oesophageal perforation after pneumatic balloon dilatation for achalasia {Online}. EuroRAD URL: http://www.eurorad.org/case.php?id=13193
23. Tonolini M (2014) EuroRAD Case 12399. Intraluminal bleeding and gastric mural perforation after diagnostic upper digestive endoscopy {Online}. URL: http://www.eurorad.org/case.php?id=12399

24. Tonolini M, Rizzi A, Gambitta P (2015) EuroRAD case 12684. Pedunculated liver hemangioma: a challenging imaging diagnosis with potential danger {Online}. URL: http://www.eurorad.org/case.php?id=12684

25. Ha CD, Kubumoto SM, Whetstone B et al (2013) Pedunculated hepatic hemangiomas often misdiagnosed despite their typical findings. Open Surg J 7:1–5

26. Liang RJ, Chen CH, Chang YC et al (2002) Pedunculated hepatic hemangioma: report of two cases. J Formos Med Assoc 101:437–441

27. Moon HK, Kim HS, Heo GM et al (2011) A case of pedunculated hepatic hemangioma mimicking submucosal tumour of the stomach. Kor J Hepatol 17:66–70

28. Vilgrain V, Boulos L, Vullierme MP et al (2000) Imaging of atypical hemangiomas of the liver with pathologic correlation. Radiographics 20:379–397

29. Vivarelli M, Gazzotti F, D'Alessandro L et al (2010) Image of the month. Emergency presentation of a giant pedunculated liver haemangioma. Dig Liver Dis 42:456

30. Solbiati L, Livraghi T, De Pra L et al (1985) Fine-needle biopsy of hepatic hemangioma with sonographic guidance. AJR Am J Roentgenol 144:471–474

31. Eloubeidi MA, Tamhane A (2008) Prospective assessment of diagnostic utility and complications of endoscopic ultrasound-guided fine needle aspiration. Results from a newly developed academic endoscopic ultrasound program. Digest Dis (Basel Switzerland) 26:356–363

32. Gambitta P, Armellino A, Forti E et al (2014) Endoscopic ultrasound-guided fine-needle aspiration for suspected malignancies adjacent to the gastrointestinal tract. World J Gastroenterol 20:8599–8605

33. O'Toole D, Palazzo L, Arotcarena R et al (2001) Assessment of complications of EUS-guided fine-needle aspiration. Gastrointest Endosc 53:470–474

34. tenBerge J, Hoffman BJ, Hawes RH et al (2002) EUS-guided fine needle aspiration of the liver: indications, yield, and safety based on an international survey of 167 cases. Gastrointest Endosc 55:859–862

35. Catalano MF, Sial S, Chak A et al (2002) EUS-guided fine needle aspiration of idiopathic abdominal masses. Gastrointest Endosc 55:854–858

36. Eloubeidi MA, Chen VK, Eltoum IA et al (2003) Endoscopic ultrasound-guided fine needle aspiration biopsy of patients with suspected pancreatic cancer: diagnostic accuracy and acute and 30-day complications. Am J Gastroenterol 98:2663–2668

37. Eloubeidi MA, Tamhane A, Varadarajulu S et al (2006) Frequency of major complications after EUS-guided FNA of solid pancreatic masses: a prospective evaluation. Gastrointest Endosc 63:622–629

38. Eloubeidi MA, Black KR, Tamhane A et al (2010) A large single-center experience of EUS-guided FNA of the left and right adrenal glands: diagnostic utility and impact on patient management. Gastrointest Endosc 71:745–753

39. Eloubeidi MA, Gress FG, Savides TJ et al (2004) Acute pancreatitis after EUS-guided FNA of solid pancreatic masses: a pooled analysis from EUS centers in the United States. Gastrointest Endosc 60:385–389

40. Eloubeidi MA, Jhala D, Chhieng DC et al (2003) Yield of endoscopic ultrasound-guided fine-needle aspiration biopsy in patients with suspected pancreatic carcinoma. Cancer 99:285–292

41. Eloubeidi MA, Varadarajulu S, Eltoum I et al (2006) Transgastric endoscopic ultrasound-guided fine-needle aspiration biopsy and flow cytometry of suspected lymphoma of the spleen. Endoscopy 38:617–620

42. Fernandez-Esparrach G, Gines A, Garcia P et al (2007) Incidence and clinical significance of hyperamylasemia after endoscopic ultrasound-guided fine-needle aspiration (EUS-FNA) of pancreatic lesions: a prospective and controlled study. Endoscopy 39:720–724

Brice Malgras, Athur Berger, Paul Bazeries,
Christophe Aubé, and Philippe Soyer

4.1 Introduction

Oesophageal and gastroduodenal stents are pre-dominantly used in patients with oesophageal or gastroduodenal carcinoma who are not candi-dates to curative surgery. However, in selected cases, oesophageal and gastroduodenal stents can be used in patients with benign conditions.

The purpose of this chapter was to provide an overview of indications and techniques for

B. Malgras, MD (✉)
Department of Surgical Oncology,
Hôpital Lariboisière, AP-HP, 2, rue Ambroise-Paré,
Paris cedex 10 75475, France

Sorbonne Paris Cité, Université Diderot-Paris 7,
10, avenue de Verdun, Paris 75010, France

UMR Inserm 965, Hôpital Lariboisière,
2, rue Ambroise-Paré, Paris 75010, France
e-mail: bricemalgras@hotmail.com

A. Berger, MD
Department of Gastroenterology and Hepatology,
CHU d'Angers, Angers 49933, France

P. Bazeries, MD • C. Aubé, MD, PhD
Department of Radiology, CHU d'Angers,
Angers 49933, France

P. Soyer, MD, PhD
Sorbonne Paris Cité, Université Diderot-Paris 7,
10, avenue de Verdun, Paris 75010, France

UMR Inserm 965, Hôpital Lariboisière,
2, rue Ambroise-Paré, Paris 75010, France

Department of Abdominal and Interventional
Imaging, Hôpital Lariboisière, AP-HP, 2,
rue Ambroise-Paré, Paris cedex 10 75475, France

oesophageal and gastroduodenal stents with a special emphasis on potential complications along with their imaging appearances.

4.2 Oesophageal Stents

Less than 50 % of patients with oesophageal car-cinoma are potential candidates to surgical resec-tion. By contrast, the majority of patients with oesophageal carcinoma have an advanced disease with local extent or distant metastases. In such patients, dysphagia is the main clinical symptom and so that palliative treatment is needed. However, palliative treatment can also improve survival time [1].

4.2.1 Indications

4.2.1.1 Malignant Strictures

Currently, self-expandable metallic stent (SEMS) placement is the most common proce-dure for palliation of dysphagia in patients with oesophageal cancer who are beyond the reach of curative surgery [2, 3]. SEMS placement is safe and effective for dysphagia palliation by comparisons with other potential options [3]. In the same time, high-dose intraluminal brachy-therapy is a suitable alternative that results in lowering the need for reintervention and pro-vides clear benefits in terms of survival rate and a better quality of life [3, 4]. The combination of stent insertion and brachytherapy seems to be a feasible and safe palliative option in patients with inoperable oesophageal carcinoma [5]. However, there are still no evidence-based recommendations for the appropriate timing of SEMS insertion when performed in combination with other modalities because of conflicting results. Two nonrandomised studies have reported discrepant results regarding the complication rate of SEMS insertion in patients who have previously received radiochemotherapy [6, 7]. In addition, two studies have reported an increased rate of stent-related complications after SEMS insertion in patients previously treated with radiochemotherapy [8, 9].

The use of oesophageal stents in patients receiving neoadjuvant therapy before surgery has been studied but is still debated because the treatment of dysphagia is not always sufficient to improve the nutritional status of the patients and is associated with non-negligible morbidity [10]. Since the 1990s, oesophageal intubation with stents has gradually developed with high rates of complete closure of tracheo-oesophageal–broncho-oesophageal fistula and improvement in symptoms of respiratory tract and quality of life [11–13]. In a retrospective analysis, SEMS improved the overall survival in such patients [14]. Malignant oesophageal fistula and strictures due to villous tumours with budding are the main indications of partially covered stents because the migration rate is low and also because removal is generally not possible because of tissue embedding, restricting the use to patients for whom definitive placement is anticipated [15]. In case of external oesophageal compression, SEMS can be inserted, but it is generally less effective than for intraluminal lesions [16].

4.2.1.2 Benign Strictures

After preliminary experience in malignant stenosis, the use of oesophageal stents has been extended to benign strictures. Benign oesophageal strictures are generally caused by caustic ingestion, oesophageal surgery and radiotherapy [17, 18]. Stents have been proposed in refractory stenosis (i.e. that remains symptomatic with dysphagia) after up to five repeated endoscopic

dilations [19, 20]. Oesophageal stents are proposed especially for long stenosis (>2 cm) and stenting is based on the concept of temporary, progressive, sustained and large-diameter dilation. In case of benign oesophageal strictures, stents are left in place for a given period of time and systematically removed. Initially, plastic stents were used (Polyflex®, Boston Scientific, Marlborough, MA, USA), but later the use of partially and fully covered SEMS was the favoured option. Indeed, stents have to be removed between 4 and 16 weeks after insertion and between 4 and 8 weeks for fully or partially covered metallic stents in order to avoid epithelial hyperplasia and stent incarceration [21]. Uncovered metallic stents should not be used because of a high risk of incarceration [22].

Stents have also been used for rupture or anastomotic leak of the oesophagus after surgery and are currently the treatment of choice (Fig. 4.1) [23–25]. A high percentage of clinical success for stent placement has been reported in a series of 267 patients [26]. In this series, healing of the perforation or leaking site was obtained in 85 % of patients, with a mean time for healing of 7 weeks, with no significant differences between the various type of stents (plastic, fully or partially covered stents) [26].

4.2.2 Technique

Some researchers observed that the Polyflex® oesophageal stent was the least preferable option compared to Ultraflex® (Boston Scientific) or the Niti-S® stent (Taewoong Medical, Seoul, South Korea) [27]. This is because the Polyflex® stent is more technically demanding and associated with a higher rate of migration after placement [27].

Covered metallic stents result in effective and rapid relief of dysphagia with significantly reduced requirement for repeat interventions for recurrent dysphagia compared to uncovered metallic stents [28]. Covered metallic stents may also help maintain general patient condition and nutritional status during chemotherapy and radiotherapy. Uncovered or partially covered stents can lead to recurrent dysphagia secondary to

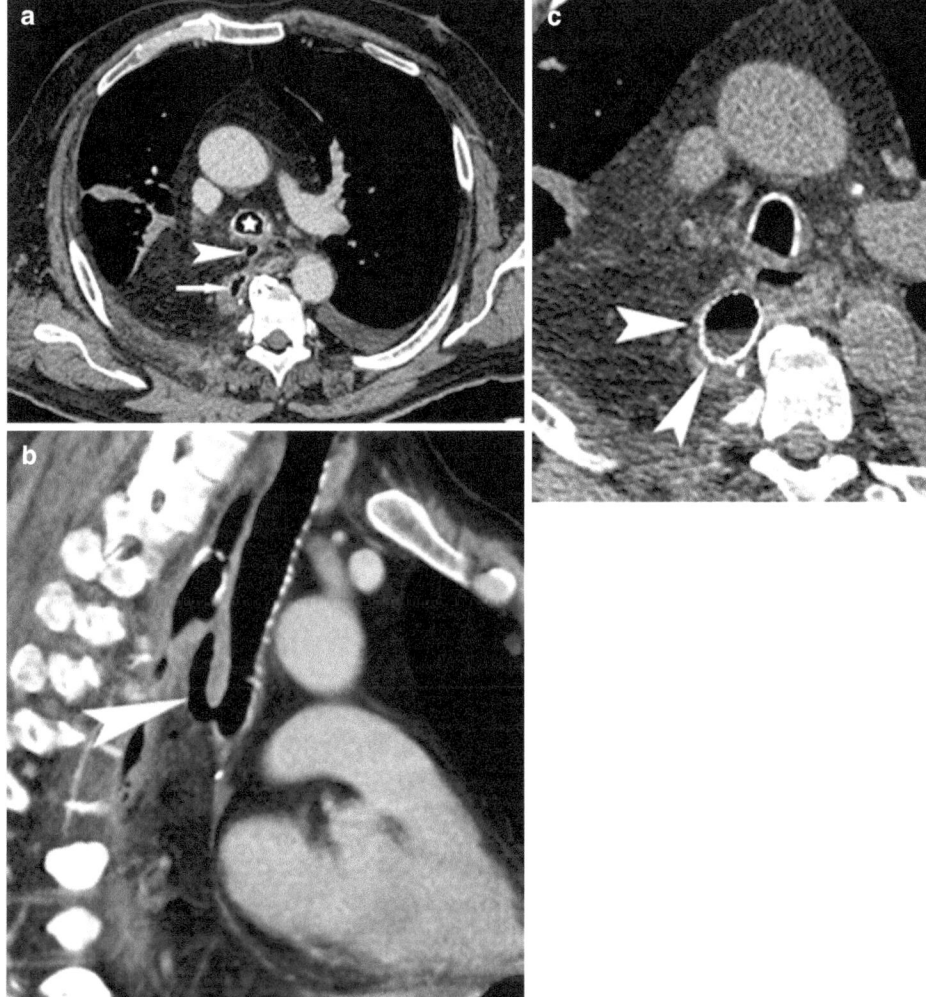

Fig. 4.1 A 58-year-old man who developed oesophago-tracheal fistula after a Lewis-Santy operation for advanced adenocarcinoma localised to the gastric cardia involving the lower third of the oesophagus. Axial MDCT image (**a**) *showed* fistula track (*arrowhead*) between the trachea (*) and the oesophagus (*arrow*), confirmed in sagittal (**b**) image. *Further axial images* (**c**) showed covered metallic stent in the oesophagus with optimal placement and satisfactory deployment (*arrowhead*)

epithelial hyperplasia [22]. In addition, epithelial hyperplasia prevents from stent removal [22].

Several antireflux stents are available for palliating dysphagia with complication rates and quality of life that are equivalent to those of conventional SEMS. Although some of the stents appear more effective in reducing gastroesophageal reflux, further research is required to confirm this favourable outcome [29–34]. During the start of radiotherapy, dysphagia often increases due to mucositis and oesophagitis. SEMS can interfere with radiotherapy dose planning and delivery scheduling because of metallic content [35]. Because the main supporting structure of biodegradable stents lacks metallic material, they do not interfere with radiotherapy. Also the tumour may shrink with therapy so that metallic stent may migrate to the stomach and may require additional procedure for removal [36, 37].

Potential benefits of using biodegradable stents include the avoidance of gastrostomy or nasoenteric feeding tubes and improvement of quality of life due to possible oral nutrition. The usual 6–8-week duration of courses of radiotherapy corresponds to the life span of the biodegradable stent [38]. However, if a biodegradable stent migrates during neoadjuvant therapy, there is no significant clinical impact due to its biodegradable properties, and if it has not migrated, it has substantially dissolved at the time of surgical resection [39].

Biodegradable stents have been used in patients with benign, refractory oesophageal strictures in a prospective series involving 21 patients [40]. In this series, 45 % of patients were dysphagia-free at the end of the study. These biodegradable stents allow obviating stent removal and have a stable expansion force during 5 weeks [40].

Self-expanding plastic stents have been successfully used in oesophageal cancer in order to reduce the risk of stent incarceration secondary to epithelial hyperplasia. But because of its cylindric shape and smooth covering, it increases the risk of stent migration compared to SEMS (29 %, 3 % and 12 %, respectively, for plastic, partially or fully covered stents) [27, 41]. Also, plastic stent delivery system is wider and stiffer than SEMS delivery system, often requiring dilation before stent deployment leading to high complication rates such as perforation and haemorrhage. Of note, haemorrhage occurs in 9 % of procedures with plastic stent and in only 3 % with metallic stents [15, 41]. They exert a higher radial force than their metallic counterparts, which can lead to patient discomfort, early migration, ulceration and rarely fistulisation [42].

4.2.3   Results

Stent placement provides rapid and effective palliation of dysphagia, but late recurrence of dysphagia leads to future complications that require further endoscopic treatments [43, 44]. Mariette et al. reported that SEMS, as a bridge to surgery, has a negative impact on outcome in patients with oesophageal carcinoma, resulting in less R0 resections, earlier recurrences, a decreased 3-year overall survival and an increased 3-year locoregional recurrence rate [45].

The technical success rate of covered stent in thoracic and abdominal oesophagus is >95 %. The mortality rate ranges between 0.5 % and 2 %.

Stents in cervical oesophagus have usually been associated with high risks of perforation, inhalation, proximal stent migration and poor tolerance. However, Verschuur et al. found similar morbidity and recurrent dysphagia in patients with cervical and thoracic/abdominal oesophageal stents [46]. Specific stents have been designed for the cervical oesophagus, for example, the "Ultraflex" (Boston Scientific) with a low radial expansion force [47], with a small proximal collar (5 mm) to reduce gastroesophageal reflux [48] or with a proximal delivery system in order to secure correct positioning of the stent (MITech Co, Pyeongtaek, South Korea) [49]. Only a few rare cases of tracheal compression due to oesophageal stent have been reported [50]. It has been suggested that high radial force and anatomic location of the stent above the carina are favouring factors for tracheal compression.

The results of plastic stent (Polyflex®) placement for benign stenosis have been studied in more than 160 patients [19], with a technical success rate of about 95 %, either for insertion or removal.

4.2.4   Complications

Early morbidity rate of oesophageal stent placement is about 20 % and may be due to technical problems in 5.3 % of cases (misplacement 0.3 %, expansion/deployment failure in 3.9/0.8 %, stent migration in 0.3 %) or related to patients in 14.6 % of cases (pain 12 %, perforation 0.6 %, haemorrhage 0.6 %, mortality 1.4 %). Late morbidity can also be due to technical problems (stent occlusion secondary to tissue in and/or overgrowth in 11.3 %, stent migration in 7 %) or related to patients (gastroesophageal reflux in 3.7 %, recurrent dysphagia in 8.2 %, oesophageal fistula in 2.8 %, haemorrhage in 3.9 %, oesophageal perforation in 0.8 % and 30-day mortality in 7.4 %) [51, 52]. Oesophageal stent migration is more common when stents are placed near the gastroesophageal junction [53]. The actual mechanism of haemorrhage after placement of oesophageal stent is controversial (pressure necrosis of the tumour and of the oesophageal wall is one of these). Some authors found that bleeding occurred more frequently in patients whose stents extended to or above the level of the aortic arch, because at this level, the left subclavian artery and the aortic arch have close relationships with the posterior wall of the oesophagus [54]. In case of dysphagia and tracheo-oesophageal fistula, the technical success of stenting ranges between 70 % and 100 % [46]. Epithelial hyperplasia is very low with plastic stents, facilitating its removal, but high rates of migration have been reported (between 47 % and 64 %) especially for proximal or distal stent location and peptic stenosis [42, 55]. Some authors reported a low migration rate after slight oversizing of stent diameter [56]. Other authors proposed a proximal fixation of the stent on the oesophageal mucosa by a clip to prevent stent migration [57]. Delayed migration could be, at least in some cases, the inevitable consequence of the dilating efficacy of the plastic stents [58]. Dysphagia is generally improved rapidly but long-term efficacy is small (between 6 % and 40 % at 1 year) especially for anastomotic strictures [59].

A meta-analysis found that clinical success (for dysphagia) was about 46.2 % with a median follow-up of 74 weeks and was better for plastic stents (55 % versus 21 %, $P=0.02$), but only two studies used metallic stents for caustic stenosis [21]. The migration rate was about 26.4 %, with a mean delay of 17 days, and 87 % of stents were removed between 4 and 8 weeks. The perforation rate was 1.5 % [21].

4.2.5 Imaging Features

MDCT is usually performed using oral water. The use of oral positive contrast material is restricted to patients with clinical suspicion of oesophageal perforation, fistula of extraluminal collection [60]. Usually, unenhanced MDCT examination of the thorax and abdomen is performed first to best evaluate stent position and location. Then MDCT is obtained with intravenous administration of iodinated contrast material and oral contrast (Fig. 4.2). The use of automated exposure control and iterative reconstruction is recommended to minimise radiation dose given to the patient [61–64].

Complications of oesophageal stenting can be classified into early complications (i.e. occurring less than 7 days following the procedure) and late complications (i.e. occurring more than 7 days after the procedure) [60]. Complications include stent misplacement, haemorrhage, perforation, tracheal compression [54], stent migration, stent fracturing, tumour ingrowth and/or tumour overgrowth, fistula formation and bolus impaction.

Oesophageal perforation on MDCT manifests as perioesophageal gas bubbles, mediastinal fluid collection and extraluminal leakage of oral contrast material [60, 65]. Left pleural effusion is often present and does not necessarily indicate oesophageal perforation.

More rarely, pneumomediastinum is observed. Pneumomediastinum indicates oesophageal perforation. It is more frequently observed after

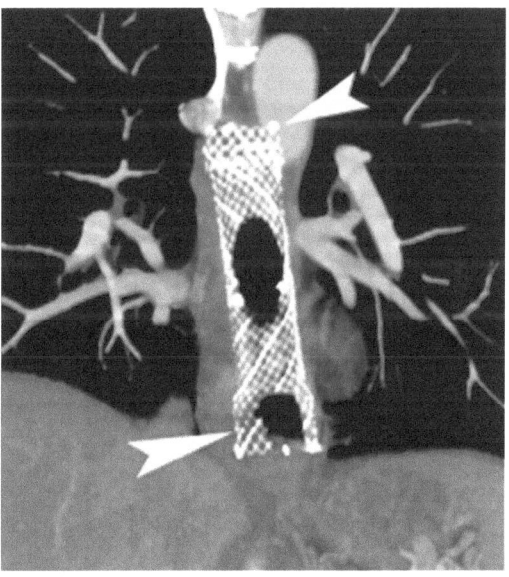

Fig. 4.2 A 53-year-old woman with unresectable T 4 epidermoid cancer of the oesophagogastric junction presented with dysphagia. The patient underwent endoluminal metallic stent placement and systemic chemotherapy. Coronal MDCT image showed correct placement of metallic stent in the oesophagus with satisfactory deployment (*arrowheads*)

oesophageal balloon dilation and can be associated with subcutaneous emphysema that is best evidenced on MDCT.

MDCT helps detect oesophageal stent leak that presents as presence of contrast material beyond the stent wall. Similarly, MDCT readily reveals stent fracture that often results in buckling and incomplete or complete oesophageal obstruction [60]. MDCT reveals oesophageal perforation with one distal tip of the stent projecting outside the oesophageal lumen. Tracheal compression by oesophageal stent is best evidenced by MDCT owing to the use of multiplanar reformations in the coronal and sagittal planes that better show the degree of luminal stenosis than transverse images alone [54].

Stent migration is best evidenced on MDCT. This is because MDCT has multiplanar capabilities (Fig. 4.3). In rare occasions, oesophageal stent may migrate into the duodenum. This is more frequent for stents placed in the gastroesophageal junction [66]. Stent migration may result in gastrointestinal perforation either at the level of the oesophagus or more distally in the duodenum [66]. Valenzuela et al. have reported oesophageal stent migration into the pleural space [60].

4.3 Gastroduodenal Stents

4.3.1 Indications

4.3.1.1 Malignant Strictures

SEMS represents the treatment of choice of gastroduodenal malignant strictures when curative surgery is not possible [67]. The most frequent indication for SEMS placement is duodenal obstruction secondary to a pancreatic cancer (up to 10–20 % of cases), usually at an advanced stage [68–70]. SEMS is also used in patients with gastroduodenal obstruction due to surrounding tumour [71]. Because of rapid efficacy, reduced morbidity and low cost compared to palliative surgery, SEMS is also used as an alternative to surgery for palliation in patients with poor life expectancy [72, 73]. Mehta et al. in a prospective randomised trial found that

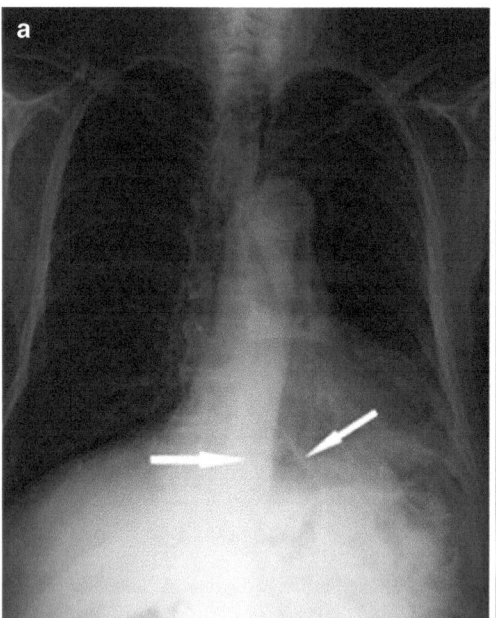
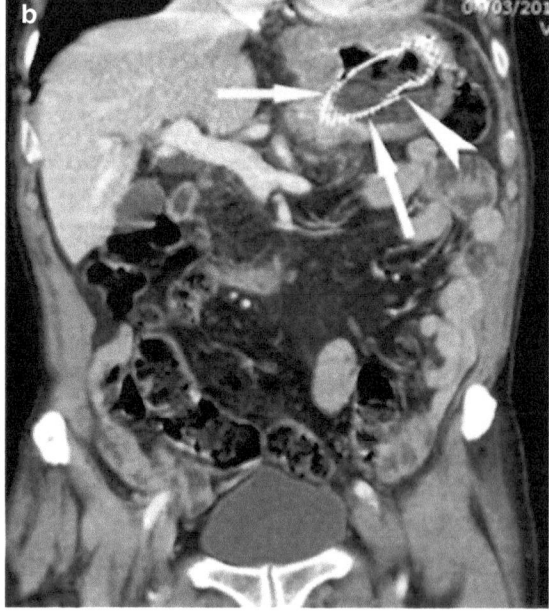

Fig. 4.3 A 77-year-old man with unresectable epidermoid carcinoma of the lower third of the oesophagus was treated with endoluminal stent placement and systemic chemotherapy. Three months later, he complained of recurrent dysphagia. Chest X-ray (**a**) showed stent migration with the stent (*arrows*) located into the stomach. Coronal MDCT image (**b**) confirmed metallic stent (*arrows*) migration into the stomach

duodenal stenting was superior to laparoscopic gastrojejunostomy for malignant gastric outflow obstruction in terms of morbidity, postoperative pain, hospital stay and 1-month quality of life [74]. These results were confirmed in a decision analysis by Siddiqui et al. who reported lower mortality–morbidity rates and a cost–benefit analysis in favour of duodenal stents compared to surgery [75]. Contraindications for duodenal SEMS include multiple stenoses or stenosis that is beyond the reach of the endoscope (e.g. in patients with peritoneal carcinomatosis or who had previous surgery), massive gastrointestinal bleeding, suspicion of perforation and haemodynamic instability.

4.3.1.2 Benign Strictures

No clear information is available concerning the use of SEMS in benign gastroduodenal stenoses, but it may be assumed that biodegradable or extractable stents would represent a good alternative in their management.

4.3.2 Results

Reported technical success rate is about 94 % and the clinical success rate (defined by relief of obstructive symptoms and reintroduction of oral feeding) is about 84 % [70, 76, 77].

Clinical success is defined by relief of clinical symptoms of obstruction, the reintroduction of oral feeding, improvement of nutritional status and a better quality of life. The clinical success of gastroduodenal stents ranges between 79 % and 91 %, with fast recovery because 60–90 % of patients are able to have oral solid food 1 day after stent insertion [70, 76]. This clinical success is prolonged with time, since 90–100 % of patients are still able to have oral feeding 3 and 6 months after stent insertion, respectively [78], with a median stent patency of 219 days [76]. In addition, it is possible to insert a second stent in the first one in case of first stent obstruction [76, 79]. Predictive factors of stent patency are chemotherapy and covered stent [80]. Studies comparing stenting with surgery for malignant stenosis of the gastroduodenal tract showed that stent was associated with a reduced

time for oral nutrition, a reduced hospital stay, a reduced cost but with a short time for recurrent obstruction and second endoscopic treatment [72, 81–83]. Indeed, surgery yields better long-term efficacy better than endoluminal stenting, which is the preferred option in case of life expectancy greater than 2 months [83]. In patients, with obstructive jaundice, biliary drainage can be performed endoscopically before duodenal stent placement [84, 85].

4.3.3 Complications

The morbidity rate of gastroduodenal stents is between 11 % and 43 % [78]. Early complications include migration, obstruction, biliary obstruction (in case of a covered stent), perforation, haemorrhage (Fig. 4.4) and misplacement [86]. Delayed complications include migration, perforation, obstruction, duodenal fistula or stent fracture and can be treated with a new stent. Migration rate for covered stent is about 25 % [76], and obstruction of non-covered stent is about 15 % [87]. Risk factor for early uncovered

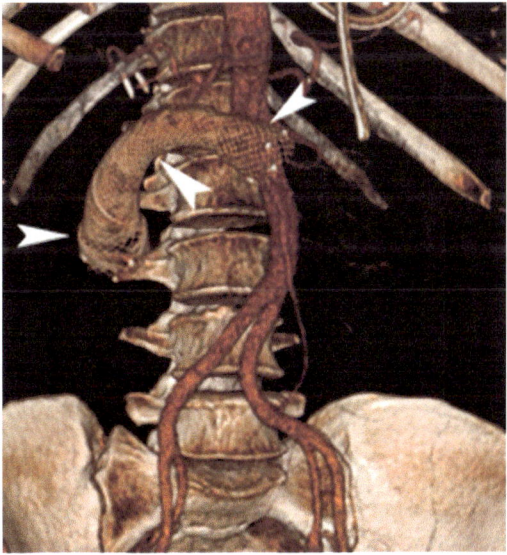

Fig. 4.4 A 56-year-old woman with unresectable gastroduodenal adenocarcinoma was palliated with metallic stent placement. Three-dimensional reconstruction from MDCT data confirmed optimal stent (*arrowheads*) deployment

stent obstruction is stenosis of a gastrojejunal or a gastroduodenal anastomosis [88]. Risk factors for perforation are previous dilation, attempt to pass the stenosis with the endoscope, use of rigid guidewire and concomitant corticosteroid therapy/chemotherapy/radiotherapy.

4.3.4   Imaging Features

MDCT is the modality of choice to confirm appropriate stent placement. Multiplanar reformations and three-dimensional images (Fig. 4.4) help confirm optimal stent placement and deployment. MDCT is usually performed using oral water. The use of oral positive contrast material is restricted to patients with clinical suspicion of gastroduodenal perforation, fistula of extraluminal collection [60].

Duodenal stent placement may result in perforation that manifests as retroperitoneal or intraperitoneal free air depending on the site of perforation. Rarely, perforation may manifest with more subtle findings and free gas is only observed adjacent to the distal tip of the stent. Extraduodenal leak of contrast material is a specific finding for the diagnosis of duodenal perforation. Similar to oesophageal stent, other complications of duodenal stents include stent misplacement, haemorrhage, perforation, stent migration, stent fracturing, tumour ingrowth and

tumour overgrowth, fistula formation and bolus impaction.

MDCT helps detect duodenal stent leak that presents as presence of contrast material beyond the stent wall. Similarly, MDCT readily reveals stent fracture that often results in buckling and incomplete or complete duodenal obstruction [60]. MDCT reveals duodenal perforation with distal tip of the stent projecting outside the duodenal lumen.

MDCT is also useful for elucidating the cause of duodenal bleeding after duodenal stent placement (Fig. 4.5) [89]. In patients presenting with duodenal bleeding after stent placement, MDCT must be performed during the arterial phase after IV administration of iodinated contrast material to depict active bleeding.

Conclusion

Currently stent insertion is well codified regarding technical, material aspects and indications. Except for emergencies, stent insertion has to be discussed during a multidisciplinary cancer conference in order to define its use in a multimodal treatment. Caution must be taken concerning oncologic outcomes of stent insertion in malignant strictures. Also, benign strictures are more and more treated with stents even if low efficacy and high morbidity rates reduce its use in such indications.

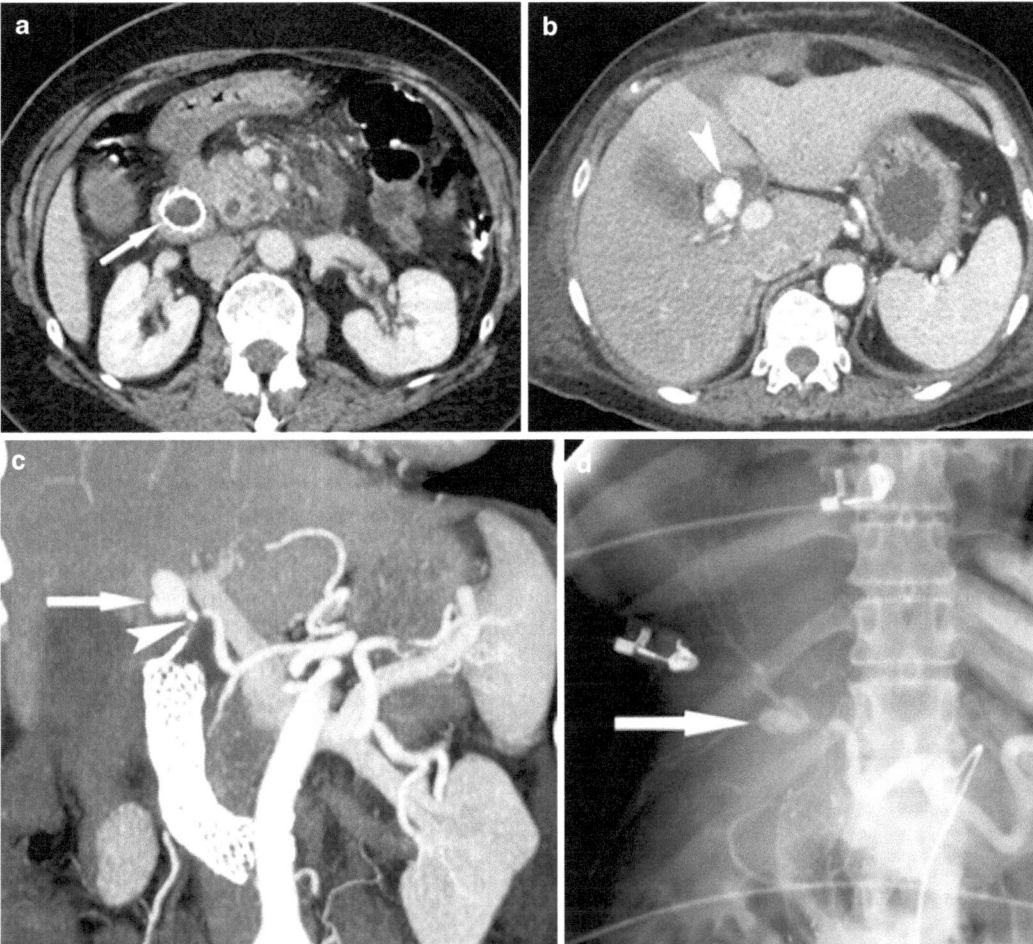

Fig. 4.5 A 70-year-old woman had unresectable adeno-carcinoma of the pancreatic head causing major dilatation of the jejunum and was palliated with non-covered self-expandable metallic stent (Hanarostent). Axial MDCT image (**a**) *showed* metallic stent (*arrow*) in the duodenum and confirmed correct its placement with satisfactory deployment. Two weeks after stent placement, the patient presented with haematemesis and haemodynamic instability. Axial MDCT image (**b**) obtained during the arterial phase after IV administration of iodinated contrast material and coronal thick-slab maximum intensity projection (MIP) reconstruction (**c**) showed pseudoaneurysm (*arrowhead*) originating from the right branch of the hepatic artery. A portion of metallic stent (*arrowhead* in **c**) was seen adjacent to hepatic artery and pseudoaneurysm suggesting arterial injury due to the stent. Angiogram (**d**) confirmed pseudoaneurysm (*arrow*) that was subsequently excluded using intra-arterial covered stent

References

1. Polednak AP (2003) Trends in survival for both histo-logic types of esophageal cancer in US surveillance, epidemiology and end results areas. Int J Cancer 105:98–100
2. Katsanos K, Sabharwal T, Adam A (2010) Stenting of the upper gastrointestinal tract: current status. Cardiovasc Intervent Radiol 33:690–705
3. Dai Y, Li C, Xie Y, Liu X, Zhang J, Zhou J et al (2014) Interventions for dysphagia in oesophageal cancer. Cochrane Database Syst Rev (10):CD005048
4. Homs MYV, Steyerberg EW, Eijkenboom WM, Tilanus HW, Stalpers LJ, Bartelsman JF et al (2004) Single-dose brachytherapy versus metal stent placement for the palliation of dysphagia from oesophageal cancer: multicentre randomised trial. Lancet 364: 1497–1504
5. Bergquist H, Johnsson E, Nyman J, Rylander H, Hammerlid E, Friesland S et al (2012) Combined stent insertion and single high- dose brachytherapy in patients with advanced esophageal cancer—results of a prospective safety study. Dis Esophagus 25:410–415
6. Kozarek RA, Raltz S, Brugge WR, Schapiro RH, Waxman I, Boyce HW et al (1996) Prospective

multicenter trial of esophageal Z-stent placement for malignant dysphagia and tracheoesophageal fistula. Gastrointest Endosc 44:562–567

7. Raijman I, Siddique I, Lynch P (1997) Does chemoradiation therapy increase the incidence of complications with self-expanding coated stents in the management of malignant esophageal strictures? Am J Gastroenterol 92:2192–2196

8. Shenfine J, McNamee P, Steen N, Bond J, Griffin SM (2009) A randomized controlled clinical trial of palliative therapies for patients with inoperable esophageal cancer. Am J Gastroenterol 104:1674–1685

9. Siersema PD, Hop WC, Dees J, Tilanus HW, van Blankenstein M (1998) Coated self-expanding metal stents versus latex prostheses for esophago-gastric cancer with special reference to prior radiation and chemotherapy: a controlled, prospective study. Gastrointest Endosc 47:113–120

10. Adler DG, Fang J, Wong R, Wills J, Hilden K (2009) Placement of Polyflex stents in patients with locally advanced esophageal cancer is safe and improves dysphagia during neoadjuvant therapy. Gastrointest Endosc 70:614–619

11. Hu Y, Zhao YF, Chen LQ, Zhu ZJ, Liu LX, Wang Y et al (2009) Comparative study of different treatments for malignant tracheoesophageal/broncho-esophageal fistulae. Dis Esophagus 22:526–531

12. Shin JH, Song HY, Ko GY, Lim J-O, Yoon HK, Sung KB (2004) Esophagorespiratory fistula: long-term results of palliative treatment with covered expandable metallic stents in 61 patients. Radiology 232:252–259

13. Balazs A, Galambos Z, Kupcsulik PK (2009) Characteristics of esophagorespiratory fistulas resulting from esophageal cancers: a single center study on 243 cases in a 20-year period. World J Surg 33:994–1001

14. Chen YH, Li SH, Chiu YC, Lu HI, Huang CH, Rau KM et al (2012) Comparative study of esophageal stent and feeding gastrostomy/jejunostomy for tracheoesophageal fistula caused by esophageal squamous cell carcinoma. PLoS One 7:e42766

15. Seven G, Irani S, Ross AS, Gan SI, Gluck M, Low D et al (2013) Partially versus fully covered self-expanding metal stents for benign and malignant esophageal conditions: a single center experience. Surg Endosc 27:2185–2192

16. Bethge N, Sommer A, Vakil N (1998) Palliation of malignant esophageal obstruction due to intrinsic and extrinsic lesions with expandable metal stents. Am J Gastroenterol 93:1829–1832

17. Spechler SJ (1999) AGA technical review on treatment of patients with dysphagia caused by benign disorders of the distal esophagus. Gastroenterology 117:233–254

18. Cook IJ, Kahrilas PJ (1999) AGA technical review on management of oropharyngeal dysphagia. Gastroenterology 116:455–478

19. Siersema PD (2009) Stenting for benign esophageal strictures. Endoscopy 41:363–373

20. Kochman ML, McClave SA, Boyce HW (2005) The refractory and the recurrent esophageal stricture: a definition. Gastrointest Endosc 62:474–475

21. Thomas T, Abrams KR, Subramanian V, Mannath J, Ragunath K (2011) Esophageal stents for benign refractory strictures: a meta- analysis. Endoscopy 43:386–393

22. Mayoral W, Fleischer D, Salcedo J, Roy P, Al-Kawas F, Benjamin S (2000) Nonmalignant obstruction is a common problem with metal stents in the treatment of esophageal cancer. Gastrointest Endosc 51:556–559

23. Amrani L, Ménard C, Berdah S, Emungania O, Soune PA, Subtil C et al (2009) From iatrogenic digestive perforation to complete anastomotic disunion: endoscopic stenting as a new concept of "stent-guided regeneration and re-epithelialization". Gastrointest Endosc 69:1282–1287

24. Hünerbein M, Stroszczynski C, Moesta KT, Schlag PM (2004) Treatment of thoracic anastomotic leaks after esophagectomy with self-expanding plastic stents. Ann Surg 240:801–807

25. Dai YY, Gretschel S, Dudeck O, Rau B, Schlag PM, Hünerbein M (2009) Treatment of oesophageal anastomotic leaks by temporary stenting with self-expanding plastic stents. Br J Surg 96:887–891

26. Van Boeckel PG, Sijbring A, Vleggaar FP, Siersema PD (2011) Systematic review: temporary stent placement for benign rupture or anastomotic leak of the oesophagus. Aliment Pharmacol Ther 33:1292–1301

27. Verschuur EM, Repici A, Kuipers EJ, Steyerberg EW, Siersema PD (2008) New design esophageal stents for the palliation of dysphagia from esophageal or gastric cardia cancer: a randomized trial. Am J Gastroenterol 103:304–312

28. Vakil N, Morris AI, Marcon N, Segalin A, Peracchia A, Bethge N et al (2001) A prospective, randomized, controlled trial of covered expandable metal stents in the palliation of malignant esophageal obstruction at the gastroesophageal junction. Am J Gastroenterol 96:1791–1796

29. Homs MY, Wahab PJ, Kuipers EJ, Steyerberg EW, Grool TA, Haringsma J et al (2004) Esophageal stents with antireflux valve for tumors of the distal esophagus and gastric cardia: a randomized trial. Gastrointest Endosc 60:695–702

30. Power C, Byrne PJ, Lim K, Ravi N, Moore J, Fitzgerald T et al (2007) Superiority of antireflux stent compared with conventional stents in the palliative management of patients with cancer of the lower esophagus and esophago-gastric junction: results of a randomized clinical trial. Dis Esophagus 20:466–470

31. Sabharwal T, Gulati MS, Fotiadis N, Dourado R, Botha A, Mason R et al (2008) Randomised comparison of the FerX Ella antireflux stent and the ultraflex stent: proton pump inhibitor combination for prevention of post-stent reflux in patients with esophageal carcinoma involving the esophago-gastric junction. J Gastroenterol Hepatol 23:723–728

32. Shim CS, Jung IS, Cheon YK, Ryu CB, Hong SJ, Kim JO et al (2005) Management of malignant stricture of

the esophago-gastric junction with a newly-designed self-expanding metal stent with an antireflux mechanism. Endoscopy 37:335–339

33. Wenger U, Johnsson E, Arnelo U, Lundell L, Lagergren J (2006) An antireflux stent versus conventional stents for palliation of distal esophageal or cardia cancer: a randomized clinical study. Surg Endosc 20:1675–1680

34. Blomberg J, Wenger U, Lagergren J, Arnelo U, Agustsson T, Johnsson E et al (2010) Antireflux stent versus conventional stent in the palliation of distal esophageal cancer. A randomized, multicenter clinical trial. Scand J Gastroenterol 45:208–216

35. Li XA, Chibani O, Greenwald B, Suntharalingam M (2002) Radiotherapy dose perturbation of metallic esophageal stents. Int J Radiat Oncol Biol Phys 54:1276–1285

36. Shin JH, Song HY, Kim JH, Kim SB, Lee GH, Park SI et al (2005) Comparison of temporary and permanent stent placement with concurrent radiation therapy in patients with esophageal carcinoma. J Vasc Interv Radiol 16:67–74

37. Song HY, Lee DH, Seo TS, Kim SB, Jung HY, Kim JH et al (2002) Retrievable covered nitinol stents: experiences in 108 patients with malignant esophageal strictures. J Vasc Interv Radiol 13:285–293

38. Griffiths EA, Gregory CJ, Pursnani KG, Ward JB, Stockwell RC (2012) The use of biodegradable (SX-ELLA) oesophageal stents to treat dysphagia due to benign and malignant oesophageal disease. Surg Endosc 26:2367–2375

39. Stivaros SM, Williams LR, Senger C, Wilbraham L, Laasch HU (2010) Woven polydioxanone biodegradable stents: a new treatment option for benign and malignant oesophageal strictures. Eur Radiol 20:1069–1072

40. Repici A, Vleggaar FP, Hassan C, Van Boeckel PG, Romeo F, Pagano N et al (2010) Efficacy and safety of biodegradable stents for refractory benign esophageal strictures: the BEST (Biodegradable Esophageal Stent) study. Gastrointest Endosc 72:927–934

41. Conio M, Repici A, Battaglia G, De Pretis G, Ghezzo L, Bittinger M et al (2007) A randomized prospective comparison of self-expandable plastic stents and partially covered self-expandable metal stents in the palliation of malignant esophageal dysphagia. Am J Gastroenterol 102:2667–2677

42. Ott C, Ratiu N, Endlicher E, Rath HC, Gelbmann CM, Schölmerich J et al (2007) Self-expanding Polyflex plastic stents in esophageal disease: various indications, complications, and outcomes. Surg Endosc 21:889–896

43. Song HY, Do YS, Han YM, Sung KB, Choi EK, Sohn KH et al (1994) Covered, expandable esophageal metallic stent tubes: experiences in 119 patients. Radiology 193:689–695

44. Hindy P, Hong J, Lam-Tsai Y, Gress F (2012) A comprehensive review of esophageal stents. Gastroenterol Hepatol 8:526–534

45. Mariette C, Gronnier C, Duhamel A, Mabrut J-Y, Bail JP, Carrere N et al (2015) Self-expanding covered metallic stent as a bridge to surgery in esophageal cancer: impact on oncologic outcomes. J Am Coll Surg 220:287–296

46. Verschuur EM, Kuipers EJ, Siersema PD (2007) Esophageal stents for malignant strictures close to the upper esophageal sphincter. Gastrointest Endosc 66:1082–1090

47. Siersema PD (2008) Esophageal cancer. Gastroenterol Clin North Am 37:943–964

48. Shim CS, Jung IS, Bhandari S, Ryu CB, Hong SJ, Kim JO et al (2004) Management of malignant strictures of the cervical esophagus with a newly-designed self-expanding metal stent. Endoscopy 36:554–557

49. Choi EK, Song HY, Kim JW, Shin JH, Kim KR, Kim JH et al (2007) Covered metallic stent placement in the management of cervical esophageal strictures. J Vasc Interv Radiol 18:888–895

50. Libby ED, Fawaz R, Leano AM, Hassoun PM (1999) Airway complication of expandable stents. Gastrointest Endosc 49:136–137

51. Ramirez FC, Dennert B, Zierer ST, Sanowski RA (1997) Esophageal self-expandable metallic stents – indications, practice, techniques, and complications: results of a national survey. Gastrointest Endosc 45:360–364

52. Homs MY, Steyerberg EW, Kuipers EJ, van der Gaast A, Haringsma J, van Blankenstein M et al (2004) Causes and treatment of recurrent dysphagia after self-expanding metal stent placement for palliation of esophageal carcinoma. Endoscopy 36:880–886

53. Schoppmann SF, Langer FB, Prager G, Zacherl J (2013) Outcome and complications of long-term self-expanding esophageal stenting. Dis Esophagus 26:154–158

54. Wang MQ, Sze DY, Wang ZP, Wang ZQ, Gao YA, Dake MD (2001) Delayed complications after esophageal stent placement for treatment of malignant esophageal obstructions and esophagorespiratory fistulas. J Vasc Interv Radiol 12:465–474

55. Dormann AJ, Eisendrath P, Wigginghaus B, Huchzermeyer H, Devière J (2003) Palliation of esophageal carcinoma with a new self- expanding plastic stent. Endoscopy 35:207–211

56. Repici A, Conio M, De Angelis C, Battaglia E, Musso A, Pellicano R et al (2004) Temporary placement of an expandable polyester silicone-covered stent for treatment of refractory benign esophageal strictures. Gastrointest Endosc 60:513–519

57. Vanbiervliet G, Filippi J, Karimdjee BS, Venissac N, Iannelli A, Rahili A et al (2012) The role of clips in preventing migration of fully covered metallic esophageal stents: a pilot comparative study. Surg Endosc 26:53–59

58. Repici A, Hassan C, Sharma P, Conio M, Siersema P (2010) Systematic review: the role of self-expanding plastic stents for benign oesophageal strictures. Aliment Pharmacol Ther 31:1268–1275

59. Evrard S, Le Moine O, Lazaraki G, Dormann A, El Nakadi I, Devière J (2004) Self-expanding plastic stents for benign esophageal lesions. Gastrointest Endosc 60:894–900

60. Valenzuela DM, Behr SC, Coakley FV, Wang ZJ, Webb EM, Yeh BM (2014) Computed tomography of iatrogenic complications of upper gastrointestinal endoscopy, stenting, and intubation. Radiol Clin North Am 52:1055–1070

61. Gervaise A, Osemont B, Louis M, Lecocq S, Teixeira P, Blum A (2014) Standard dose versus low-dose abdominal and pelvic CT: comparison between filtered back projection versus adaptive iterative dose reduction 3D. Diagn Interv Imaging 95:47–53

62. Gervaise A, Teixeira P, Villani N, Lecocq S, Louis M, Blum A (2013) CT dose optimisation and reduction in osteoarticular disease. Diagn Interv Imaging 94:371–388

63. Greffier J, Fernandez A, Macri F, Freitag C, Metge L, Beregi J-P (2013) Which dose for what image? Iterative reconstruction for CT scan. Diagn Interv Imaging 94:1117–1121

64. Burckel LA, Defez D, Chaillot PF, Douek P, Boussel L (2015) Use of an automatic recording system for CT doses: evaluation of the impact of iterative reconstruction on radiation exposure in clinical practice. Diagn Interv Imaging 96:265–272

65. Young CA, Menias CO, Bhalla S, Prasad SR (2008) CT features of esophageal emergencies. Radiographics 28:1541–1553

66. Kim HC, Han JK, Kim TK, Do KH, Kim HB, Park JH et al (2000) Duodenal perforation as a delayed complication of placement of an esophageal stent. J Vasc Interv Radiol 11:902–904

67. Dormann A, Meisner S, Verin N, Wenk Lang A (2004) Self-expanding metal stents for gastroduodenal malignancies: systematic review of their clinical effectiveness. Endoscopy 36:543–550

68. Adler DG, Baron TH (2002) Endoscopic palliation of malignant gastric outlet obstruction using self-expanding metal stents: experience in 36 patients. Am J Gastroenterol 97:72–78

69. Lopera JE, Brazzini A, Gonzales A, Castaneda-Zuniga WR (2004) Gastroduodenal stent placement: current status. Radiographics 24:1561–1573

70. Van Hooft JE, Uitdehaag MJ, Bruno MJ, Timmer R, Siersema PD, Dijkgraaf MG et al (2009) Efficacy and safety of the new WallFlex enteral stent in palliative treatment of malignant gastric outlet obstruction (DUOFLEX study): a prospective multicenter study. Gastrointest Endosc 69:1059–1066

71. Del Piano M, Ballarè M, Montino F, Todesco A, Orsello M, Magnani C et al (2005) Endoscopy or surgery for malignant GI outlet obstruction? Gastrointest Endosc 61:421–426

72. Jeurnink SM, Steyerberg EW, van Hooft JE, van Eijck CH, Schwartz MP, Vleggaar FP et al (2010) Surgical gastrojejunostomy or endoscopic stent placement for the palliation of malignant gastric outlet obstruction (SUSTENT study): a multicenter randomized trial. Gastrointest Endosc 71:490–499

73. Fiori E, Lamazza A, De Cesare A, Bononi M, Volpino P, Schillaci A et al (2004) Palliative management of malignant rectosigmoidal obstruction. Colostomy vs endoscopic stenting. A randomized prospective trial. Anticancer Res 24:265–268

74. Mehta S, Hindmarsh A, Cheong E, Cockburn J, Saada J, Tighe R et al (2006) Prospective randomized trial of laparoscopic gastrojejunostomy versus duodenal stenting for malignant gastric outflow obstruction. Surg Endosc 20:239–242

75. Siddiqui A, Spechler SJ, Huerta S (2007) Surgical bypass versus endoscopic stenting for malignant gastroduodenal obstruction: a decision analysis. Dig Dis Sci 52:276–281

76. Gaidos JK, Draganov PV (2009) Treatment of malignant gastric out- let obstruction with endoscopically placed self-expandable metal stents. World J Gastroenterol 15:4365–4371

77. Diamantopoulos A, Sabharwal T, Katsanos K, Krokidis M, Adam A (2015) Fluoroscopic-guided insertion of self-expanding metal stents for malignant gastroduodenal outlet obstruction: immediate results and clinical outcomes. Acta Radiol 56:1373–1379

78. Masci E, Viale E, Mangiavillano B, Contin G, Lomazzi A, Buffoli F et al (2008) Enteral self-expanding metal stent for malignant luminal obstruction of the upper and lower gastrointestinal tract: a prospective multicentric study. J Clin Gastroenterol 42:389–394

79. Flug JA, Garnet DJ, Widmer J, Stavropoulos S, Gidwaney R, Katz DS et al (2013) Advanced gastrointestinal endoscopic procedures: indications, imaging findings, and implications for the radiologist. Clin Imaging 37:624–630

80. Cho YK, Kim SW, Hur WH, Nam KW, Chang JH, Park JM et al (2010) Clinical outcomes of self-expandable metal stent and prognostic factors for stent patency in gastric outlet obstruction caused by gastric cancer. Dig Dis Sci 55:668–674

81. Maetani I, Tada T, Ukita T, Inoue H, Sakai Y, Nagao J (2004) Comparison of duodenal stent placement with surgical gastrojejunostomy for palliation in patients with duodenal obstructions caused by pancreaticobiliary malignancies. Endoscopy 36:73–78

82. Mittal A, Windsor J, Woodfield J, Casey P, Lane M (2004) Matched study of three methods for palliation of malignant pyloroduodenal obstruction. Br J Surg 91:205–209

83. Jeurnink SM, Steyerberg EW, Hof VG, van Eijck CH, Kuipers EJ, Siersema PD (2007) Gastrojejunostomy versus stent placement in patients with malignant gastric outlet obstruction: a comparison in 95 patients. J Surg Oncol 96:389–396

84. Vanbiervliet G, Demarquay J-F, Dumas R, Caroli-Bosc F-X, Piche T, Tran A (2004) Endoscopic insertion of biliary stents in 18 patients with metallic duodenal stents who developed secondary malignant obstructive jaundice. Gastroenterol Clin Biol 28:1209–1213

85. Mutignani M, Tringali A, Shah SG, Perri V, Familiari P, Iacopini F et al (2007) Combined endoscopic stent insertion in malignant biliary and duodenal obstruction. Endoscopy 39:440–447

86. Nassif T, Prat F, Meduri B, Fritsch J, Choury AD, Dumont JL et al (2003) Endoscopic palliation of malignant gastric outlet obstruction using self-expandable metallic stents: results of a multicenter study. Endoscopy 35:483–489

87. Nevitt AW, Vida F, Kozarek RA, Traverso LW, Raltz SL (1998) Expandable metallic prostheses for malignant obstructions of gastric outlet and proximal small bowel. Gastrointest Endosc 47:271–276

88. Kim GH, Kang DH, Lee DH, Heo J, Song GA, Cho M et al (2004) Which types of stent, uncovered or covered, should be used in gastric outlet obstructions? Scand J Gastroenterol 39:1010–1014

89. Dohan A, Eveno C, Dautry R, Guerrache Y, Camus M, Boudiaf M et al (2015) Role and effectiveness of percutaneous arterial embolization in hemodynamically unstable patients with ruptured splanchnic artery pseudoaneurysms. Cardiovasc Intervent Radiol 38:862–870

Part II

Complications of Percutaneous Endoscopic Gastrostomy

Complications of Percutaneous Endoscopic Gastrostomy (PEG)

5

Alessandra Dell'Era

5.1 Percutaneous Endoscopic Gastrostomy: An Overview

Percutaneous endoscopic gastrostomy (PEG) was first introduced by Ponsky and Gauderer in 1980 [1]. Since its introduction in medicine, its use has progressively grown, and now it is a widely used method for providing nutritional support to patients with various contraindications to oral feeding [2, 3].

5.1.1 Indications

PEG tube insertion has two main indications: feeding and gut decompression [4].

Enteral nutrition support is indicated for patients with impossible oral intake due to neurological conditions, oropharyngeal dysfunction or pathologies, short bowel syndrome, major trauma and burns, generally if the condition would prevent eating for more than 30 days.

Although PEG feeding can be beneficial, growing evidence shows that in some patients it

can be futile and even dangerous. In patients with advanced dementia, for instance, it has been shown that PEG does not provide survival benefit or improvement of the nutritional status [5] while increasing the risk of aspiration pneumonia, infection, leakage and diarrhoea.

In patients with advanced abdominal malignancies causing chronic obstruction/ileus, PEG tubes can be used to decompress the gastrointestinal tract [4].

5.1.2 Patient- and Procedure-Related Risk Factors and Contraindications

Contraindications of PEG placement are the same of upper GI endoscopy plus the inability to transilluminate the abdominal wall (as we will see necessary to identify the site of PEG placement).

Patient-related risk factors for complications or PEG placement failure are coagulopathy, portal hypertension, moderate or severe ascites, peritoneal dialysis and neoplastic or inflammatory diseases of the abdominal wall [6]. In case of obstruction of the pharynx or of the oesophagus, deterioration of the clinical status of the patients intraprocedurally and development of haematoma at the gastrostomy site [7], PEG placement may fail. Previous surgery that has altered the oesophageal, gastric or bowel anatomy may lead to ineffective or difficult PEG placement.

A. Dell'Era, PhD
Gastroenterology Unit, "Luigi Sacco" University Hospital, Via G.B. Grassi 74, Milan 20157, Italy

Department of Clinical and Medical Sciences, Università degli Studi di Milano, Via G.B. Grassi 74, Milan 20157, Italy
e-mail: alessandra.dellera@unimi.it

© Springer International Publishing Switzerland 2016
M. Tonolini (ed.), *Imaging Complications of Gastrointestinal and Biliopancreatic Endoscopy Procedures*, DOI 10.1007/978-3-319-31211-8_5

43

5.1.3 The Procedure

The most commonly used PEG placement technique is the "pull" method [1, 8]. The sedated patient is in the supine position, and the abdomen is disinfected. A complete upper gastrointestinal endoscopy is performed in order to rule out oesophageal, gastric or duodenal pathologies that can contraindicate the PEG placement. The stomach is then insufflated, causing its close apposition to the abdominal wall. The point which will be chosen for PEG placement is the point in the mid-epigastrium where maximal transillumination is seen, and indentation of the gastric lumen (seen by the endoscopist) is observed during direct pressure with the finger. Local anaesthesia is injected in the identified area and a small incision is made. A large bore needle is inserted in the same point under endoscopic observation. A guidewire is threaded through the needle, grasped by the endoscopist with a snare and withdrawn from the stomach through the mouth with the endoscope. The tapered end of the gastrostomy tube is then secured to the guidewire and pulled back to the stomach. The correct placement of the internal bumper, snug against the gastric wall, is confirmed by a second endoscopy. An external bumper is used to secure the PEG tub in place and prevent distal migration of the internal bumper.

During the following days, the PEG site should be cleaned with mild soap and water (hydrogen peroxide should not be used as it can irritate the skin and contribute to stomal leaks). Cut drain sponges should be placed over, and not under, the external bumper so as not to apply excessive tension to the PEG site. Occlusive dressings should not be used as they can lead to peristomal skin maceration and breakdown.

The overall success rate for PEG placement is about 94–98 % [7, 9].

5.2 PEG-Related Complications

Complications have been known to occur after PEG placement, with a stable overall complication rate of 4–23.8 % [7, 10, 11].

Complications of PEG placement can be due to the upper GI endoscopy performed and

Table 5.1 Complications of percutaneous endoscopic gastrostomy

Complication	Prevalence (%)
Aspiration	0.3–1.0
Haemorrhage	0–2.5
Peritonitis	0.5–1.3
Fistulous tracts	0.3–6.7
Ileus	1–2
Peristomal infection	5.4–30
Stomal leakage	1–2
Buried bumper syndrome	0.3–2.4
Inadvertent removal	1.6–4.4
Tumour seeding	<1
Death	0–2.1

sedation (0.1 %) including perforation, haemorrhage, aspiration, hypoxia and hypotension [12].

Other complications are specific for PEG placement. Of these, only a minority are major complications (3–4 %) that need surgical intervention and/or are life threatening [7, 10, 13–15], while in about 7.4–20 % of cases, minor complications can occur [7, 10, 13–16] (see Table 5.1).

Pneumoperitoneum is a common finding after oral PEG placement [14–17], and as we will see, it should not be considered a complication.

Death after PEG placement is mainly due to comorbidities, with immediate and 30-day procedure-related death rates of 0–2 % and 1.5–2.1 %, respectively [10, 18].

5.2.1 Aspiration

Aspiration during PEG placement has been reported in 0.3–1 % of cases [7, 19].

Risk factors for intraprocedural aspiration include supine position, sedation, neurological impairment and advanced age [6].

Prevention: this complication can be minimised by avoiding oversedation, minimising air insufflation in the stomach and aspirating the gastric contents before the procedure [6].

Clinical and laboratory manifestations and diagnosis: the patient presents with symptoms and signs of pneumonia, with consistent chest X-ray appearances, particularly lung-base consolidation.

Treatment options: treatment with broad-spectrum antibiotics should be instituted.

5.2.2 Haemorrhage and Haematoma

Bleeding due to PEG placement can be distinguished in intraprocedural and post-procedural. *Acute bleeding during PEG placement* occurs in approximately 1 % of cases [20] and is due to the puncture of an abdominal wall vessel. Significant bleeding following PEG for aortic perforation, gastric artery perforation and a retroperitoneal haemorrhage are reported as case reports [21]. The development of a haematoma at the PEG site complicates about 1 % of cases [22].

Risk factors include anticoagulation and previous anatomic alteration [23]. *Post-procedural bleeding* is reported in 0.3–1.2 % of cases [7, 24]. It is usually caused by peptic ulcer disease, traumatic erosion of the gastric wall opposite the internal bumper or ulceration beneath the internal bumper. To reduce risk of ulcerations at the gastrostomy site, excessive lateral traction on the tube should be avoided. During endoscopy, the mucosa under the internal bolster should be visualised by externally manipulating the PEG [25].

Clinical and laboratory manifestations: post-PEG placement bleeding is manifested by haemorrhage around the PEG insertion site, evidence of blood in the PEG tube or melaena.

Diagnosis: the diagnosis is made by clinical observation of the bleeding around the PEG insertion site in case of abdominal vessel puncture or by endoscopy in case of post-procedural bleeding.

Treatment options: antisecretory therapy should be instituted in case of peptic disease. In case of minor bleeding from PEG tract, the treatment consists in tightening the external bolster against the skin for a maximum of 48 h to avoid mucosal necrosis. In case of a more important bleeding, standard resuscitation procedure and treatment according to the source of bleeding found should be instituted.

5.2.3 Pneumoperitoneum

Transient subclinical pneumoperitoneum can be observed in up to 56 % of PEG placement procedures and, if not associated to a specific clinic (see below) generally, is not of any clinical significance [14]. It is probably due to air that escapes through the opening in the stomach during the time interval between needle puncture and PEG placement [15].

Clinical and laboratory manifestations: if no gastric perforation is associated, it is usually asymptomatic. The issue of post-procedural pneumoperitoneum is further discussed in Chap. 6.

Treatment options: pneumoperitoneum is usually self limiting, and it is clinically concerning in case of worsening and/or associated signs of peritonitis [14].

5.2.4 Perforation

Perforation during PEG placement occurs in 0.5–1.3 % of cases [7, 22] and is one of the more threatened complications of this procedure due to its significant morbidity and mortality if not treated promptly [25].

Clinical and laboratory manifestations: the patient presents with symptoms and signs of peritonitis (abdominal pain, leucocytosis, ileus and fever).

Diagnosis: at plain films of the abdomen, pneumoperitoneum can be seen, but it is of limited utility (see below) [14]. Some authors suggest obtaining fluoroscopic imaging of the PEG tube with infusion of water-soluble contrast, in order to evaluate visceral integrity in patients in whom peritonitis is a concern [26]. As further discussed in Chap. 6, imaging (particularly with CT) allows confirming clinical diagnosis of peritonitis.

Treatment options: if active leakage of contrast is identified in a patient with clinical signs of peritonitis, broad-spectrum antibiotics and surgical exploration (in patients fit for surgery) are usually indicated.

5.2.5 Fistulous Tracts/Migration of the Tube

A rare complication of PEG placement is the occurrence of a (gastro)-colo-cutaneous fistula which may occur when the colon is inadvertently punctured and traversed during PEG placement or, less commonly, with subsequent erosion of the tube into juxtaposed colon.

Prevention: this complication can be prevented by using the so-called safe track technique [25], that is, using an aspirating syringe during anaesthesia to identify intervening bowel between the skin and the stomach: if air bubbles appear in the syringe prior to endoscopic visualisation of the needle in the gastric lumen, colonic interposition should be suspected.

Clinical and laboratory manifestations: patients may present acutely with sign and symptoms of colonic perforation or obstruction. More commonly, patients present with stool leaking around the PEG tube and diarrhoea resembling nutritional formula. Plain radiographs and, better, CT allow assessment of device migration.

Treatment options: management consists of removing the tube and allowing the fistula to close [27]. If the patient has developed signs of peritonitis or the fistula does not close, surgery is required.

5.2.6   Prolonged Ileus

After PEG placement, tube feeding may start as soon as after 3 h [28]. However, in 1–2 % of cases prolonged, ileus may follow PEG placement [7].

Clinical and laboratory manifestations: the patient presents with abdominal distension, nausea and vomiting.

Diagnosis: the diagnosis is clinical revealing abdominal distension, absence of bowel sounds.

Treatment options: post-PEG ileus should be managed conservatively, with supportive therapy and gastric decompression by uncapping the PEG tube. PEG feeding should be withheld until the ileus resolves.

5.2.7   Skin Infection

Infection of the PEG site is the most common complication of PEG placement, being reported in as much as 30 % of cases [29]. Fortunately, only the minority of these infections (less than 1.6 %) requires aggressive medical and/or surgical treatment [30]. A rare but potentially

life-threatening complication is the development of necrotising fasciitis.

Risk factors for peristomal infection are diabetes mellitus, chronic renal failure, obesity, poor nutritional status, alcoholism and chronic corticosteroid therapy [31, 32]. Another recognised risk factor is the excessive pressure between the PEG's external and internal bumper that causes ischaemia [33]; therefore, it is important to maintain only a loose contact of the outer bolster with the skin to appose the gastric and abdominal wall.

Prevention: the administration of prophylactic antibiotics prior to PEG placement has been shown to be beneficial [30] and cost-effective [34]. The standard practice is to administer a single dose of a first- or third-generation cephalosporin 30 min prior to the procedure. Prophylaxis is not necessary in those patients already receiving comparable antibiotics for other reasons at the time of PEG placement.

Another strategy shown to reduce skin infection is to practise an adequate skin incision, 1–2 mm larger than the feeding tube, to allow egression of bacteria and gastric secretions.

Clinical and laboratory manifestations: reddening and swelling of the peristomal skin may be evident. Blood analysis may show signs of inflammatory response.

Diagnosis: clinical evidence of the signs described above may give the diagnosis. Skin swabs may be useful to identify the pathogen.

Treatment options: if diagnosed early, oral broad-spectrum antibiotics for 5–7 days may be all that is required for a PEG site infection. If there are more systemic signs, intravenous broad-spectrum antibiotics coupled with local wound care are necessary. In case the patient shows also signs of peritonitis, surgical intervention may be required. In case of necrotising fasciitis is diagnosed, broad-spectrum intravenous antibiotics and aggressive surgical debridement are mandatory.

5.2.8   PEG Leakage

The reported incidence of leakage of tube feeding formula and/or gastric contents around the PEG site is of 1–2 % [35].

Risk factors include infection of the site, increased gastric acid secretion, excessive cleansing with hydrogen peroxide, buried bumper syndrome, side torsion on the PEG tube and the absence of an external bolster to stabilise the tube [13]. Patient risk factors associated with peristomal leakage are those that hinder wound healing: diabetes, malnutrition and immunodeficiency.

Clinical and laboratory manifestations: the feeding formula and gastric content are seen to leak around the PEG tube causing chemical burns of the peristomal skin.

Diagnosis: evaluation of a leaking PEG site should include examination for evidence of infection, ulceration or a buried bumper.

Treatment options: the optimisation of glycaemic control and nutritional status is the first step. Patients should also start gastric acid suppression, with proton pump inhibitor therapy. Side torsion of the PEG resulting in ulceration and enlargement of the tract may be corrected with a clamping device to stabilise the tube or replacing the PEG with a low-profile button device. The replacement of the gastrostomy tube with a larger one is usually ineffective and can result in continued leakage around an even larger stoma [26].

After the primary cause of the stomal leakage has been addressed, stoma adhesive powder or zinc oxide can be applied to the site to prevent local skin irritation. Foam dressing rather than gauze can help to reduce local skin irritation caused by gastric contents (foam lifts the drainage away from the skin while gauze tends to trap it). Local fungal skin infections may also be associated with leakage and can be treated with topical antifungals. Referral to evaluation of ostomy nurses is recommended.

In refractory cases, the PEG tube must be removed for several days to allow the stoma to approximate the tube more closely, and a new PEG can be placed through the same site [36]. Occasionally the tube must be removed, and a new PEG should be placed at a new site [36].

5.2.9 Gastric Outlet Obstruction

Gastric outlet obstruction is a rare complication caused by the migration of the distal part of the PEG tube in the pylorus, causing its complete or partial obstruction. It is due to the absence of the external bumper that allows PEG dislocation.

Clinical and laboratory manifestations: the patient presents with abdominal cramps and intermittent vomiting.

Diagnosis: upper gastrointestinal study or upper gastrointestinal will confirm the suspicion.

Treatment options: the treatment consists in the retrieval of the internal bumper by endoscopy.

5.2.10 Buried Bumper Syndrome

This complication occurs in 0.3–2.4 % of patients with PEG. It is caused by the growth of gastric mucosa to cover, completely or partially, the internal bumper; the bumper may then migrate through the gastric wall and may lodge anywhere along the PEG tract [7, 37].

Risk factors include excessive tension between the internal and external bolsters, malnutrition, poor wound healing and significant weight gain secondary to successful enteral nutrition [13]. Fatal cases have been reported.

Prevention consists in slackening the external bolster once the fistula is mature; rotate and push the PEG tube once a week, and adjust the external bolster if the patient puts on weight.

Clinical and laboratory manifestations: peritubal leakage or infection, immobile catheter or abdominal pain or resistance with formula infusion.

Diagnosis: the buried bumper should be suspected when the PEG can't be pushed easily [26] and may be confirmed endoscopically or radiographically. Endoscopy may show an irregular crevice or a raised mound with a central concave area of mucosa without ulceration or oedema [37]. The buried bumper may be localised by CT imaging, as discussed in Chap. 6.

Treatment options: buried bumpers should be removed even if the patient is asymptomatic, due to the high risk of tube impaction in the abdominal wall and/or perforation. The key principle is to use a technique that minimises trauma to the PEG tract. Computed tomography, ultrasonography and endoscopic ultrasound may be used to localise the bumper and decide if an endoscopic, surgical or combined approach should be used [37]. If the bumper is completely covered by gastric mucosa, electrosurgical incisions may be necessary to access and remove the bumper endoscopically.

5.2.11 Inadvertent Removal

The reported prevalence of accidental PEG tube removal is 1.6–4.4 % [3, 7, 24]. An important *risk factor* is a confused patient who pulls on the feeding tube.

Clinical and laboratory manifestations: the clinical and laboratory manifestations vary according to the moment in which the removal occurs. In early removal signs of peritonitis can be present since the apposition of the stomach to the abdominal wall may not be complete. In late removals no clinical signs can be present. PEG removal can be complete (complete displacement of the internal bumper) or incomplete (i.e. the internal bumper is outside the gastric wall but in the peritoneum). If this latter case in not recognised, nutritional formula would be given intra-peritoneally causing serious peritonitis.

Diagnosis: once the PEG has been removed, CT scan is useful to determine the degree of peritoneal contamination, a key factor to decide the subsequent management.

Treatment options: the most worrisome period in which PEG removal can occur is the first 7–10 days (but may be delayed up to 4 weeks in the presence of malnutrition, ascites or corticosteroid treatment) because the apposition of gastric wall to abdominal wall may be incomplete, and PEG removal may cause free perforation. If PEG removal occurs in the timeframe, PEG should be replaced under fluoroscopic guidance or endoscopically (keeping air insufflation to the minimum); the blind reinsertion of a PEG tube may lead to its placement in the peritoneal cavity. If recognised immediately, a new PEG tube may be placed through, or near, the original PEG site, sealing the stomach against the anterior abdominal wall [38]. If recognition is delayed, management consists of nasogastric suction, broad-spectrum antibiotics and repeat PEG placement in 7–10 days [39]. Surgical exploration is reserved for patients with signs of peritonitis.

If PEG removal occurs more than 1 month after placement, stoma tract maturation can be assumed, and the replacement of the tube can be done without endoscopy. It is important to remember that the tract would close within 24 h, so the PEG tube has to be replaced as soon as possible, or a Foley catheter should be inserted, to keep the fistula patent, aiming at replacing it in the shortest possible time.

In patients prone to pulling at tubes, an abdominal binder can secure the PEG tube in place. Also consider cutting the tube down to 6–8 in. to decrease the likelihood that the tube is inadvertently caught on another object. Finally, an initial placement of low-profile device (button) may be beneficial.

5.2.12 Tumour Seeding

In patients with head or neck cancer, placement of prophylactic gastrostomy feeding tubes has been shown to be beneficial [40]; however, implantation of head and neck cancer at the stoma site has been reported with an incidence <1 % [41]. The mechanism of implantation is most likely direct seeding of tumour at the PEG site after the tube shears tumour cells as it passes through the aerodigestive tract [42].

The *prevention* of this occurrence can be placing the PEG using the introducer technique, in which the PEG is placed directly through the abdominal wall.

Clinical and laboratory manifestations and diagnosis: tumour implantation should be suspected in patients with head and neck cancer who develop unexplained skin changes at the PEG site.

Treatment options: should a patient develop tumour at the gastrostomy site, no treatment is usually given, but palliative radiotherapy has been reported in one case [43, 44].

References

1. Ponsky JL, Gauderer MW (1981) Percutaneous endoscopic gastrostomy: a nonoperative technique for feeding gastrostomy. Gastrointest Endosc 27(1):9–11
2. Gauderer MW (1999) Twenty years of percutaneous endoscopic gastrostomy: origin and evolution of a

concept and its expanded applications. Gastrointest Endosc 50(6):879–883

3. Dwyer KM, Watts DD, Thurber JS et al (2002) Percutaneous endoscopic gastrostomy: the preferred method of elective feeding tube placement in trauma patients. J Trauma 52:26–32

4. McClave SA, Ritchie CS (2006) The role of endoscopically placed feeding or decompression tubes. Gastroenterol Clin North Am 35:83–100

5. Finucane TE, Christmas C, Travis K (1999) Tube feeding in patients with advanced dementia: a review of the evidence. JAMA 282(14):1365–1370

6. Safadi BY, Marks JM, Ponsky JL (1998) Percutaneous endoscopic gastrostomy. Gastrointest Endosc Clin N Am 8:551–568

7. Larson DE, Burton DD, Schroeder KW et al (1987) Percutaneous endoscopic gastrostomy. Indications, success, complications, and mortality in 314 consecutive patients. Gastroenterology 93:48–52

8. Gauderer MW, Ponsky JL, Izant R Jr (1980) Gastrostomy without laparotomy: a percutaneous endoscopic technique. J Pediatr Surg 15:872–875

9. Taylor CA, Larson DE, Ballard DJ et al (1992) Predictors of outcome after percutaneous endoscopic gastrostomy: a community-based study. Mayo Clin Proc 67:1042–1049

10. Loser C, Wolters S, Folsch UR (1998) Enteral long-term nutrition via percutaneous endoscopic gastrostomy in 210 patients: a four-year prospective study. Dig Dis Sci 43:2549–2557

11. Lockett MA, Templeton ML, Byrne TK et al (2002) Percutaneous endoscopic gastrostomy complications in a tertiary-care center. Am Surg 68:117–120

12. Kavic SM, Basson MD (2001) Complications of endoscopy. Am J Surg 181:319–332

13. McClave SA, Chang WK (2003) Complications of enteral access. Gastrointest Endosc 58:739–751

14. Wojtowycz MM, Arata JA Jr, Micklos TJ et al (1988) CT findings after uncomplicated percutaneous gastrostomy. Am J Radiol 151:307–309

15. Gottfried EB, Plumser AB, Clair MR (1986) Pneumoperitoneum following percutaneous endoscopic gastrostomy: a prospective study. Gastrointest Endosc 32:397–399

16. Stassen WN, McCullough AJ, Marshall JB et al (1984) Percutaneous gastrostomy: another cause of "benign" pneumoperitoneum. Gastrointest Endosc 30:296–298

17. Hillman KM (1982) Pneumoperitoneum: a review. Crit Care Med 10:476–481

18. Davis JB Jr, Bowden TJ, Rives DA (1990) Percutaneous endoscopic gastrostomy. Do surgeons and gastroenterologists get the same results? Am Surg 56:47–51

19. Grant JP (1993) Percutaneous endoscopic gastrostomy. Initial placement by single endoscopic technique and long-term follow-up. Ann Surg 217:168–174

20. Petersen TI, Kruse A (1997) Complications of percutaneous endoscopic gastrostomy. Eur J Surg 163:351–356

21. Schurink CA, Tuynman H, Scholten P et al (2001) Percutaneous endoscopic gastrostomy: complications and suggestions to avoid them. Eur J Gastroenterol Hepatol 13:819

22. Rabeneck L, Wray NP, Petersen NJ (1996) Long-term outcomes of patients receiving percutaneous endoscopic gastrostomy tubes. J Gen Intern Med 11:287–293

23. Hament JM, Bax NM, van der Zee DC et al (2001) Complications of percutaneous endoscopic gastrostomy with or without concomitant antireflux surgery in 96 children. J Pediatr Surg 36:1412–1415

24. Rimon E (2001) The safety and feasibility of percutaneous endoscopic gastrostomy placement by a single physician. Endoscopy 33:241–244

25. Fang JC (2007) Minimizing endoscopic complications in enteral access. Gastrointest Endosc Clin N Am 17:179–196

26. Schapiro GD, Edmundowicz SA (1996) Complications of percutaneous endoscopic gastrostomy. Gastrointest Endosc Clin N Am 6:409–422

27. Rino Y, Tokunaga M, Morinaga S et al (2002) The buried bumper syndrome: an early complication of percutaneous endoscopic gastrostomy. Hepatogastroenterology 49:1183–1184

28. Choudhry U, Barde CJ, Markert R et al (1996) Percutaneous endoscopic gastrostomy: a randomized prospective comparison of early and delayed feeding. Gastrointest Endosc 44:164–167

29. Hull MA, Rawlings J, Murray FE et al (1993) Audit of outcome of longterm enteral nutrition by percutaneous endoscopic gastrostomy. Lancet 341:869–872

30. Gossner L, Keymling J, Hahn EG et al (1999) Antibiotic prophylaxis in percutaneous endoscopic gastrostomy (PEG): a prospective randomized clinical trial. Endoscopy 31:119–124

31. Lee JH, Kim JJ, Kim YH et al (2002) Increased risk of peristomal wound infection after percutaneous endoscopic gastrostomy in patients with diabetes mellitus. Dig Liver Dis 34:857–861

32. Greif JM, Ragland JJ, Ochsner MG et al (1986) Necrotising fasciitis complicating percutaneous endoscopic gastrostomy. Gastrointest Endosc 32:292–294

33. Chung RS, Schertzer M (1990) Pathogenesis of complications of percutaneous endoscopic gastrostomy: a lesson in surgical principles. Am Surg 56:134–137

34. Kulling D, Sonnenberg A, Fried M et al (2000) Cost analysis of antibiotic prophylaxis for PEG. Gastrointest Endosc 51:152–156

35. Lin HS, Ibrahim HZ, Kheng JW et al (2001) Percutaneous endoscopic gastrostomy: strategies for prevention and management of complications. Laryngoscope 111:1847–1852

36. Tsang TK, Eaton D, Falconio MA (1989) Percutaneous ostomy dilation: a technique for dilating the closed percutaneous endoscopic gastrostomy sites and reinserting gastrostomies. Gastrointest Endosc 35:336

37. Venu RP, Brown RD, Pastika BJ et al (2002) The buried bumper syndrome: a simple management approach in two patients. Gastrointest Endosc 56:582–584

38. Yamazaki T, Sakai Y, Hatekeyama K et al (1999) Colocutaneous fistula after percutaneous endoscopic gastrostomy in a remnant stomach. Surg Endosc 13:280–282

39. Galat SA, Gerig KD, Porter JA et al (1990) Management of premature removal of percutaneous gastrostomy. Am Surg 56:733–736

40. Lynch CR, Fang JC (2004) Prevention and management of complications of percutaneous endoscopic gastrostomy (PEG) tubes. Pract Gastroenterol 28:66–76

41. Romano M, McLaughlin M, Scolapio J (2000) PEG tube placement in head and neck cancer patients prior to radiation therapy [abstract]. JPEN 24:S25

42. Cruz I, Mamel JJ, Brady PG et al (2005) Incidence of abdominal wall metastasis complicating PEG tube placement in untreated head and neck cancer. Gastrointest Endosc 62:708–711

43. Mincheff TV (2005) Metastatic spread to a percutaneous gastrostomy site from head and neck cancer: case report and literature review. J Soc Laparoendosc Surg 9:466–471

44. Laccourreye O, Chabardes E, Merite-Drancy A et al (1993) Implantation metastasis following percutaneous endoscopic gastrostomy. J Laryngol Otol 107:946–949

Imaging of Percutaneous Endoscopic Gastrostomy (PEG)-Related Complications

6

Massimo Tonolini

6.1 Introduction

6.1.1 Percutaneous Endoscopic Gastrostomy: Indications and Technical Basics

Enteral nutrition is needed in those individuals with normal intestinal function but unable to take oral feeding and is commonly administered through nasoenteric tubes in patients who are expected to resume oral nutrition within a month. Traditionally, long-term enteral nutrition required surgical gastrostomy or jejunostomy. Since its initial description by Gauderer et al. in 1980, percutaneous endoscopic gastrostomy (PEG) has increasingly gained acceptance and has replaced surgical gastrostomy as a safe, rapid and effective means of establishing an enteral access. Currently PEG represents the preferred minimally invasive technique to provide long-term nutrition support and prevent lung aspiration [1–4].

The commonest indications for PEG positioning include dysphagia or swallowing disorders from neurological conditions such as amyotrophic lateral sclerosis and stroke, and upper aerodigestive tract tumours undergoing chemoradiotherapy. Furthermore, PEG is often adopted in intensive

care units (ICU), particularly in patients with cerebral injuries requiring long-term hospitalisation. According to the most recent guidelines from the American Society for Gastrointestinal Endoscopy (ASGE), absolute contraindications include severe coagulopathy, pharyngeal or oesophageal obstruction and inability to bring the anterior gastric wall in apposition with the abdominal wall. Relative contraindications include ascites and neoplastic, inflammatory or infiltrative diseases of the stomach and abdominal wall [1–4].

The most widely used PEG technique is the "pull" method. Basically, PEG positioning begins with endoscopic access to the upper gastrointestinal tract, insufflation of the stomach and detection of an area of maximum transillumination at the anterior abdominal wall. After sterile preparation and local anaesthesia, a tapered cannula is introduced over the needle through the abdominal wall into the gastric lumen and grasped with the endoscopic loop snare. After needle withdrawal, a long guidewire is introduced into the stomach and withdrawn through the mouth along with the endoscope so that its distal end is left to protrude through the anterior abdominal wall. The gastrostomy tube is then secured to the proximal end of the loop and tractioned through the upper gastrointestinal tract to the exit site. Some endoscopists perform a repeat endoscopy to confirm correct placement of the internal bumper. Previous gastric resection, hepatomegaly and obesity may hinder or impede PEG placement [3, 5].

M. Tonolini
Radiology Department, "Luigi Sacco" University Hospital, Via G.B. Grassi 74, Milano 20157, Italy
e-mail: mtonolini@sirm.org

© Springer International Publishing Switzerland 2016
M. Tonolini (ed.), *Imaging Complications of Gastrointestinal and Biliopancreatic Endoscopy Procedures*, DOI 10.1007/978-3-319-31211-8_6

6.1.2 Percutaneous Endoscopic Gastrostomy: Overview of Complications

PEG has a high technical success rate and may be easily replaced when malfunction occurs. However, PEG is associated with a non-negligible risk of complications, which may result from insertion, from devices left in place for a long time or during replacement, and is favoured by associated comorbidities. The overall PEG complication rate ranges from 4.9 % to 21 %, irrespective to the technique used. Reported to occur in approximately 3–4 % of cases, major complications are more frequent in patients with malignancies, often require urgent surgery and are associated with a significant mortality (approaching 17 % of cases). The commonest immediate (arising during or just after the PEG positioning) and early (occurring within 4 weeks) complications include respiratory depression, aspiration pneumonia, visceral perforation and peritonitis, misplacement, leakage, occasional abdominal wall or gastric haemorrhage. The all-cause short-term (30 days) mortality approaches 10–15 % of patients but is mostly attributed to the severity of underlying disease. However, PEG has a non-negligible direct procedure-related mortality which is estimated at 0.7–2 % [1, 3, 4, 6–8].

After the early post-procedural period, late adverse events occur in 18–21 % of cases and include peristomal infection as the commonest occurrence (which may occasionally give rise to abdominal wall abscesses or necrotising fasciitis), diarrhoea, inadvertent removal, tube dysfunction or obstruction, leakage and device dislodgement [1, 3, 4, 6–8].

6.1.3 Aim

Despite the high technical success rate, improved instrumentation and growing experience, due to the steady increase in referrals for PEG positioning for enteral feeding and palliation, over the last decade, clinicians and radiologists are increasingly faced with suspected acute post-procedural and long-term PEG-related complications [1, 2, 7–9].

This chapter reviews and illustrates the role of conventional radiographs and computed tomography (CT) studies in the elucidation of post-PEG complications, aiming to provide radiologists with an increased familiarity with normal and abnormal imaging appearances. In our experience, multidetector CT provides a comprehensive assessment of the entire PEG device between the exit site and the stomach, may be complemented by administration of water-soluble contrast medium (CM) if needed and allows prompt and reliable assessment of the PEG device positioning and function [10–12]. Therefore, in most patients, CT proves helpful to elucidate most complications requiring external, endoscopic or surgical treatment. Furthermore, radiologists interpreting routine CT studies in patients with a PEG should carefully assess the device, its position and surrounding structures, to detect possible unsuspected complications [7, 10–12].

6.2 Post-PEG Imaging: Techniques and Normal Appearances

6.2.1 Role of Physical Findings

Patient history and physical examination by specifically trained nurses and physicians remains the mainstay for clinical PEG assessment, which is more extensively discussed in the previous Chap. 5. Within a few days after positioning, local pain and guarding around the PEG exit site are commonly observed and generally managed with delayed initiation of feeding (beyond the usual 24 h) plus broad-spectrum antibiotics. External leakage of gastric contents and persistent inflammatory signs around the PEG exit site usually suggest a peristomal infection. Conversely, early onset of abdominal pain and physical signs consistent with peritonitis often herald visceral damage and should prompt urgent imaging investigation and surgical consultation. Furthermore, pain during feeding and PEG malfunction with impaired ability to administer fluids suggest partial or complete dislodgement, which usually requires feeding suspension and appropriate investigation [1–4, 7].

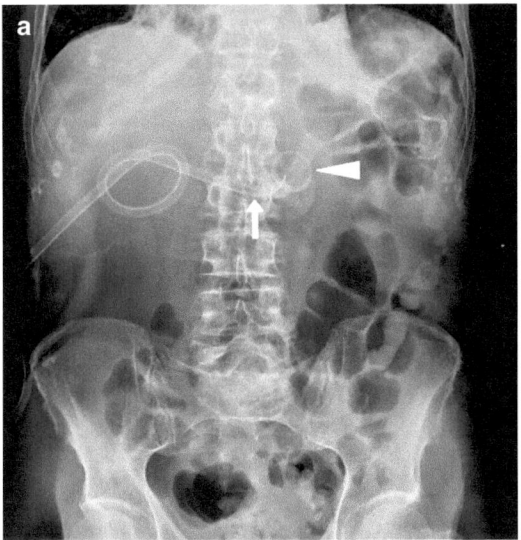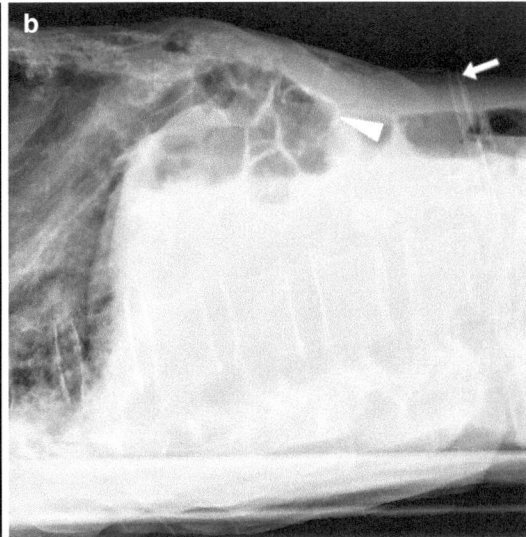

Fig. 6.1 Normal radiographic appearance of a percutaneous endoscopic gastrostomy (*PEG*) on supine (**a**) and tangential (**b**) plain abdominal radiographs. The faintly radio-opaque device tube (*arrows*) and circular internal bumper (*arrowheads*) are recognisable. The latter is located at the transition between gastric body and antrum, correctly adherent to the internal layer of the anterior abdominal wall (**b**)

Unfortunately, patients with altered mental status, on long-term sedation/analgesia and ventilatory support, have unreliable physical findings. Furthermore, fever, ileus and laboratory changes suggesting sepsis are common in ICU patients. Therefore, in most patients, diagnostic imaging is helpful to complement the clinical and endoscopic assessment of PEG device positioning and function [1–4, 7].

6.2.2 Imaging Techniques and Normal Appearances

Plain abdominal radiographs are routinely performed after PEG positioning at some centres in order to detect misplacement. Radiographically, the internal bumper should be usually located in the body of the stomach (Fig. 6.1). The injection of water-soluble CM such as meglumine diatrizoate sodium (Gastrografin®, Schering) or iopromide (Ultravist®, Schering) under fluoroscopy ("PEG-gram") rapidly allows confirming the correct device positioning and patency of the PEG tube (Fig. 6.2). Furthermore, plain films may be helpful for detection and monitoring of post-procedural pneumoperitoneum [11].

Compared to radiographs, multidetector CT provides a much more comprehensive assessment of the entire PEG device between the exit site and the stomach, including information on all anatomical structures and abnormalities located along the PEG tract. The anatomical region to be scanned should include the lung bases along with the abdomen and pelvis. Routinely complemented with multiplanar image reconstructions, CT allows an easy confirmation of the correct positioning of internal bumper, which should adhere to the anterior wall of the gastric body (Fig. 6.3) and of the device's integrity and structure (Fig. 6.4). Alternatively, the PEG internal bumper may be located in the gastric antrum, a situation which does not impede feeding but may predispose to tube migration into the duodenum (Figs. 6.4 and 6.5). In case of uncertainty, the correct device placement and function may be verified with repeated CT after administration of diluted CM through the external PEG access (Figs. 6.6 and 6.7); the same technique allows to detect or exclude any extraluminal CM leakage [10–13].

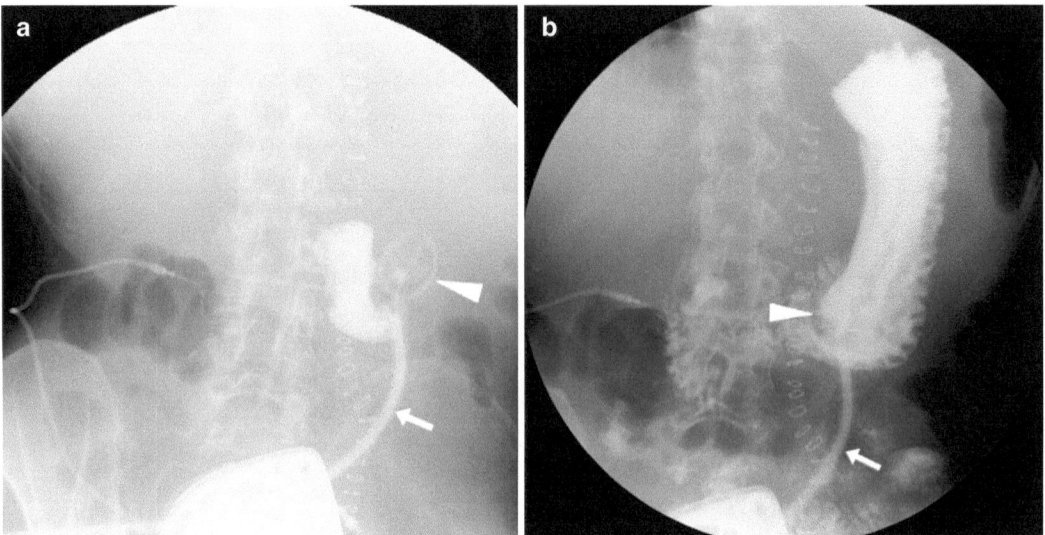

Fig. 6.2 Fluoroscopic study ("PEG-gram") with injection of water-soluble contrast medium (*CM*) showing normal positioning of PEG device in a 63-year-old female with HIV infection, algoneurodystrophy and severe polyneuropathy, currently hospitalised because of neurological worsening with severe dysphagia and wasting syndrome. The internal PEG bumper is indicated by *arrowheads*. CM administration through the PEG external access allowed opacification of the tube (*arrows*) and of the gastric fundus and body, thus confirming its patency and correct positioning. Extraluminal CM leakage was excluded

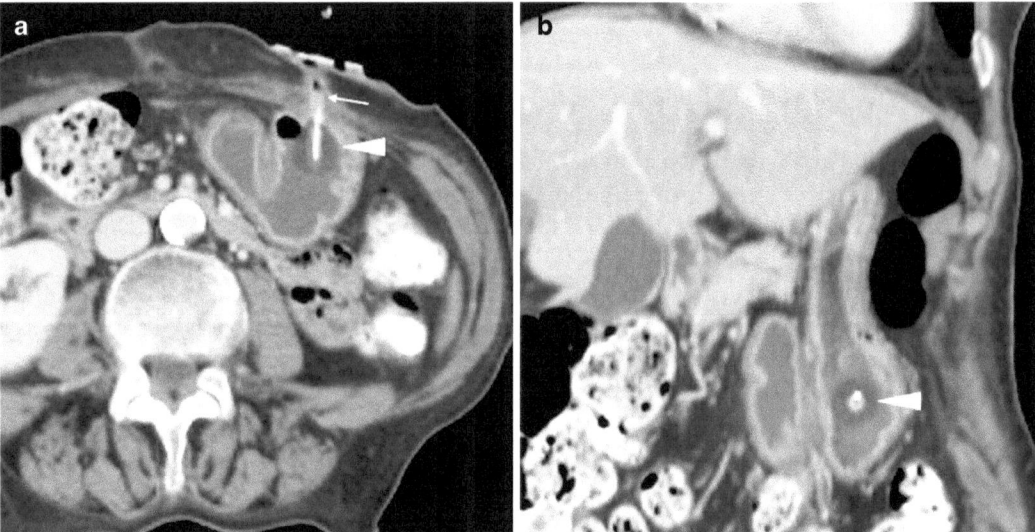

Fig. 6.3 Normal multidetector CT appearance of the PEG, positioned to palliate severe dysphagia in an elderly 83-year-old female with recurrent squamocellular carcinoma of the tongue after previous surgery, chemotherapy and radiotherapy. Contrast-enhanced axial (**a**) and coronal (**b**) CT images showed normally positioned internal bumper (*arrowheads*) in the fluid-filled gastric body. Note the absence of "peritoneal gap" between greater curvature of the stomach and posterior aspect of anterior abdominal wall and of abnormal thickening or inflammatory changes in the anterior abdominal wall muscles and subcutaneous fat traversed by the PEG tube (*thin arrow* in **a**)

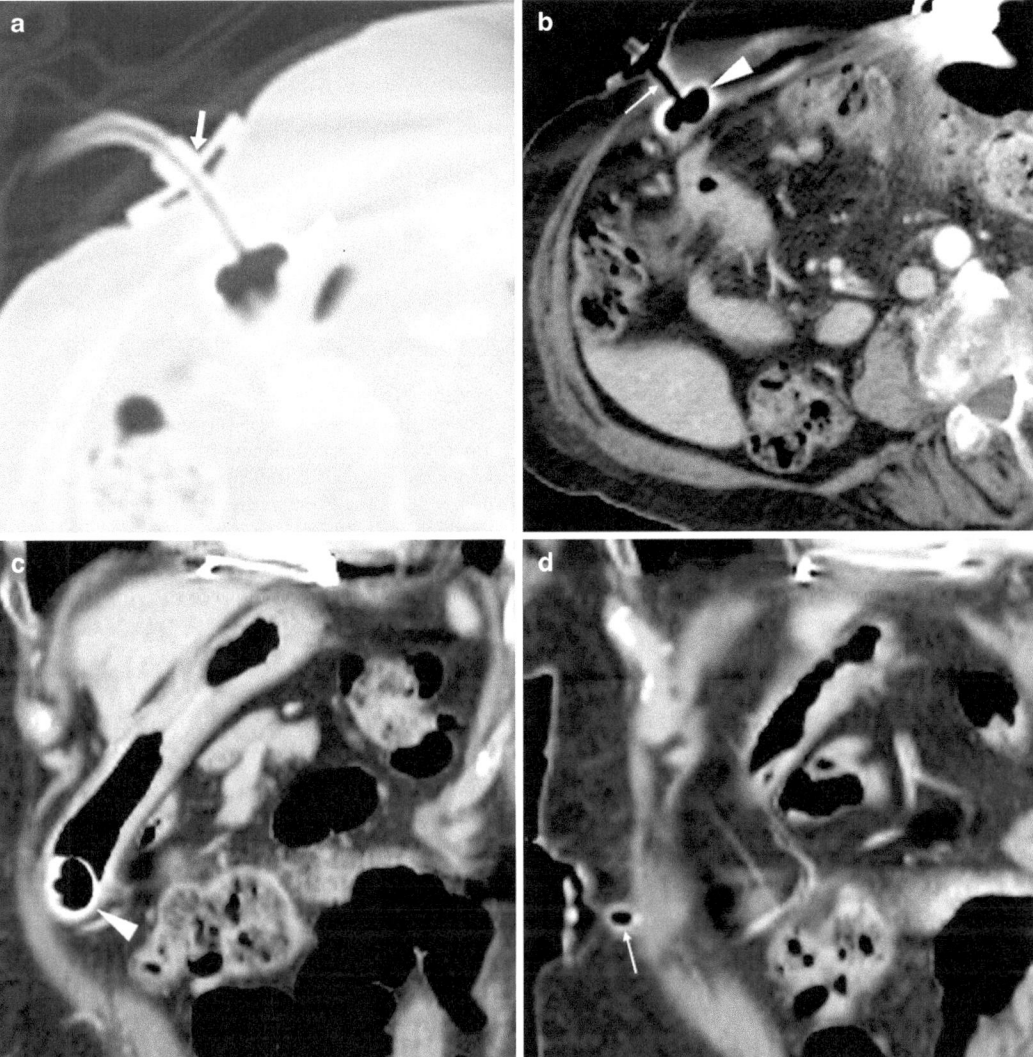

Fig. 6.4 Right-sided PEG positioning with the internal bumper in the gastric antrum. An unenhanced detail axial CT image viewed at lung window settings (**a**) shows the entire structure of the PEG device, including the external fixation "bolster" device (*arrow*), tube (*thin arrow*) and internal bumper (*arrowheads*). The latter, as seen in mul- tiplanar CT images viewed at soft tissue window settings (**b–d**), is located distally in the prepyloric region. Note the absent "peritoneal gap" between anterior gastric wall and posterior aspect of anterior abdominal wall (**b**) and the normal appearance of abdominal wall muscles and subcu- taneous fat traversed by the PEG tube (*thin arrows*)

Furthermore, radiologists should bear in mind the high risk of aspiration pneumonia when interpreting plain radiographs and CT studies in patients with a PEG: the lung bases should be carefully scrutinised to detect infiltrates or consolidations, even without clin- ical or laboratory data suggesting infection [10–13].

6.2.3 The "Peritoneal Gap"

Multidetector CT is the only technique that can assess the thickness and structural changes of subcutaneous fat and abdominal wall muscles and that allows detection and measurement of the "peritoneal gap" (Figs. 6.5 and 6.7) which may develop when the stomach is not closely anchored

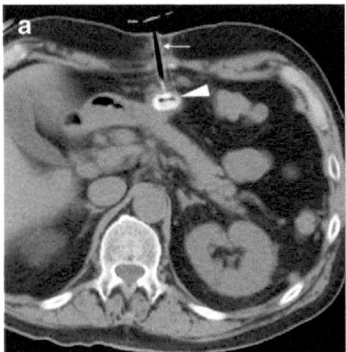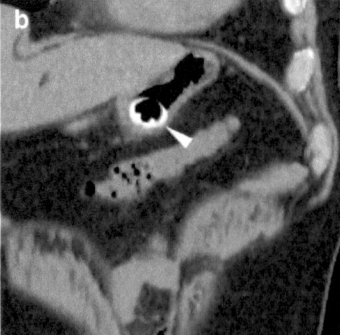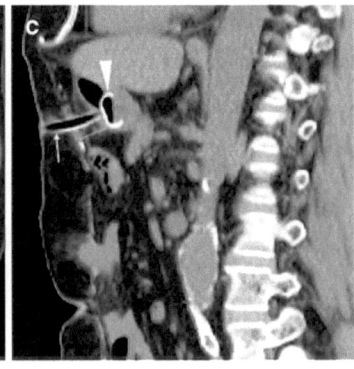

Fig. 6.5 A 66-year-old male patient had past history of Hodgkin's lymphoma (treated with splenectomy and chemoradiotherapy) and of recurrent laryngeal squamocellular carcinoma after laryngectomy 14 months earlier. Three weeks after PEG positioning, he suffered from septic fever. Detail multiplanar images from unenhanced CT (**a–c**) showed the internal bumper (*arrowheads*) positioned in the gastric antrum, a normal course of the PEG tube (*thin arrows*) through the anterior gastric wall, a moderate (nearly 1 cm) "peritoneal gap" (*dotted line*) between the greater gastric curvature and the posterior aspect of anterior abdominal wall, and the subcutaneous fat without appreciable inflammatory changes and abnormal collections. Pneumoperitoneum and signs of local infection and peritoneal effusion were excluded. The PEG device was tractioned, and the patient received intensive antibiotic treatment for *Pseudomonas* infection cultured from tracheal secretions

to the anterior abdominal wall. A study reported peritoneal gaps between 0.5 and 1.0 cm, between 1.0 and 2.0 cm, and greater than 2.0 cm in 24.6 %, 10.5 %, and 7 % of patients respectively, with mean ± SD values of 0.59 ± 0.70 cm (range, 0–2.35 cm). Notably, the presence of peritoneal gap is undetected by physical, endoscopic and radiographic examinations, but generally dictates external traction and is associated with need for PEG repositioning if significant (exceeding 0.5–1 cm) [3, 10, 13].

6.2.4 Post-procedural Pneumoperitoneum: Worrisome or Not?

Pneumoperitoneum is commonly observed after PEG positioning, particularly at hospitals that routinely acquire post-procedural chest and abdomen radiographs in all patients. The reported detection rates of post-PEG pneumoperitoneum vary from 16 to 56 % according to the imaging modality used. For instance, pneumoperitoneum was detected radiographically three hours after PEG positioning in 38 % of patients. Plain radiographs are considered relatively sensitive for pneumoperitoneum, provided that upright films are acquired after standing for at least 5–10 min or in the left lateral decubitus, at mid-inspiration or in expiratory phase. Conversely, CT has absolute (100 %) sensitivity as it detects even minimal amounts of extraluminal air. Pneumoperitoneum may be grossly quantified as small, moderate or large, and its absence is consistently reported as highly predictive of technical success and complication-free procedure (negative predictive value 100 %) [5, 12, 14–19].

However, the clinical significance of pneumoperitoneum remains debated. The classically worrisome identification of subphrenic air may lead radiologists to suggest the possibility of a visceral perforation and therefore an underlying surgical emergency. Conversely, after PEG positioning, limited or moderate free peritoneal gas is commonly considered a benign finding, secondary to air insufflated during endoscopy that escapes the gastric lumen and enters the peritoneal cavity through the puncture site in the gastric wall [12, 15–19].

According to some authors, the vast majority (85 %) of post-PEG pneumoperitoneum are benign self-limiting occurrences which typically resolve within 2–3 days and may sometimes last up to 2 weeks. In a cohort of patients with uncomplicated follow-up after PEG positioning, the

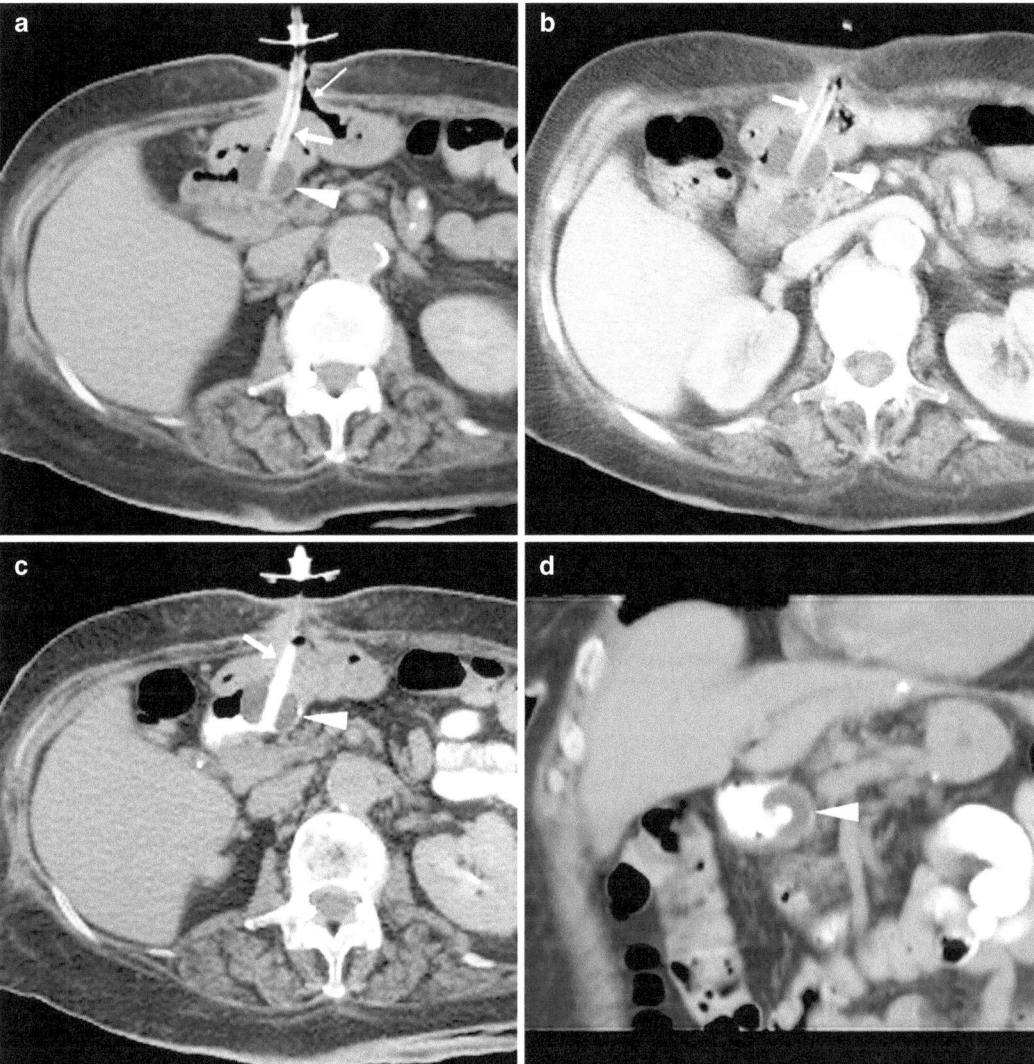

Fig. 6.6 Three months after PEG positioning, a 73-year-old female with previous surgery and irradiation of maxillary antrum carcinoma was brought to emergency department due to clinical suspicion of peristomal infection. The patient was found in a satisfactory nutritional status with inflamed, purulent, easily bleeding peristomal skin, a functioning PEG device and external leakage of gastric material. Initially, unenhanced (**a**) and post-contrast (**c**) CT acquisitions showed unclear position of the internal PEG bumper (*arrowheads*) relative to the pylorus, air (*thin arrows*) leaking from the stomach along the left side of the device tube. Repeated CT acquisition after introduction of water-soluble CM (**c, d**) opacified the PEG tube (*arrow*) and the prepyloric region, confirming the antral position of the internal bumper (*arrowheads*). Following these CT findings, surgical or endoscopic treatments were deemed unnecessary. Infection and leakage were treated by local toilette and medications with clinical improvement

systematic use of CT revealed pneumoperitoneum ranging in volume up to 130 ml in more than half (56 %) of cases. Interestingly, no complications requiring treatment occurred in patients with pneumoperitoneum; conversely those events requiring treatment (including dislodgement, transcolonic placement and upper gastrointestinal bleeding) were radiographically undetected. Therefore, post-procedural pneumoperitoneum does not represent a true complication and does not warrant exploratory laparotomy, provided that (a) signs and symptoms of peritoneal

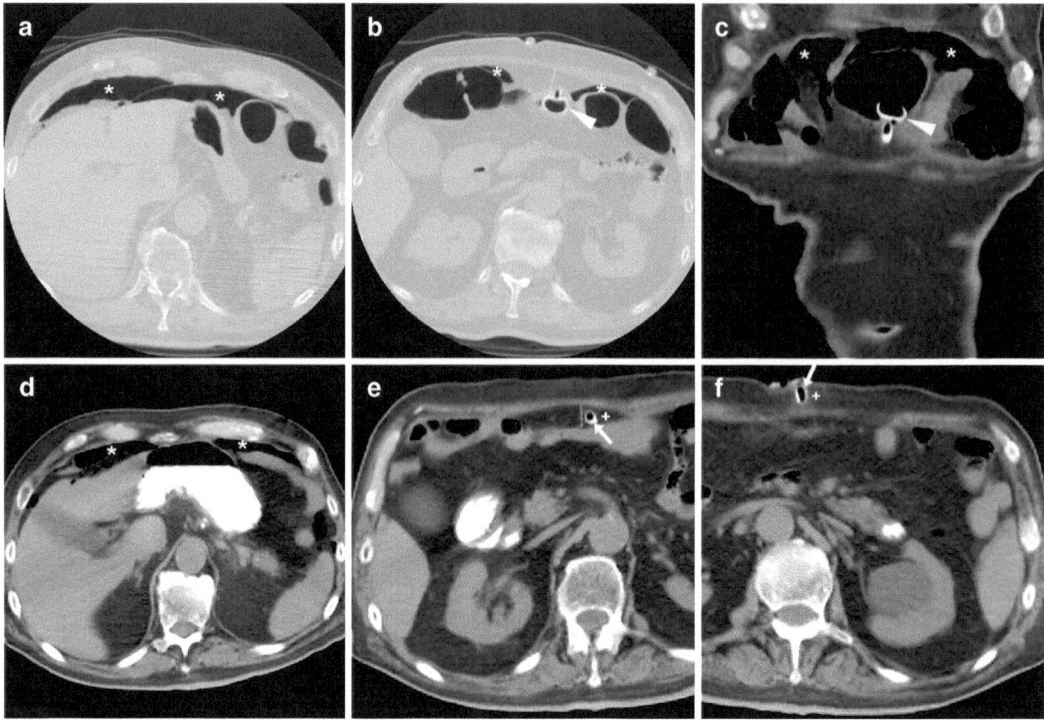

Fig. 6.7 Post-procedural pneumoperitoneum in an 86-year-old male with severe Alzheimer's disease and impossible feeding. After PEG positioning with the "pull" technique without immediate complications, the patient experienced high fever. Forty-eight hours after the procedure, unenhanced CT (**a, b**) viewed at both bone and standard window settings showed moderate pneumoperitoneum (*), normally positioned PEG bumper (*arrowheads*) in the gastric body and moderate peritoneal gap (*dotted line*). After conservative treatment, 4 days later repeated unenhanced CT including water-soluble CM administration (**c–f**) showed decreased pneumoperitoneum (*), normal course of PEG tube with unchanged peritoneal gap (*dotted line*) and unremarkable surrounding fat planes (+). After tube traction, the patient started enteral feeding and did well

inflammation or systemic infection are absent and (b) the correct PEG device placement is verified by the use of CT (Fig. 6.7). Occasionally, shortly after PEG positioning, air may track upwards giving rise to pneumomediastinum (Fig. 6.8) [12, 15–19].

6.3 Imaging of PEG-Related Complications

6.3.1 Misplacement, Visceral Perforation and Peritonitis

Alternatively, post-procedural pneumoperitoneum may herald potentially serious early complications. In a large systematic review of PEGs in ICU patients, the presence of pneumoperitoneum was associated with an increased likelihood for complications requiring emergent surgical intervention and early (within 30 days) mortality [14].

Unfortunately, the differentiation of benign pneumoperitoneum from underlying visceral injury often represents a diagnostic dilemma because signs of peritoneal irritation are unreliable in patients with impaired mental status. Exceptionally, the PEG tube is inadvertently misplaced into or through the transverse colon during tube placement. In our experience, the rare stomach or bowel injuries should be suspected when pneumoperitoneum is massive or does not resolve within 72 h, particularly if associated with peritoneal effusion and/or serosal thickening suggesting peritonitis (Figs. 6.8 and 6.9). Subcutaneous emphysema and ascites should be considered abnormal findings which suggest external leakage of

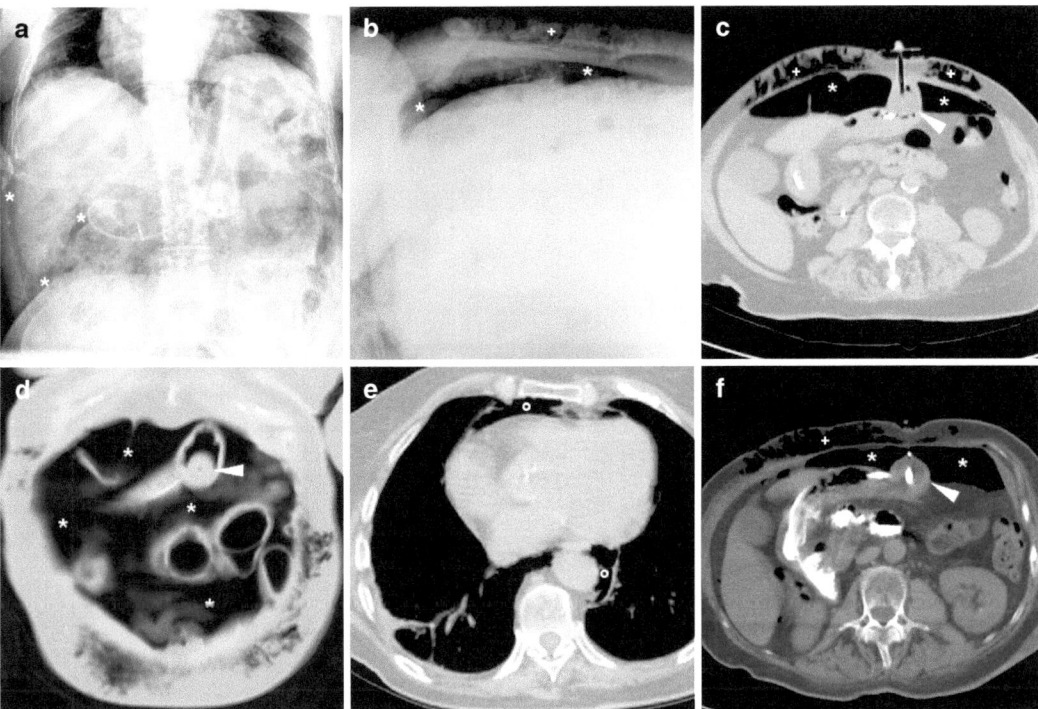

Fig. 6.8 A 76-year-old female with severe mental impairment in Alzheimer's disease, previous cerebral stroke and diabetes mellitus underwent positioning of PEG jejunostomy to prevent recurrent aspiration pneumonia. Supine (**a**) and lateral (**b**) radiographs showed abundant pneumoperitoneum (*) and subcutaneous emphysema (+) immediately after the procedure (note guidewire in the stomach) and persisted at further investigation with CT 24 h later (**c–e**). The internal PEG bumper (*arrowhead*) was located in the stomach. Additionally, pneumomediastinum (o in **e**) was detected. Without clinical signs of sepsis and peritonitis, the patient started enteral nutrition. Seven days later, repeated CT (**f**) including water-soluble CM showed absent CM leakage, moderately decreased subcutaneous emphysema (+) and pneumoperitoneum (*), and detachment of the gastric greater curvature from the anterior abdominal wall (compare images **f** and **c**) which required PEG repositioning

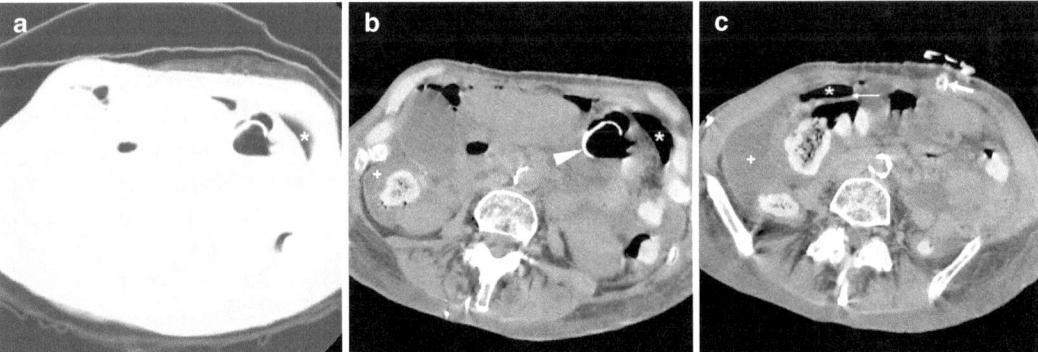

Fig. 6.9 After repeated PEG positioning, within 24 h, the same patient in Fig. 6.4 suffered from acute abdomen with physical findings consistent with peritonitis. Emergency unenhanced CT viewed at both lung (**a**) and standard (**b**, **c**) window settings showed moderate pneumoperitoneum (*) associated with abundant peritoneal effusion (+), forming air–fluid levels (*thin arrow*). Note position of internal PEG bumper (*arrowheads*) in the stomach and course of device tube (*arrow*). Surgical exploration confirmed iatrogenic gastric perforation and mixed peritonitis from enteral nutrition leakage, with *Enterococcus* and *Pseudomonas* infection. A gastric laceration was sutured and the PEG was consolidated

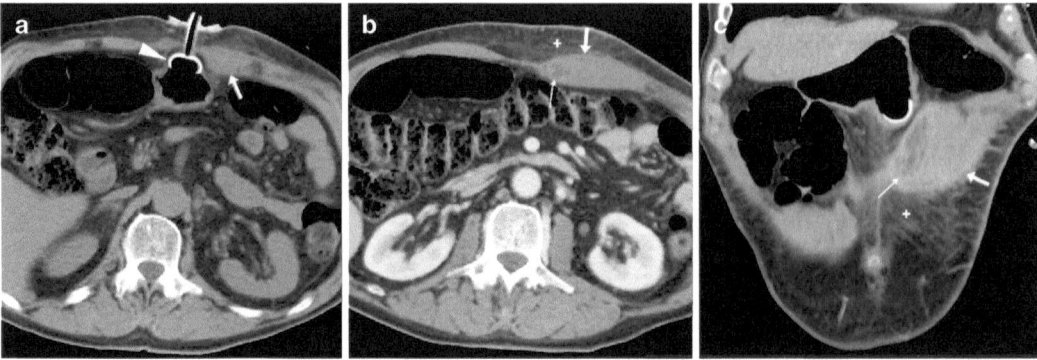

Fig. 6.10 Abdominal wall infection in a 78-year-old male who suffered from intermittent fever since PEG positioning 3 weeks earlier to relieve dysphagia following severe ischaemic cerebral stroke. Clinically, palpable inflamed swelling was appreciated nearby the PEG exit site and digital compression yielded pus. Unenhanced (**a**) and post-contrast (**b**, **c**) CT images showed PEG with internal bumper (*arrowheads*) in the gastric antrum, inflammatory-type increased attenuation of the subcutaneous fat (+) and thickened left rectus abdominis muscle (*arrows*) containing low-attenuation regions with peripheral enhancement suggesting abscess. The attending surgeon opted for incision, drainage and toilette plus intensive antibiotics

gastric content [5, 12, 19]. Intra-abdominal leakage, peritonitis, visceral injury and PEG misplacement represent the commonest complications requiring emergency surgical repair [7].

6.3.2 Abdominal Wall Haematoma, Infection and Leakage

Abdominal wall haematoma in the site of PEG external access is not uncommon and may develop in up to one-third of patients, without a significant association with anticoagulation. However, it very seldom represents a life-threatening complication. Borrowing from experience with anticoagulated patients, rectus abdominis haematoma is heralded by variable muscle thickening compared to the contralateral side with the characteristic hyperattenuation (40–75 Hounsfield units) on unenhanced CT images [9, 12].

Infection is a common occurrence which may occur in up to 10–20 % of patients with cancer, cirrhosis and radiation therapy as the key risk factors. The majority of cases are uncomplicated wound infections (cellulitis) at the anterior abdominal wall which generally respond well to antibiotic treatment. Clinically, periostomy infection is usually heralded by soft tissue thickening and inflammatory changes at the PEG exit site. Diagnostic

imaging is often not required, unless the clinician suspects the presence of an underlying abscess. CT appearances consistent with infection include skin indentation at PEG exit site, increased attenuation of the subcutaneous fat planes, soft tissue thickening of the anterior abdominal wall and rectus muscle encasing the PEG tube. In oncologic patients, infectious and haemorrhagic changes should not be misinterpreted as metastatic tumour seeding by taking into consideration the appropriate clinical information. Occasionally, peristomal air/enteral leakage may be visualised by CT (Fig. 6.5). Sometimes, peristomal infection may be complicated with extensive abdominal wall involvement, abscess (Fig. 6.10) or necrotising fasciitis. The use of CT allows depicting the extent of infectious involvement and therefore choosing the appropriate treatment between prolonged antibiotics, PEG removal, percutaneous or surgical abscess drainage [9–11, 13].

6.4 Cases Presentations

6.4.1 Buried Bumper Syndrome

An 84-year-old woman with recurrent squamocellular carcinoma of the oral cavity infiltrating the mandible was admitted to the emergency

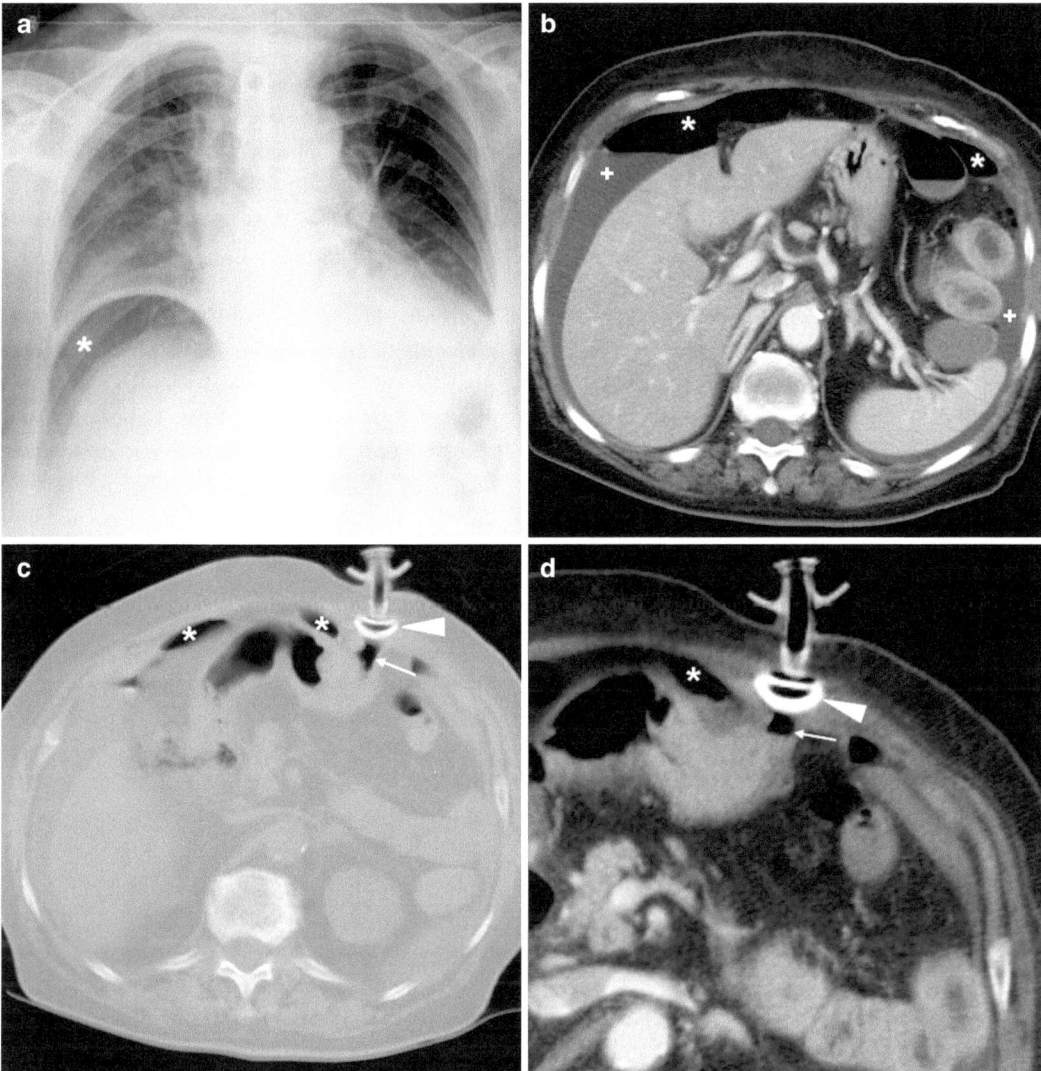

Fig. 6.11 Semi-erect plain radiograph (**a**) obtained with the bedridden patient showed right subphrenic air crescent (*) indicating pneumoperitoneum, bilateral basal lung opacities consistent with atelectasis, and tracheostomy in place. The PEG bumper was not clearly seen. Multidetector CT images viewed at abdominal (**b**), and bone (**c**) window settings confirmed the presence of pneumoperitoneum (*) associated with fluid-attenuation ascites (+). Detail view (**d**) showed the PEG device externally dislocated, with the internal bumper (*arrowheads*) outside the stomach in the anterior abdominal wall within the thickened left rectus muscle. Air (*thin arrow*) was seen along the PEG migration tract (Partially reproduced with permission from Tonolini [20])

department because of fever, abdominal pain and inability to pass stools. Two months earlier at another Institution, she had positioning of PEG and permanent tracheostomy.

Pneumoperitoneum and lung base atelectasis were detected radiographically (Fig. 6.11a). Afterwards, the patient's clinical conditions rapidly worsened with altered mental state,

hypotension, metabolic decompensation and oliguria.

Urgent CT (Fig. 6.11b–d) confirmed pneumoperitoneum, associated with fluid-attenuation ascites. The PEG device was seen dislocated externally, with the internal bumper clearly outside the collapsed stomach and located in the anterior abdominal wall within the thickened left rectus muscle.

These findings were interpreted as consistent with "buried bumper syndrome" (BBS).

Emergency laparotomic surgical exploration confirmed biliary ascites and gastric perforation from PEG dislodgement, which was repaired and anchored to the abdominal wall. Unfortunately, the patient could not recover from her critical conditions [20].

A rare PEG-related complication (incidence 0.3–2.4 %), BBS corresponds to progressive migration of the tightly juxtaposed internal bumper through the gastric wall along the PEG tract, leading to bleeding, difficult feeding and abdominal pain. The name refers to the endoscopic appearance of the internal bumper hardly seen, "buried" into a large ulceration. Generally considered a late event, BBS may sometimes present within 2 months from PEG positioning. Delayed recognition and treatment are associated with severe morbidity and death [1, 4, 6–8, 21]

As this case exemplifies, CT allows localisation of the buried internal bumper between the gastric and abdominal wall, demonstrating its migration path and assessing the presence and severity of inflammation, abscess collections, extraluminal air or effusion. Alternatively, long-term migration may give rise to gastric herniation, in which a portion of the stomach protrudes ventrally along the PEG tract. Therefore, CT findings are highly valuable for a correct therapeutic choice including surgical, manual or endoscopic removal (either out of the abdominal wall or back in the stomach), and replacement with a new feeding tube [10, 13, 21].

6.4.2 Device Migration

A 77-year-old male with history of post-radiation distal colonic stricture following rectal resection and radiotherapy and worsening Parkinson's disease symptoms underwent PEG positioning to relieve dysphagia, without immediate post-procedural complications. Twenty-four hours later, he complained of abdominal pain and distension.

Massive pneumoperitoneum and associated posterior pneumomediastinum were detected by plain abdominal radiographs (Fig. 6.12a–c) and confirmed by CT (Fig. 6.12d–f). Furthermore, CT verified the correct positioning of the PEG bumper in the stomach and excluded misplacement and infection. Since fever and clinical signs of peritonism were absent, the patient started enteral nutrition 2 days after PEG positioning and was discharged.

Three weeks later, the patient suffered from diarrhoea, abdominal pain and profound asthenia, without clinical evidence of peritoneal irritation. Two litres of enteral nutrition-like fluid were drained through a rectal tube. Laboratory tests revealed severe hypokalaemia and moderately increased C-reactive protein. Repeated radiographs (Fig. 6.13a–c) and CT (Fig. 6.13d–f) showed persistent pneumoperitoneum and posterior pneumomediastinum, appearance of abundant fluid in the distended large bowel, and the PEG bumper located within haustra in the distal transverse colon.

After endoscopic confirmation of absent internal bumper in the stomach, laparotomic surgery was performed including removal of PEG device which had migrated through a gastrocolic fistula, gastrostomy, and left hemicolectomy with colostomy [22].

Generally, the incorrect PEG position may result from misplacement or from subsequent migration secondary to tension on the gastrostomy tube. A correct initial placement does not guarantee against an eventual dislodgement beyond the gastric lumen, including advancement into the duodenum and proximal jejunum. Occasionally device migration from the stomach to the transverse colon may occur weeks after PEG insertion, secondary from excessive tension leading to dislodgement and gastrocolic fistulisation. Unfortunately, device migration and fistula formation represent late complications commonly requiring surgical treatment. As in this case, this exceedingly rare complication may be facilitated by interposition of the colon between the stomach and the anterior abdominal wall and manifests with sudden diarrhoea and abdominal cramping pain [7, 11, 23–26].

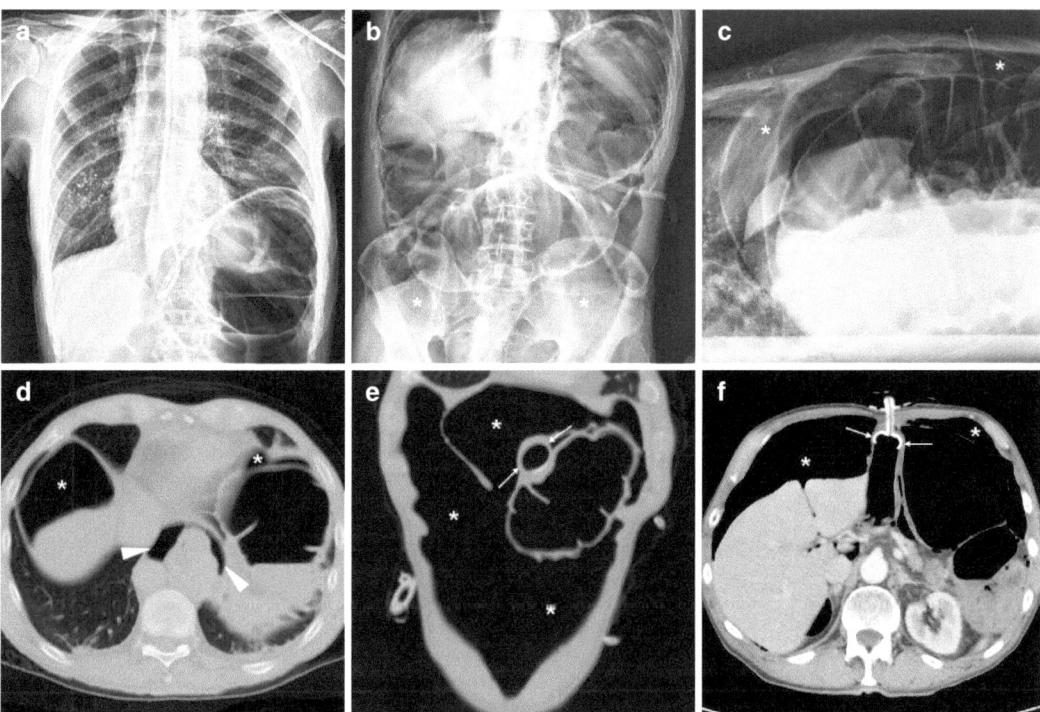

Fig. 6.12 Pre-procedural plain chest radiograph (**a**) showed nasogastric tube in place with its distal tract coiled within the collapsed stomach, marked gaseous colonic distension secondary to known distal colonic post-radiation stenosis. Hours after PEG positioning, supine (**b**) and tangential (**c**) abdominal radiographs show appearance of pneumoperitoneum (*) and persistent colonic hyperinflation. Unenhanced (**d**) and post-contrast (**e, f**) CT images confirmed pneumoperitoneum (*) associated with posterior pneumomediastinum (*arrowheads* in **d**). The internal PEG bumper (*thin arrows*) was correctly located in the stomach, retracted ventrally towards the anterior abdominal wall and abutting the distended left colonic flexure (Adapted with permission from Pagani & Tonolini [22])

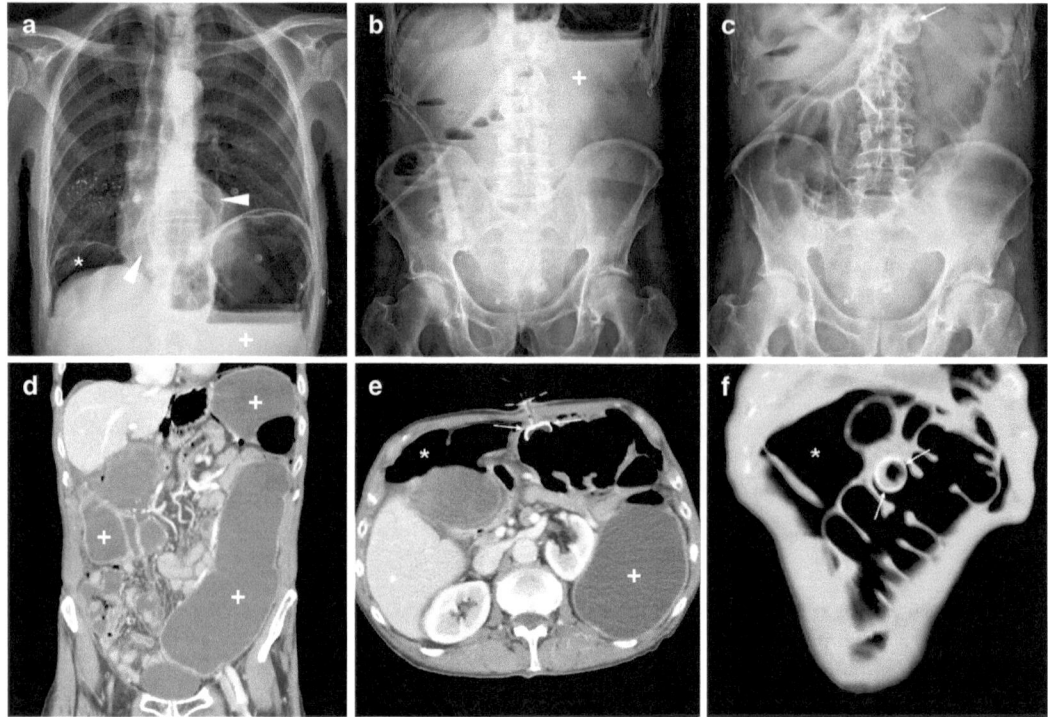

Fig. 6.13 Plain chest (**a**) and abdomen (**b** upright, **c** supine) radiographs showed decreased pneumoperitoneum (*), persistent posterior pneumomediastinum (*arrowheads* in **a**) and abundant fluid (+) in the distended colon with prominent air–fluid level at the left flexure. The PEG bumper (*thin arrow* in **c**) was seen abutting the distended large bowel. Contrast-enhanced multidetector CT (**d–f**) confirmed abundant endoluminal colonic fluid (+) and residual pneumoperitoneum (*). The PEG bumper (*thin arrows*) was now located within haustra in the distal transverse colon (Adapted with permission from Pagani & Tonolini [22])

References

1. Ermis F, Ozel M, Oncu K et al (2012) Indications, complications and long-term follow-up of patients undergoing percutaneous endoscopic gastrostomy: a retrospective study. Wien Klin Wochenschr 124: 148–153
2. Gomes CA Jr, Lustosa SA, Matos D et al (2012) Percutaneous endoscopic gastrostomy versus nasogastric tube feeding for adults with swallowing disturbances. Cochrane Database Syst Rev (3):CD008096
3. Jain R, Maple JT, Anderson MA et al (2011) The role of endoscopy in enteral feeding. Gastrointest Endosc 74:7–12
4. Vanis N, Saray A, Gornjakovic S et al (2012) Percutaneous endoscopic gastrostomy (PEG): retrospective analysis of a 7-year clinical experience. Acta Inform Med 20:235–237
5. Milanchi S, Allins A (2007) Early pneumoperitoneum after percutaneous endoscopic gastrostomy in intensive care patients: sign of possible bowel injury. Am J Crit Care 16:132–136
6. Blomberg J, Lagergren J, Martin L et al (2012) Complications after percutaneous endoscopic gastrostomy in a prospective study. Scand J Gastroenterol 47:737–742
7. Schulenberg E, Schule S, Lehnert T (2010) Emergency surgery for complications related to percutaneous endoscopic gastrostomy. Endoscopy 42:872–874
8. Wirth R, Voss C, Smoliner C et al (2012) Complications and mortality after percutaneous endoscopic gastrostomy in geriatrics: a prospective multicenter observational trial. J Am Med Dir Assoc 13:228–233
9. Richter-Schrag HJ, Richter S, Ruthmann O et al (2011) Risk factors and complications following percutaneous endoscopic gastrostomy: a case series of 1041 patients. Can J Gastroenterol 25:201–206
10. Chang WK, Huang WC, Yu CY et al (2011) Long-term percutaneous endoscopic gastrostomy: characteristic computed tomographic findings. Abdom Imaging 36:684–688
11. Levine CD, Handler B, Baker SR et al (1995) Imaging of percutaneous tube gastrostomies: spectrum of normal and abnormal findings. AJR Am J Roentgenol 164:347–351
12. Wojtowycz MM, Arata JA Jr, Micklos TJ et al (1988) CT findings after uncomplicated percutaneous gastrostomy. AJR Am J Roentgenol 151:307–309

13. Wax BN, Katz DS, Badler RL et al (2006) Complications of abdominal and pelvic procedures: computed tomographic diagnosis. Curr Probl Diagn Radiol 35:171–187

14. Nazarian A, Cross W, Kowdley GC (2012) Pneumoperitoneum after percutaneous endoscopic gastrostomy among adults in the intensive care unit: incidence, predictive factors, and clinical significance. Am Surg 78:591–594

15. Alley JB, Corneille MG, Stewart RM et al (2007) Pneumoperitoneum after percutaneous endoscopic gastrostomy in patients in the intensive care unit. Am Surg 73:765–767; discussion 768

16. Blum CA, Selander C, Ruddy JM et al (2009) The incidence and clinical significance of pneumoperitoneum after percutaneous endoscopic gastrostomy: a review of 722 cases. Am Surg 75:39–43

17. Roberts PA, Wrenn K, Lundquist S (2005) Pneumoperitoneum after percutaneous endoscopic gastrostomy: a case report and review. J Emerg Med 28:45–48

18. Dulabon GR, Abrams JE, Rutherford EJ (2002) The incidence and significance of free air after percutaneous endoscopic gastrostomy. Am Surg 68:590–593

19. Wiesen AJ, Sideridis K, Fernandes A et al (2006) True incidence and clinical significance of pneumoperitoneum after PEG placement: a prospective study. Gastrointest Endosc 64:886–889

20. Tonolini M (2013) EuroRAD case 11442. A lethal case of buried bumper syndrome with gastric perforation. {Online} URL: http://www.eurorad.org/case.php?id=11442

21. Lee TH, Lin JT (2008) Clinical manifestations and management of buried bumper syndrome in patients with percutaneous endoscopic gastrostomy. Gastrointest Endosc 68:580–584

22. Pagani A, Tonolini M (2014) EuroRAD case 11713. Pneumoperitoneum after percutaneous endoscopic gastrostomy: worrisome or not? {Online} URL: http://www.eurorad.org/case.php?id=11713

23. Lenzen H, Weismuller T, Bredt M et al (2012) Education and imaging. Gastrointestinal: PEG feeding tube migration into the colon; a late manifestation. J Gastroenterol Hepatol 27:1254

24. Ward M, Rees C, Asthana AK et al (2011) Colonic perforation during percutaneous endoscopic gastrostomy tube insertion with subsequent bumper migration into colon. Clin Gastroenterol Hepatol 9, e128

25. Huang SY, Levine MS, Raper SE (2005) Gastrocolic fistula with migration of feeding tube into transverse colon as a complication of percutaneous endoscopic gastrostomy. AJR Am J Roentgenol 184:S65–S66

26. Liu SY, Ng SS, Yip HC et al (2010) Migration of a percutaneous endoscopic gastrostomy tube into the transverse colon: a forgotten cause of refractory diarrhea. Endoscopy 42(Suppl 2):E324–E325

Complications of Endoscopic Retrograde Cholangiopancreatography and Endoscopic Biliopancreatic Interventions

Complications of Endoscopic Retrograde Cholangiopancreatography (ERCP)

7

Emilia Bareggi

7.1 ERCP: An Overview

Introduced in 1968, endoscopic retrograde cholangiopancreatography (ERCP) was soon accepted as a safe and direct technique for evaluating biliary and pancreatic disease. Since then, ERCP has become a widely available procedure [1].

With the subsequent introduction of sphincterotomy in 1974, therapeutic biliopancreatic endoscopy began. Afterwards, since the development of diagnostic techniques such as US, TC, magnetic resonance imaging (MRI) and echoendoscopy (EUS), ERCP progressively evolved from a diagnostic towards an almost exclusively therapeutic procedure [2, 3].

The diagnostic and therapeutic roles of ERCP have well been demonstrated for a variety of disorders, including management of common bile duct stones (choledocholithiasis), diagnosis and management of biliary malignancies and of pancreatic diseases [4].

In order to accurately assess the appropriate clinical use of ERCP, it is essential to have a thorough understanding of the potential complications of this procedure.

In approximately 5–10 % of cases, ERCP itself causes adverse events; however, significant ERCP-specific complications occur in 1.8 % of all ERCPs performed, with an overall mortality of 0.6 % [5].

Despite the potential benefits of ERCP, the procedure is operator dependent and patients are at risk for developing complications secondary to biliary and pancreatic manipulations or related to endoscopy [7, 8]. Complication rates are lower with increased experience of endoscopist [6].

7.1.1 Technique, Indications and Contraindications

ERCP is performed with intravenous sedation and analgesia (opioid–sedative combination); fasting is required for at least 6–8 h before the procedure. The patient is initially placed in left lateral decubitus position, followed by prone position for the procedure [7].

The endoscopist should have appropriate training and expertise, in particular must be competent to perform therapeutic interventions at the time of ERCP. Pre-procedural coagulation studies are necessary, particularly in patients with a history of coagulopathy or with prolonged cholestasis. Antibiotic prophylaxis is indicated in the setting of suspected biliary obstruction, pancreatic pseudocysts or ductal leaks or in every case with high risk of septic complication [8].

ERCP allows obtaining radiographic images of biliary and pancreatic tree, by approaching it

E. Bareggi
Gastroenterology Unit, "Luigi Sacco" University Hospital, Via G.B. Grassi 74, Milan 20157, Italy
e-mail: bareggi.emilia@gmail.com

© Springer International Publishing Switzerland 2016
M. Tonolini (ed.), *Imaging Complications of Gastrointestinal and Biliopancreatic Endoscopy Procedures*, DOI 10.1007/978-3-319-31211-8_7

from the duodenal lumen. The procedure is performed thanks to the use of a side-viewing endoscope, with light source and image-processing unit. The procedure must be performed in a dedicated room, with all protections for the use of fluoroscopy [7].

ERCP is particularly useful in the management of patients with obstruction of biliary tract caused by stones or less common by benign or malign strictures. ERCP should be the first approach, only in those patients who need quickly a therapeutic indication for the resolution of the obstruction; conversely in the majority of cases, MR cholangiopancreatography (MRCP) or EUS allows pre-procedural diagnosis and ERCP is required only as therapeutic approach. In selected cases, ERCP is useful to assess the benign or malign nature of biliary obstruction, through the use of brushings or biopsies [2].

Sphincterotomy and stone extraction, with the help of Fogarty-type balloons or wire baskets, represent the usual procedures to resolve biliary obstruction and are successful in 90 % of cases. Sometimes preliminary lithotripsy is necessary for fragmentation of large stones. When primary biliary cannulation fails, pre-cut papillotomy or a combined percutaneous or endoscopic approach may be necessary. Urgent ERCP for biliary decompression is indicated in patient with acute cholangitis and severe gallstone pancreatitis.

Benign biliary strictures include postsurgical strictures, dominant strictures in primary sclerosing cholangitis (PSC) and biliary strictures secondary to chronic pancreatitis; their treatment include dilatation with hydrostatic balloons or graduated catheter passed over a guidewire and stent placement, sometimes multiple, if it is necessary to maintain patency [9]. Dominant strictures in PSC should undergo endoscopic assessment by brushing and biopsy, to exclude the presence of malignancy. In malignant biliary obstructions, endoscopic stent placement provides effective palliation of jaundice, either as a long-term palliation or as a temporary procedure before surgical treatment.

ERCP is also useful for other indications, such as the resolution of symptoms in patients with sphincter of Oddi dysfunction and recurrent acute pancreatitis caused by microlithiasis or by congenital abnormalities of pancreas such as pancreas divisum and annular pancreas, the treatment of pancreatic stones or strictures in chronic pancreatitis, the treatment of both biliary and pancreatic duct strictures caused by pancreatic cancer, and the diagnosis and treatment of pancreatic fluid collections such as acute pseudocysts, chronic pseudocysts and pancreatic necrosis [10].

Absolute contraindications of ERCP include pharyngeal or oesophageal obstruction, active coagulopathy and anaphylactic reaction to contrast medium. Relative contraindications include portal hypertension with oesophageal and or gastric varices, acute pancreatitis (except gallstone pancreatitis), recent myocardial infarction and severe cardiopulmonary disease. Patients with previous Roux-en-Y anastomosis, Billroth II surgical reconstruction or pancreaticoduodenectomy can not undergo traditional ERCP and are at high risk for procedure due to altered anatomy [11].

7.2 Complications of ERCP

Specific complications of ERCP which can occur also in expert hands include infections, pancreatitis, haemorrhage and perforation. Several factors, such as patients' comorbidities, operator skill and complexity of the intervention, can add to the intrinsic risks of ERCP. In a prospective 2-year study of 2,347 patients of 17 institutions, 9.8 % had post-ERCP complications, and the most common were pancreatitis (5.4 %) and haemorrhage (2 %) [6, 12].

7.2.1 Post-ERCP Pancreatitis

Post-ERCP pancreatitis (PEP) is the most common complication. The consensus definition of PEP is new or worsened abdominal pain, serum amylase three or more times the upper limits of normal, more than 24 h after the procedure and new or prolongation of hospitalisation for at least 2 days [13, 14].

Transient elevation post procedure of amylase is common (30–70 % of patients), but does not, by itself, constitute pancreatitis [15].

Table 7.1 Risk factors associated with PEP

Factors related to patients	Factors related to technique
Sphincter of Oddi dysfunction	Difficult cannulation (prolonged or repeated attempts)
Pre-existing pancreatitis	Increased manipulation around the papilla and multiple contrast injections of pancreatic duct
Prior history of PEP	Pre-cut sphincterotomy
Female gender	Pancreatic sphincterotomy
Younger age <70	Balloon sphincter dilatation
Normal size bile duct or small common bile duct <10 mm	Biliary sphincteroplasty
Normal serum bilirubin	
History of PEP	

Using the consensus definition of PEP, its incidence in a meta-analysis of 21 prospective studies was about 3.5 %, but varied according to the selection of patients [10].

Several parameters are related to the risk of developing pancreatitis: factors related to experience of the operator (low case volume), factors related to selection of patients and factors related to technique (Table 7.1) [16–19].

Clinically, PEP is classified into mild (amylase at least three times more of normal at more than 24 h after procedure and requiring hospitalisation of 2–3 days), moderate (requiring hospitalisation of 4–10 days) and severe acute pancreatitis [19].

In 90 % of cases, it is mild to moderate and resolves with simple measures of hydration and analgesia [20]. The minority of patients develops severe pancreatitis and requires prolonged hospitalisation for more than 10 days in an intensive care unit; for the onset of haemorrhagic pancreatitis, phlegmon or pseudocyst; or for necessity of intervention (percutaneous drainage or surgery).

Normally the treatment of severe PEP is the same of severe pancreatitis from other causes.

Understanding and recognition of risk factors for PEP have allowed endoscopists to provide more accurate preventive measures in appropriate clinical situation to reduce the risk of this complication: for example, appropriate patients selection is fundamental to reduce PEP and prefer other type of approach when possible.

In order to reduce the risk of PEP, it is also important that both endoscopist and endoscopy assistants have adequate training and competence, adequate case volume to acquire experience and maintain competence, avoid diagnostic ERCP and prefer other methods for a diagnostic purpose, limit time for cannulation to avoid trauma to papilla, limit injection number and volume of contrast, avoid cannulation of pancreatic duct when not necessary and use stent in pancreatic duct for pancreatic sphincterotomy [19].

Multiple prospective studies have shown the benefits of temporary pancreatic duct stents in lowering the risk and severity of pancreatitis in high-risk population. Also from a meta-analysis, the use of wire-guided cannulation before contrast injection seems to result in greater success of biliary cannulation and lower risk of pancreatitis. Numerous therapeutic agents have been tried as prophylaxis to reduce PEP (such as somatostatin, octreotide, gabexate mesilate, etc.), but none of them has gained universal acceptance [10].

7.2.2 Haemorrhage

Gastrointestinal bleeding is essentially a complication of sphincterotomy rather than diagnostic ERCP.

Significant haemorrhage is defined as clinical evidence of melaena or haematemesis associated with haemoglobin drop of at least 2 g/dl or the need for blood transfusion [6].

The most recent studies have shown that bleeding post-endoscopic sphincterotomy has an incidence around 2 % with a mortality of 0.1 % [21].

Post-sphincterotomy bleeding can occur immediately (within 24 h) or be delayed (after 24 h) after the procedure and can be arterial or venous [20]. Approximately 50 % of bleeding occurs immediately after sphincterotomy. However, sometimes significant bleed may occur up to 10 days later [19].

Table 7.2 Risk factors associated with post-ERCP bleeding

Patient-related factors	Anatomical features	Technical-related factors
Coagulopathy	Billroth II partial gastrectomy	Limited experience of endoscopist
Use of anticoagulants within 72 h of sphincterotomy	Periampullary diverticulum	Pre-cut sphincterotomy
Acute cholangitis	Papillary stenosis	Length of sphincterotomy
Bleeding during procedure	Impacted stone in common bile duct	Extension of previous sphincterotomy
Child's grade C cirrhosis		Uncontrolled sphincterotomy
Renal failure		
Ongoing haemodialysis		

Anyway, advanced sphincterotomy techniques and increased endoscopists' experience have greatly reduced the incidence of bleeding.

Clinically, post-ERCP bleeding is classified as mild when haemoglobin drop is below 3 g/dL, moderate if four or less haemotransfusion units are required and severe when it requires transfusion of more than five units of blood, surgery or angiography. Approximately 70 % of bleeding episodes are classified as mild, and severe haemorrhage is estimated to occur in less than 1/1,000 sphincterotomies [10].

Risk factors related to post-ERCP bleeding have been identified and can be distinguished into patient-related, anatomical and technical factors (Table 7.2).

Normally post-sphincterotomy bleedings stop spontaneously. When bleeding does not stop, endoscopic therapy include spray area with adrenalin or better injection of diluted adrenaline 1:10,000, through a sclerotherapy needle, with or without association of thermal therapy (electrocautery) and endoscopic haemoclips. Argon beam coagulation has also been used, but efficacy is unclear [19].

When all previous strategies are unsuccessful, angiographic embolisation can be effective. Surgery is reserved only for refractory cases, when all other methods have failed; anyway the use of surgery has considerably declined.

Strategies to reduce the risk of bleeding during sphincterotomy require a platelet count >50,000 and INR <1.2, which are considered safe for sphincterotomy. Correction of severe coagulation disorders and preventive measures in patients with platelet dysfunction are recommended before sphincterotomy. The use of aspirin and NSAIDs 3 days pre- and post procedure is considered safe for sphincterotomy, but some recommend discontinuation when it is possible. Heparin and the newer antiplatelet drugs such as clopidogrel must be stopped before procedure. Warfarin must be discontinued 3 or 5 days before planned sphincterotomy (better avoid the use of vitamin K) and if necessary fresh frozen plasma can be used to reverse the anticoagulation effect [19].

7.2.3 Visceral Perforation

Duodenal perforation is a rare post-ERCP complication with reported rate of 0.3–1 %. More recently the incidence seems decreased to less than 0.5 %, perhaps due to improved experience and skill of endoscopists [22].

Perforations complicating endoscopic sphincterotomy can be of three distinct types: guidewire-induced, periampullary perforation related to sphincterotomy and distant luminal perforation.

Another classification distinguishes four types:

Type I: free bowel wall perforation
Type II: retroperitoneal duodenal perforation secondary to periampullary injury
Type III: perforation of the pancreatic or bile duct
Type IV: retroperitoneal air alone

The second type, retroperitoneal duodenal perforations, is the most common and usually is secondary to sphincterotomy that extend beyond intramural portion of bile duct. Perforation of the pancreatic or bile duct generally occurs as a consequence of dilation of strictures, forced cannulation, stent migration, guidewire insertion or difficult stone extraction. Free abdominal perforation of duodenum or jejunum is rare, and normally it occurs in patients with altered anatomy due to strictures or surgical resection such as Billroth II gastrectomy [23]. Anyway free retroperitoneal air has been seen in 29 % of asymptomatic patients on CT scan obtained within 24 h of procedure [22]. If patients are clinically asymptomatic, they may not require intervention. Gastric and oesophageal perforation and pneumomediastinum without perforation have been described.

Numerous risk factors related to patients or procedure have been identified; they include an abnormal gastrointestinal anatomy such as in Billroth II partial gastrectomy, sphincterotomy, intramural injection of contrast, prolonged duration of procedure, stenosis of upper gastrointestinal tract or bile duct, biliary stricture dilation, sphincter of Oddi dysfunction and the presence of peripapillary diverticulum [24].

Management of perforation depends on lots of factors such as clinical status and site of perforation. Early identification of a perforation is associated with decreased morbidity and mortality. Timely treatment with biliary and duodenal drainage plus broad-spectrum antibiotics can result in clinical resolution without the need of surgery [10].

Normally free abdominal perforation is always recognised immediately because of its symptoms, physical signs and radiological findings. Patients may present hours after the procedure with pain, fever and leucocytosis. Pneumomediastinum and subcutaneous emphysema have been described.

As discussed in the appropriate imaging chapter, abdominal CT is the most sensitive technique for detecting perforation and is warranted when perforation is suspected. Retroduodenal perforation is usually heralded by air or contrast in the retroperitoneal space.

Post-ERCP perforations can be clinically graded as:

- Mild: very limited leak of fluid or contrast, treated medically for 3 days or less
- Moderate: any perforation treated medically for 4–10 days
- Severe: requiring medical treatment for more than 10 days or intervention

A conservative approach is appropriate in patients with small retroperitoneal perforation following endoscopic sphincterotomy. All patients should be treated by keeping fasting, receiving hydration, nasogastric or nasoduodenal suction, and intravenous antibiotics. Anyway early surgical consultation and careful observation is mandatory, because the outcome may be poor in patients not receiving prompt and appropriate treatment. Type I perforation, free bowel wall perforation, if immediately recognised, can be treated endoscopically. Patients with oesophageal, gastric, jejunal or duodenal perforation usually require surgery [23].

The risk of perforation can be reduced if ERCP is performed by well-trained endoscopists and assistants, following simple technique principles: proper orientation of sphincterotomy between 11 and 1 o'clock, avoiding a zipper cut, step by step incision and sphincterotomy length tailored to the size of papilla or bile duct.

7.2.4 Infectious Complications

Potential infectious complications of ERCP are multiple and include ascending cholangitis, cholecystitis, infected pancreatic pseudocysts, liver abscesses, peritonitis and less common endocarditis.

The most frequent occurrence is cholangitis, defined by temperature elevation to more than 38 °C without evidence of acute cholecystitis; the diagnosis is made by the presence of pain, fever and elevated white blood cell count.

Although bacteraemia is common, occurring in 15 % of diagnostic and 27 % of therapeutic procedures, the rate of post-ERCP cholangitis is less than 1 %, and it is the most common cause of death following ERCP.

Usually cholangitis is an indication that occurs after incomplete or failed biliary drainage of an infected obstructed biliary system, and normally 87 % of these patients develop sepsis.

Risk factors include also the use of combined percutaneous–endoscopic procedures, stent placement in malignant stenosis, presence of jaundice and primary sclerosing cholangitis [10].

Post-ERCP cholangitis are classified as mild if temperature is more than 38 °C for 24/48 h, moderate when the septic state requires more than 3 days of treatment or endoscopic or percutaneous treatment and severe when septic shock is present and surgery is needed [19].

Acute cholecystitis as complication of ERCP is quite rare as it complicates approximately in 0.2–0.5 % of ERCPs; one risk factor could be the presence of gallbladder stones, so in patients with high risk, prophylactic antibiotic therapy is recommended. Also the possible filling of gallbladder with contrast during examination and the placement of self-expandable metal stents may increase the risk of cholecystitis, in particular if the stent is covered and cystic duct is obstructed.

Antibiotic prophylaxis must be considered before ERCP in patients with high risk of infective endocarditis and patients with pancreatic pseudocysts; it is also necessary in patients with known biliary obstruction in which there is the possibility that complete drainage may not be achieved, for example, in patients with strictures of the hepatic hilum or primary sclerosing cholangitis. When biliary drainage is incomplete, prosecution of antibiotic therapy after procedure is recommended [10].

In general, to prevent septic complication of ERCP, a prompt endoscopic decompression of biliary obstruction is necessary, and when definitive drainage cannot be achieved, a temporary drainage with a nasobiliary tube is mandatory till the procedure can be completed or in some cases percutaneous drainage or surgery must be considered soon, without any delay [19].

7.2.5 Post-Sphincterotomy Strictures

In the past, this complication occurred in 8 % of patients, and now it is uncommon. Fibrosis at the site of sphincterotomy was responsible of mechanical obstruction of bile flow and insurgence of cholangitis and obstructive jaundice, months after the procedure. Pancreatic duct orifice stenosis can also occur following pancreatic sphincterotomy, leading to recurrent pancreatitis and abdominal pain. Simply extending of prior sphincterotomy, or stricture dilation or insertion of biliary stents, can relieve the narrowing and resolve the symptoms [25].

7.2.6 Other Complications

Cardiopulmonary complications following ERCP are rare (<1 %), but significant and represent the leading cause of death from the procedure. They can be related to underlying morbidities or to medications used for sedation and analgesia [26]. The overall mortality rate is twice as high (0.4 %) following therapeutic ERCP as that reported after diagnostic ERCP (0.2 %). These complications include arrhythmia, hypoxaemia and aspiration.

Other rare complications include pneumothorax and pneumomediastinum and impaction of therapeutic device, such as stone retrieval baskets in presence of large stones (more present before the introduction of mechanical lithotripsy) [10].

Conclusion

ERCP is now considered a therapeutic procedure. Knowledge of potential complications, of their frequency and risk factors, is fundamental in order to be prompt to diagnose and manage them and minimise the morbidity and mortality. Considering the difficulty of the technique, it is important to remember that the experience of operator, the volume of cases and selection of patients can significantly reduce the incidence of complications. Obviously an experienced surgeon should always be consulted in the decisional process, since surgery may be required as necessary approach to manage the complication.

References

1. McCune WS, Shorb PE, Moscovitz H (1968) Endoscopic cannulation of ampulla of Vater. A preliminary report. Ann Surg 167:725–726
2. Adler DG, Baron TH, Davila RE, Egan J, Hirota WK, Leighton JA, Qureshi W, Rajan E, Zuckerman MJ, Fanelli R, Wheeler-Harbaugh J, Faigel DO; Standards of Practice Committee of American Society for Gastrointestinal Endoscopy (2005) ASGE guidelines: the role of ERCP in disease of the biliary tract and the pancreas. Gastrointest Endosc 62(1):1–8
3. NIH state-of-the-science statement on endoscopic retrograde cholangiopancreatography (ERCP) for diagnosis and therapy (2002) NIH Consens State Sci Statement 19.1–26
4. Mallery JS et al (2003) Complications of ERCP. Gastrointestinal endoscopy 57(6):633–638
5. The Victoria Surgical Consultative Council (VSCC) guidelines. Complications of ERCP; 2007
6. Freeman ML, Nelson DB, Sherman S et al (1996) Complications of endoscopic sphincterotomy. N Engl J Med 335:909–918
7. Chutkan RK, Ahmad AS et al (2006) ERCP core curriculum prepared by the ASGE training committee. Gastrointest Endosc 63:361–376
8. Hirota WK, Petersen K, Baron TH, Goldstein JL, Jacobson BC, Leighton JA et al (2003) Guidelines for antibiotic prophylaxis for GI endoscopy. Gastrointest Endosc 58:475–482
9. Costamagna G, Shah SK, Tringali A (2003) Current management of postoperative complications and benign biliary stricture. Gastrointest Endosc Clin N Am 13:635–648, ix
10. ASGE guideline. Complications of ERCP (2012) Gastrointest Endosc 75(3):467–473
11. Silviera ML, Seamon MJ, Porshinsky B et al (2009) Complication related to endoscopic retrograde cholangiopancreatography: a comprehensive clinical review. J Gastrointest Liver Dis 18(1):73–82
12. Szary NN M.D., Al-Kawas FH M.D. (2013) Complications of endoscopic retrograde cholangiopancreatography: how to avoid and manage them. Gastroenterol Hepatolol (N Y) 9(8):496–504
13. McCuneWS Shorb PE, Moscovitz H (1968) Endoscopic cannulation of the Ampulla of Vater: a preliminary report. Ann Surg 167:752–756
14. Maple JT, Ben Menachem T, Anderson MA et al (2010) The role of endoscopy in the evaluation of suspected choledocholithiasis. Gastrointest Endosc 71:1–9
15. Cotton PB, Lehman G, Vennes J, Green JE, Russell RC, Meyers WC et al (1991) Endoscopic sphincterotomy complications and their management: an attempt at consensus. Gastrointest Endosc 37:383–393
16. Freeman ML (1998) Complications of endoscopic sphincterotomy. Endoscopy 30:A216–A220
17. Freeman ML, DiSario JA, Nelson DB et al (2001) Risk factors for post-ERCP pancreatitis: a prospective, multicentre study. Gastrointest Endosc 54:425–434
18. Shimizu S, Kutsumi H, Fujimoto S, Kawai K (1999) Diagnostic endoscopic retrograde cholangiopancreatography. Endoscopy 31:74–79
19. Chapman RW. Complications of ERCP (2006) BSG Guidelines in Gastroenterology 20–25. Available at: http://f.i-md.com/medinfo/material/475/4ea7cdb844a ebf27f87d9475/4ea7cdb844aebf27f87d9479.pdf
20. Baille J (1998) Complications of ERCP. In: Jacobson IM (ed) ERCP and its applications. Lippincott-Raven, Philadelphia, pp 37–54
21. Loperfido S, Angelini G, Benedetti G et al (1998) Major early complications from diagnostic and therapeutic ERCP: a prospective multi-centre study. Gastrointest Endosc 48:1
22. Genzlinger JL, McPhee MS, Fisher JK, Jacob KM, Helzberg JH (1999) Significance of retroperitoneal air after endoscopic retrograde cholangiopancreatography with sphincterotomy. Am J Gastroenterol 94:1267–1270
23. Loperfido S, Ferrara F, Costamagna G (2015) Post-ERCP perforation. UpToDate Sep 2015
24. Enns R, Eloubeidi MA, Mergener K, Jowell PS, Branch MS, Pappas TM et al (2002) ERCP- perforations: risk factors and management. Endoscopy 34:293–298
25. Szary NM, Al-Kawas F (2013) Complications of retrograde cholangiopancreatography: how to avoid and manage them. Gastroenterol Hepatol (N Y) 9(8): 496–504
26. ASGE (2002) Guidelines for the use of deep sedation and anesthesia for gastrointestinal endoscopy. Gastrointest Endosc 56:613–617

Imaging Techniques, Expected and Reactive Appearances After Endoscopic Retrograde Cholangiopancreatography (ERCP)

Massimo Tonolini

8.1 Introduction

Due to technical improvements and widespread availability of non-invasive imaging such as magnetic resonance cholangiopancreatography (MRCP) and multidetector computed tomography (CT), endoscopic retrograde cholangiopancreatography (ERCP) has transitioned from a diagnostic tool towards a primarily therapeutic procedure. Currently, ERCP is extensively used to treat several disorders of the biliary tract, ampulla and pancreas [1–3].

The main indications for ERCP include retained or recurrent choledocholithiasis, benign and malignant biliary strictures, sphincter of Oddi dysfunction (SOD), postoperative and traumatic ductal injuries, acute gallstone and chronic pancreatitis. ERCP is generally considered a safe procedure which often obviates the need for surgery, particularly in frail patients with poor performance status. Its limited contraindications include upper aerodigestive obstruction, severe coagulopathy, oesophageal and/or gastric varices, anaphylactic reaction to iodinated contrast medium (CM), acute nonbiliary pancreatitis, severe cardiopulmonary impairment and recent myocardial infarction. ERCP is unfeasible within

patients with previous Roux-en-Y anastomosis and technically challenging after pancreaticoduodenectomy or Billroth type II surgical reconstruction. Following identification and cannulation of the ampullary orifice and CM injection under fluoroscopy, the available endoscopic equipment allows performing sphincterotomy, extraction of common bile duct (CBD) stones, lithotripsy, biliary drainage, stricture dilatation, brush cytology and biopsy [1–3].

Furthermore, biliary endoprostheses represent the ideal minimally invasive treatment of obstructive jaundice from benign and neoplastic causes, which allows relieving symptoms and signs of cholestasis and preventing the superimposition of infectious cholangitis. The endoscopic positioning of biliary stents achieves high technical (over 90 %) and clinical (approximately 80 %) success rates. Currently, plastic stents are commonly used to treat postoperative bile leaks and benign strictures such as those secondary to iatrogenic duct damage during surgical procedures, anastomotic fibrosis, sclerosing cholangitis or chronic pancreatitis. Conversely self-expanding metal stents (SEMS) generally provide effective palliation of malignant biliary obstruction [4–7].

However, ERCP is associated with a non-negligible post-procedural morbidity (estimated in the range 4–10 %), particularly in elderly patients with comorbidities and at centres with limited experience and caseloads. More or less severe cardiopulmonary problems (hypoxia,

M. Tonolini, MD
Radiology Department, "Luigi Sacco" University Hospital, Via G.B. Grassi 74, Milano 20157, Italy
e-mail: mtonolini@sirm.org

© Springer International Publishing Switzerland 2016
M. Tonolini (ed.), *Imaging Complications of Gastrointestinal and Biliopancreatic Endoscopy Procedures*, DOI 10.1007/978-3-319-31211-8_8

arrhythmia and aspiration) represent the commonest post-ERCP adverse events and are usually secondary to medications used for analgesia and sedation. Specific complications occur in a variable proportion (5–40%) of patients depending on patients' age and comorbidities, the underlying disorders and operative techniques performed. The commonest short-term (occurring within 3 days) occurrences include post-ERCP acute pancreatitis (PEAP), haemorrhage, infection and duodenal perforation (DP) in descending order of frequency [1, 8–10].

8.2 Early Post-ERCP Imaging

8.2.1 Clinical Setting and Indications for Imaging

Due to the increasing number and complexity of endoscopic biliary procedures, clinicians and radiologists are increasingly confronted with suspected post-ERCP complications which represent a serious concern and a potential cause of litigation [11]. Therefore, early recognition and appropriate intervention are essential in optimising patient management, aiming to limit the iatrogenic morbidity and avoid a fatal outcome. According to the guidelines issued by the American Society for Gastrointestinal Endoscopy (ASGE), the European Society for Gastrointestinal Endoscopy (ESGE) and the World Society of Emergency Surgery (WSES), diagnosis and management of ERCP-related complications should rely upon a combination of clinical, laboratory and imaging (particularly CT) data [8, 12–14].

In the vast majority of patients, the clinical suspicion of early iatrogenic complications results from a combination of intraprocedural findings (difficult or repeated cannulation, suspected or confirmed DP), post-procedural symptoms and physical signs (such as sudden or worsening abdominal pain, distension, fever, hemodynamic impairment) and laboratory data (decreasing haemoglobin, elevated leukocyte count, acute phase reactants, serum lipase or amylase) [8, 13, 15, 16]. However, in patients who become acutely ill hours or days after ERCP, physical findings are of limited value due to the retroperitoneal location of most iatrogenic injuries. Furthermore, most complications and particularly AP and DP have remarkably similar clinical and laboratory manifestations [1, 8, 13, 14].

Some authors suggested that the duration of ERCP procedure represents a useful surrogated marker for challenging cannulation and/or operative manoeuvres which can cause papillary oedema and compromise ductal outflow, thus resulting in an increased risk and severity of complications (particularly PEAP). According to both literature and personal experience, planned CT may be warranted in patients after prolonged ERCP procedures, particularly with sphincterotomy or multiple cannulations [15, 17].

8.2.2 CT Technique

Unless contraindicated by critical unstable clinical conditions, multidetector CT is almost invariably the preferred imaging modality to promptly assess or exclude post-procedural complications after ERCP. Albeit the gold standard technique, CT should be used with caution due to the ionising radiation dose erogated, particularly in young patients and in those requiring serial follow-up studies. To provide optimal imaging triage of complications, radiologists should become familiar with interpretation of early post-procedural studies [15, 18–20].

On the basis of our experience, the anatomic region to be scanned should include the lung bases through the entire abdomen and pelvis in at least one acquisition. A preliminary unenhanced CT acquisition without intravenous CM is warranted in most cases, as it is helpful to detect hyperattenuating (35–70 Hounsfield Units, HU) intra- or extraluminal fresh blood. Image review at lung or bone window settings reliably allows identifying or excluding extraluminal air in the peritoneal cavity or retroperitoneum [15, 18–20].

Afterwards, following standard-dose intravenous CM injection, we suggest to adopt a biphasic CT protocol including arterial-dominant (starting approximately 30–35 s after CM bolus

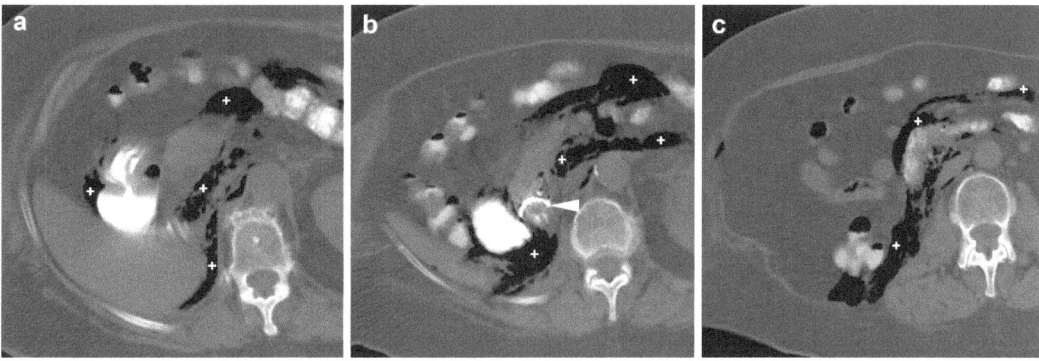

Fig. 8.1 During endoscopic retrograde cholangiopancreatography (ERCP), a 65-year-old female with sphincter of Oddi dysfunction experienced duodenal perforation (DP) which was recognised intraprocedurally and treated with endoluminal clipping. Twenty-four hours later, unenhanced multidetector CT obtained after peroral ingestion of enteral contrast medium (CM) and viewed at bone window setting (**a–c**) showed well-opacified gastroduodenal lumen without extraluminal CM leak, consistent with sealed DP. Note persistent extensive retroperitoneal air (+) and metallic clips (*arrowhead* in **b**) (Reproduced from Open Access Ref. no [15])

start) and portal venous (75–80 s delay), particularly when pancreatic necrosis and active bleeding are suspected. Otherwise, when concern exists about limiting irradiation, a single portal venous post-contrast acquisition should be performed [15, 18–20].

Additionally, in selected cases, gastroduodenal opacification by means of peroral ingestion of enteral CM such as diatrizoate meglumine (Gastrografin, Schering) may be beneficial to confirm or exclude extraluminal leakage consistent with DP (Fig. 8.1). However, the latter technique is seldom performed because of nausea, vomiting and inability to drink diluted CM, to avoid the risk of bronchial CM aspiration in bedridden patients with impaired swallowing [15].

8.2.3 Usual Post-ERCP Imaging Findings and Reactive Changes

Following ERCP the presence of air in the biliary tree is an expected, common finding. At CT, intra- and extrahepatic pneumobilia is visible in the majority of patients days or weeks from the procedure (Fig. 8.2) and may persist for months or years in patients who received sphincterotomy. Within 24–72 h after ERCP, retained CM is commonly seen in the biliary tree and gallbladder,

often with a characteristic dependent "stratified" appearance (Fig. 8.2) [15, 18–20]

Early post-ERCP CT studies commonly show limited retroperitoneal air (Fig. 8.3) in up to one-third of patients. This occurrence is attributable to excessive insufflation during endoscopy and is categorised as type IV perforation according to the classification by Stapfer (see Chap. 9, Table 2). However, we suggest not to emphasise the term "perforation" in the radiological report since it does not require treatment in absence of clinical and laboratory signs of peritonitis or sepsis [1, 15, 16, 21–23].

Similarly, peripancreatic fat stranding, minimal effusion in the pancreatic-duodenal groove and/or fluid thickening of the retroperitoneal fasciae should not be overemphasised in the CT report, since these changes do not dictate a diagnosis of PEAP in the absence of consistent clinical signs and laboratory abnormalities [15].

Multiplanar review of CT studies (Figs. 8.2, 8.3, 8.4 and 8.5) including maximum-intensity projections (MIP) reconstructions provide a thorough high-resolution visualisation of biliary endoprostheses and of their anatomical relationships. Plastic stents (Figs. 8.2 and 8.4) appear as thin straight or curved hyperdense tubes with a continuous wall, sometimes with small anchoring "claws" at their extremities. Conversely, metallic stents (Figs. 8.3 and 8.5) are wider and characterised by a "reticular" wall. Sometimes,

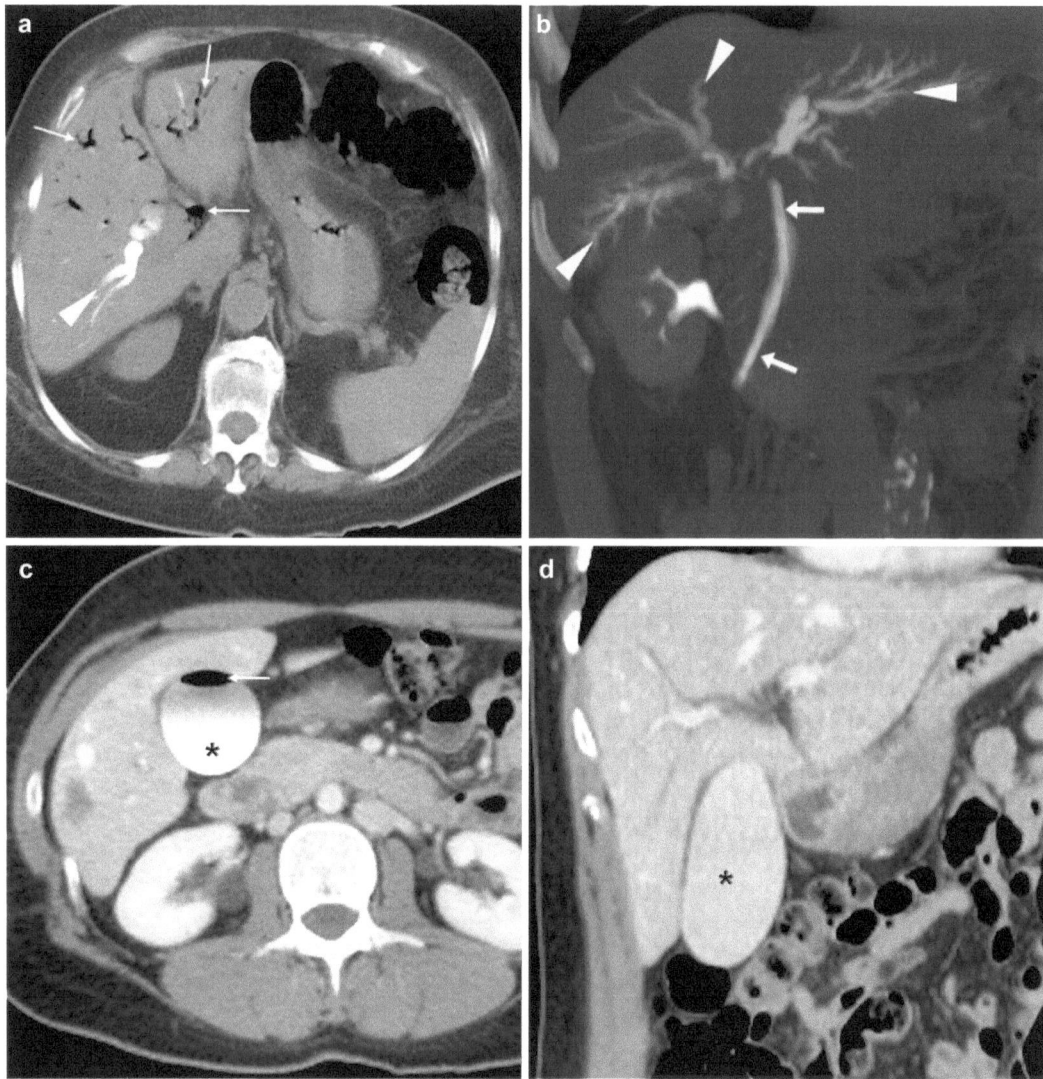

Fig. 8.2 Normal findings observed hours after operative ERCP in a 75-year-old male investigated with unenhanced CT (**a**, **b**) to verify correct placement of a plastic biliary stent, including dependent CM (*arrowheads*) and air (*thin arrows*) in the intrahepatic bile ducts. Note opacified urine in the renal collecting system. In a different patient, a 44-year-old female patient suffering from acute post-procedural pain, contrast-enhanced CT (**c**, **d**) 2 days after ERCP excluded signs of acute complications and showed stratified iodinated contrast medium (*), bile and air (*thin arrow*) in the gallbladder (Partially reproduced from Open Access Ref. no [15])

smaller-calibre stents are positioned endoscopically to relieve obstruction of the main pancreatic duct. When interpreting post-procedural studies, radiologists should describe the stent type, integrity, patency and position including proximal and distal extremities [15, 18, 24].

Finally, reversible oedematous-type mural thickening consistent with reactive acute duodenitis (see case presentation at paragraph 8.3) are sometimes observed following therapeutic ERCP [25].

8.2.4 Role of Ultrasound and Magnetic Resonance Imaging (MRI)

Compared to CT, the sonographic investigation of patients with suspected post-ERCP complications is strongly limited by the usual abdominal distension due to ileus, pneumoperitoneum or pneumoretroperitoneum and by its inability to assess pancreatic necrosis and

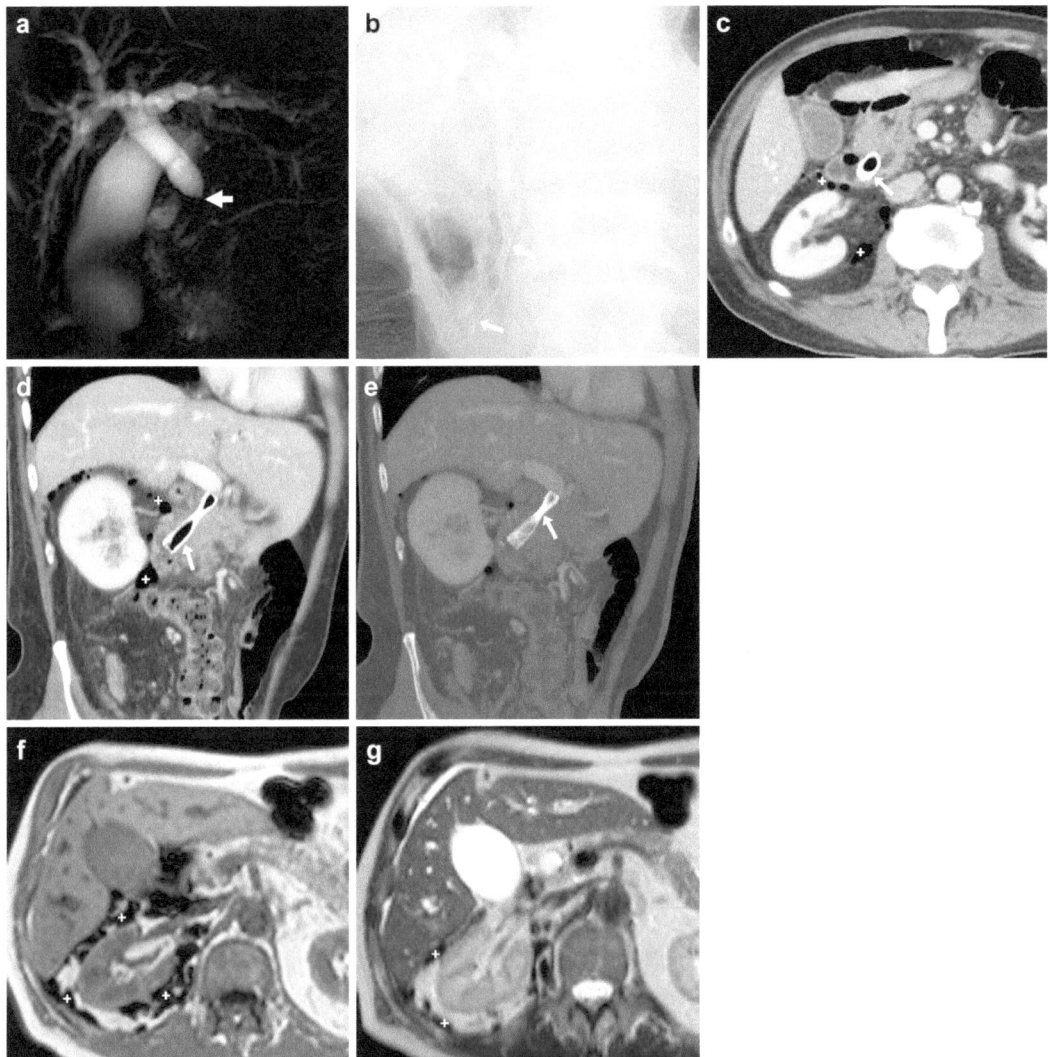

Fig. 8.3 A 69-year-old male with pancreatic head adeno-carcinoma causing CBD obstruction (*short arrow* in MRCP image **a**) underwent endoscopic positioning of a self-expanding metal stent (SEMS, *arrows* in **b**) to relieve cholestasis. Axial (**c**) and oblique (**d**) contrast-enhanced images from post-procedural CT showed decreased intrahepatic bile dilatation, SEMS in place (*arrows*) and minimal gas haemorrhage. Practically, ultrasound may be

bubbles in the right perirenal space (+). Maximum-intensity projection (MIP, **e**) reconstruction documented integrity of the SEMS with persisting constriction at its upper half. Hypointense signal from retroperitoneal air (+) was also visible in axial T1- (**f**) and T2-weighted (**g**) MRI images. With the SEMS in place, thereafter the patient successfully underwent pancreaticoduodenectomy

haemorrhage. Practically, ultrasound may be useful for rapid assessment of the gallbladder and biliary tree (with or without stents) and for follow-up of known collections, and its use is not recommended by current practice guidelines [8, 12–14].

An increasingly attractive alternative modality, MRI, can image PEAP and abnormal collections without the use of ionising radiation, and its use is particularly beneficial in younger

patients. An unenhanced protocol should include axial T1-, axial and coronal T2-weighted sequences with and without fat suppression, and standard MRCP sequences to assess the biliary and pancreatic ducts. The addition of diffusion-weighted MRI may be more sensitive in detecting cases of mild pancreas inflammation. Furthermore, a dynamic study using fat-suppressed T1-weighted gradient echo sequences during bolus intravenous gadolinium contrast

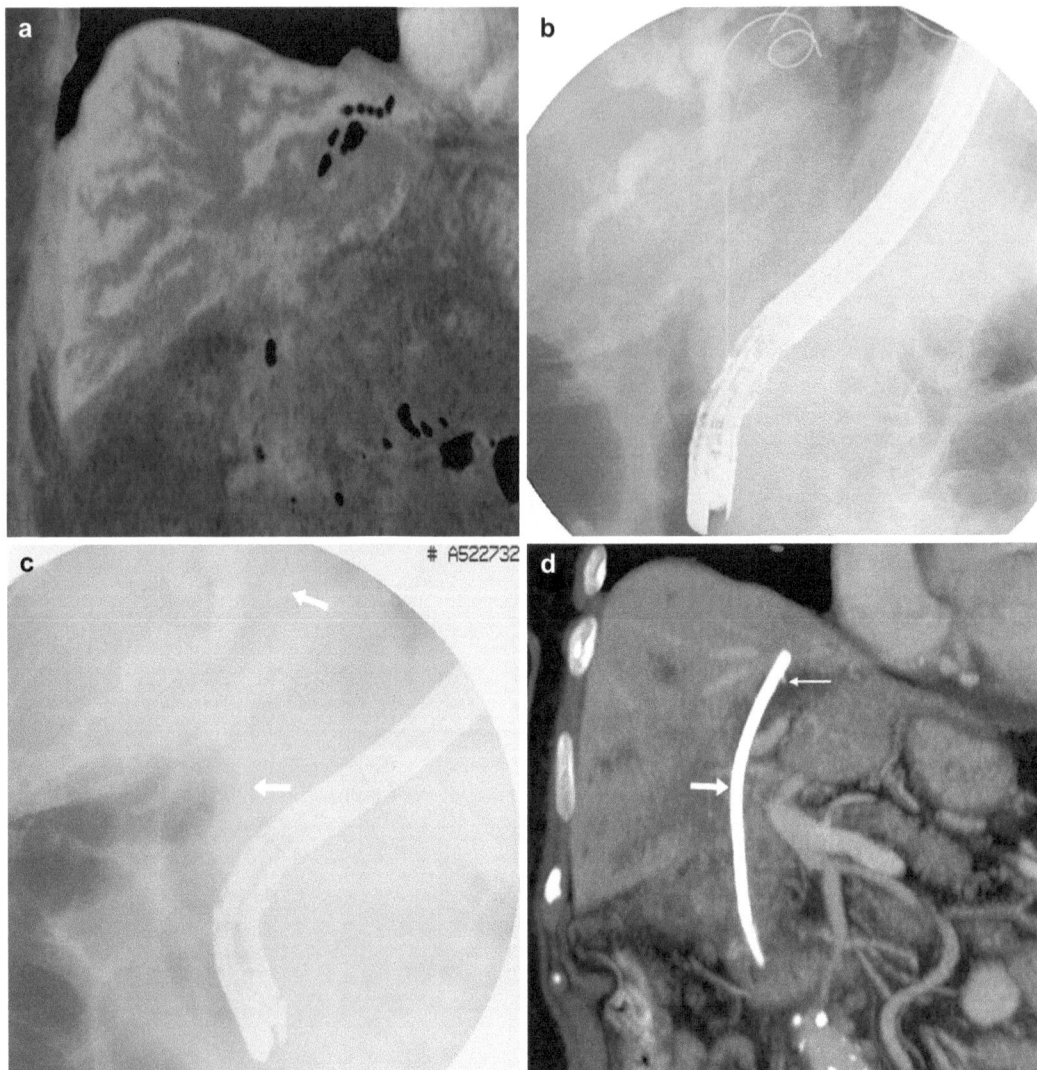

Fig. 8.4 In an elderly female with hilar (Klatskin-type) cholangiocarcinoma, pre-procedural CT including minimum-intensity projection reconstruction (**a**) depicted the degree and diffuse bilobar distribution of intrahepatic biliary obstruction. Under fluoroscopy, endoscopic cannulation of the Vaterian ampulla allowed to pass a guidewire (**b**) through the common bile duct (CBD) and above the tumour and to position a plastic endoprosthesis (*arrows* in **c**). Subsequently, the correct placement and integrity of the stent (*arrow*) was documented by means of CT including coronal MIP reconstruction (**d**). Note small anchoring "claw" (*thin arrow*) at the upper extremity of the stent

should be performed to assess the possible presence of pancreatic necrosis [26].

However, despite recent technical advancements, the use of MRI remains limited in acutely ill or uncooperative patients. Furthermore, in our experience, post-procedural MRCP sequences are commonly uninformative or confusing due to the common presence of pneumobilia which nulls the hyperintense signal of bile [15, 18, 27, 28].

8.3 Case Presentation: Acute Reversible Duodenitis Following ERCP

A 78-year-old diabetic male with diabetes mellitus was admitted because of jaundice, weight loss and intermittent upper abdominal pain. Laboratory tests disclosed anaemia (haemoglobin 9.4 mg/dL), elevated C-reactive protein,

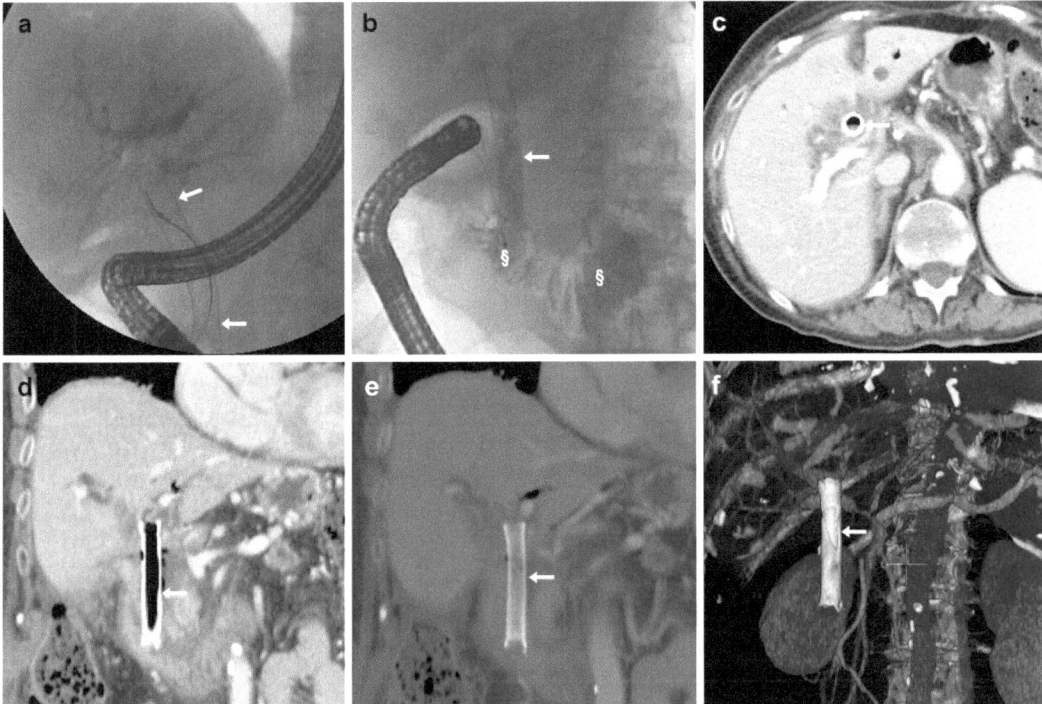

Fig. 8.5 Fluoroscopic-guided endoscopic placement (**a**, **b**) of a biliary SEMS (*arrows*) in a 79-year-old female with CBD carcinoma. Note CM in the duodenum (§ in **b**) indicating stent patency. Post-ERCP multidetector CT documented relief of intrahepatic biliary dilatation and excluded acute procedural complications. Multiplanar contrast-enhanced images (**c**, **d**) confirmed correctly placed SEMS (*arrows*) with intraluminal air. MIP (**e**), and three-dimensional volume-rendering (**f**) reconstructions documented the integrity and characteristic reticular "mesh" appearance of the stent (*arrows*)

serum bilirubin (17 mg/dl), transaminase and alkaline phosphatase (343 IU/l) levels. Following ultrasound confirmation of biliary dilatation (not shown), contrast-enhanced CT and MRCP (Fig. 8.6) depicted a concentric 12-mm long choledochal with upstream intrahepatic biliary obstruction, consistent with tumour [25].

Endoscopy showed a normal-appearing Vaterian ampulla, which was cannulated without the need for sphincterotomy. Cytological brushing ultimately diagnosed CBD adenocarcinoma. A 10-cm long, 10-French plastic biliary stent was positioned, without immediate adverse events.

Twenty-four hours later, the patient complained of acute diffuse abdominal pain, without signs of peritonitis at physical examination. Urgent CT showed correctly placed biliary stent, appearance of peritoneal effusion and marked oedematous mural changes of the duo-denum and periduodenal fat planes (Fig. 8.7) consistent with duodenitis. Imaging findings (including the normal size and homogeneous contrast enhancement of the pancreatic gland) and laboratory data (particularly serum amylase and lipase levels) were inconsistent with post-procedural acute pancreatitis, haemorrhage and duodenal perforation [25].

The patient promptly improved with conservative treatment, and jaundice was effectively relieved. Paracentesis fluid analysis excluded infection and malignancy. Three weeks later, repeated ERCP showed normal endoscopic aspect of the duodenum. To achieve long-term tumour palliation, the plastic biliary stent was removed and replaced with a SEMS. Follow-up CT 1 month later (Fig. 8.8) showed regression of biliary dilatation and of acute duodenal inflammatory changes [25].

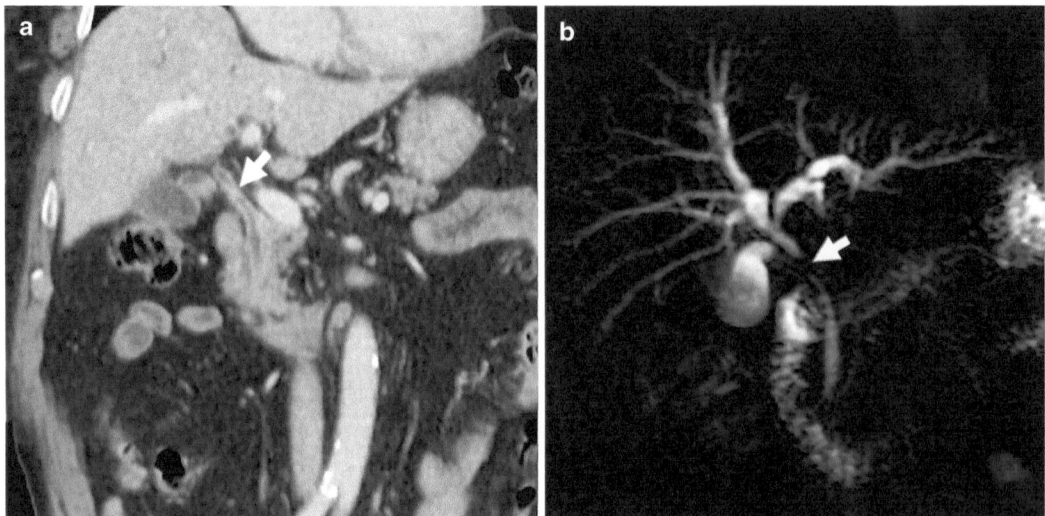

Fig. 8.6 Coronal reconstructed image from contrast-enhanced multidetector CT (**a**) and oblique-coronal MRCP (**b**) images showed common bile duct stricture (*short arrows*) with moderate upstream dilatation of common hepatic duct and intrahepatic branches (Partially reproduced with permission from Ref. no [25])

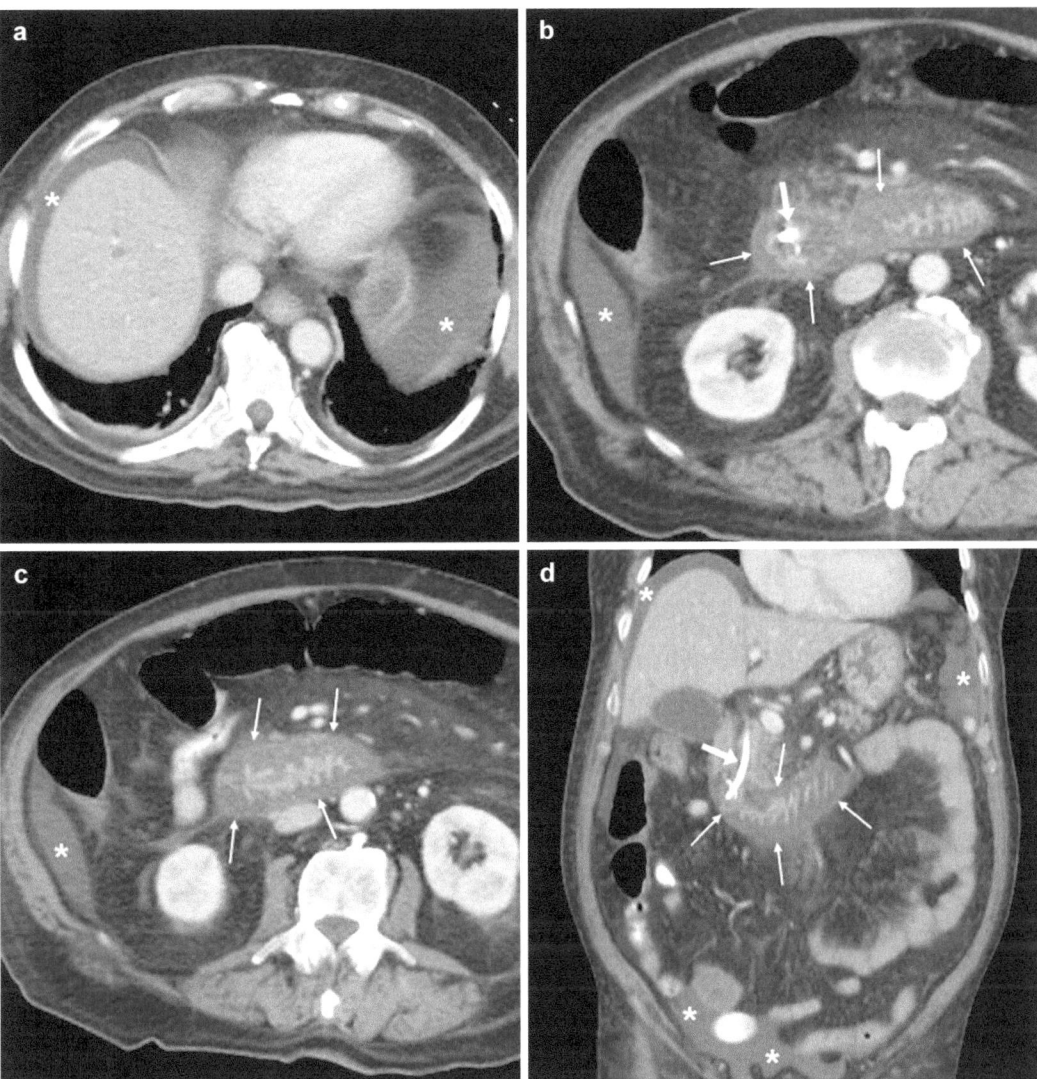

Fig. 8.7 Contrast-enhanced CT (**a–d**) after therapeutic ERCP confirmed correct positioning of plastic biliary stent (*arrows*) and detected the appearance of moderate ascites (*) and of marked circumferential mural thickening of the duodenum from the Vaterian ampulla to the Treitz angle, with stratified appearance ("target sign") due to enhancing inflamed mucosa and hypoattenuating oedematous submucosa (*arrows* in **b, c**), plus minimal associated inflammatory changes in the periduodenal fat (Partially reproduced with permission from Ref. no [25])

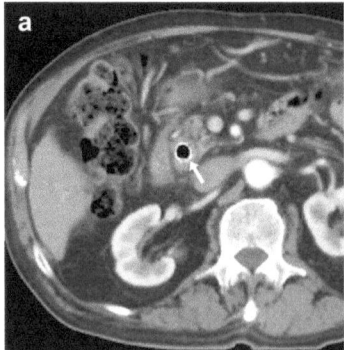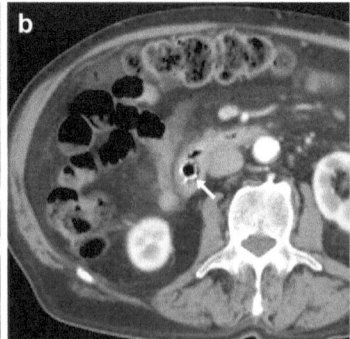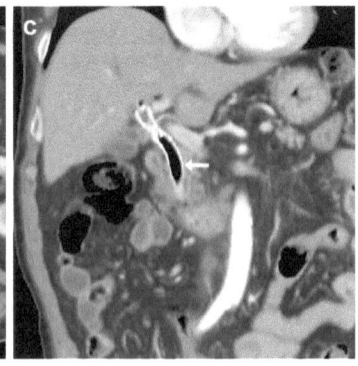

Fig. 8.8 Axial (**a**, **b**) and coronal (**c**) images from follow-up multidetector CT shows SEMS in place (*arrows*) and imaging resolution of both biliary obstruction and acute duodenal inflammatory changes (Partially reproduced with permission from Ref. no [25])

References

1. Silviera ML, Seamon MJ, Porshinsky B et al (2009) Complications related to endoscopic retrograde cholangiopancreatography: a comprehensive clinical review. J Gastrointest Liver Dis 18:73–82
2. Glomsaker TB, Hoff G, Kvaloy JT et al (2013) Patient-reported outcome measures after endoscopic retrograde cholangiopancreatography: a prospective, multicentre study. Scand J Gastroenterol 48:868–876
3. Adler DG, Baron TH, Davila RE et al (2005) ASGE guideline: the role of ERCP in diseases of the biliary tract and the pancreas. Gastrointest Endosc 62:1–8
4. van Boeckel PG, Vleggaar FP, Siersema PD (2009) Plastic or metal stents for benign extrahepatic biliary strictures: a systematic review. BMC Gastroenterol 9:96
5. Matlock J, Freeman ML (2005) Endoscopic therapy of benign biliary strictures. Rev Gastroenterol Disord 5:206–214
6. Judah JR, Draganov PV (2007) Endoscopic therapy of benign biliary strictures. World J Gastroenterol 13:3531–3539
7. Siriwardana HP, Siriwardena AK (2005) Systematic appraisal of the role of metallic endobiliary stents in the treatment of benign bile duct stricture. Ann Surg 242:10–19
8. Anderson MA, Fisher L, Jain R et al (2012) Complications of ERCP. Gastrointest Endosc 75:467–473
9. Glomsaker T, Hoff G, Kvaloy JT et al (2013) Patterns and predictive factors of complications after endoscopic retrograde cholangiopancreatography. Br J Surg 100:373–380
10. Kapral C, Duller C, Wewalka F et al (2008) Case volume and outcome of endoscopic retrograde cholangiopancreatography: results of a nationwide Austrian benchmarking project. Endoscopy 40:625–630
11. Cotton PB (2006) Analysis of 59 ERCP lawsuits; mainly about indications. Gastrointest Endosc 63:378–382; quiz 464
12. Dumonceau JM, Andriulli A, Elmunzer BJ et al (2014) Prophylaxis of post-ERCP pancreatitis: European Society of Gastrointestinal Endoscopy (ESGE) Guideline - updated June 2014. Endoscopy 46:799–815
13. Paspatis GA, Dumonceau JM, Barthet M et al (2014) Diagnosis and management of iatrogenic endoscopic perforations: European Society of Gastrointestinal Endoscopy (ESGE) Position Statement. Endoscopy 46:693–711
14. Sartelli M, Viale P, Catena F et al (2013) 2013 WSES guidelines for management of intra-abdominal infections. World J Emerg Surg 8:3
15. Tonolini M, Pagani A, Bianco R (2015) Cross-sectional imaging of common and unusual complications after endoscopic retrograde cholangiopancreatography. Insights Imag 6:323–338
16. Stapfer M, Selby RR, Stain SC et al (2000) Management of duodenal perforation after endoscopic retrograde cholangiopancreatography and sphincterotomy. Ann Surg 232:191–198
17. Woods RW, Akshintala VS, Singh VK et al (2014) CT severity of post-ERCP pancreatitis: results from a single tertiary medical center. Abdom Imaging 39:1162–1168
18. Pannu HK, Fishman EK (2001) Complications of endoscopic retrograde cholangiopancreatography: spectrum of abnormalities demonstrated with CT. Radiographics 21:1441–1453
19. Saddala P, Ramanathan S, Tirumani SH et al (2014) Complications of minimally invasive procedures of the abdomen and pelvis: a comprehensive update on the clinical and imaging features. Emerg Radiol 22:283–294
20. Wax BN, Katz DS, Badler RL et al (2006) Complications of abdominal and pelvic procedures: computed tomographic diagnosis. Curr Probl Diagn Radiol 35:171–187
21. Dubecz A, Ottmann J, Schweigert M et al (2012) Management of ERCP-related small bowel perforations: the pivotal role of physical investigation. Can J Surg 55:99–104

22. Zissin R, Shapiro-Feinberg M, Oscadchy A et al (2000) Retroperitoneal perforation during endoscopic sphincterotomy: imaging findings. Abdom Imaging 25:279–282

23. Ruiz-Tovar J, Lobo E, Sanjuanbenito A et al (2009) Case series: pneumoretroperitoneum secondary to duodenal perforation after endoscopic retrograde cholangiopancreatography. Can J Surg 52:68–69

24. Catalano O, De Bellis M, Sandomenico F et al (2012) Complications of biliary and gastrointestinal stents: MDCT of the cancer patient. AJR Am J Roentgenol 199:W187–W196

25. Tonolini M (2014) Reversible acute duodenitis as a complication of endoscopic biliary stenting. J Gastrointest Liver Dis 23:8

26. de Freitas TF, Schraibman V, Ardengh JC et al (2014) Diffusion-weighted magnetic resonance imaging indicates the severity of acute pancreatitis. Abdom Imaging 40:265–271

27. Zaheer A, Singh VK, Qureshi RO et al (2013) The revised Atlanta classification for acute pancreatitis: updates in imaging terminology and guidelines. Abdom Imaging 38:125–136

28. Sheu Y, Furlan A, Almusa O et al (2012) The revised Atlanta classification for acute pancreatitis: a CT imaging guide for radiologists. Emerg Radiol 19:237–243

Imaging Findings of Complications After Endoscopic Retrograde Cholangiopancreatography (ERCP) and Biliary Stenting

9

Massimo Tonolini and Alessandra Pagani

9.1 Introduction

As already mentioned in the Chap. 8, endoscopic retrograde cholangiopancreatography (ERCP) is associated with a non-negligible post-procedural morbidity. Following ERCP complications occur in a variable proportion (5–40 %) of patients depending on the complexity of the procedure, the underlying diagnoses, patients' age and comorbidities. The risk of complications is further increased by operative techniques such as use of balloons and dilating catheters, tissue sampling, mechanical lithotripsy and wire baskets for stone retrieval and placement of plastic and metallic biliary stents [1–4].

Apart from cardiorespiratory adverse events resulting from use of medications for analgesia and sedation, the commonest short-term (occurring within 3 days) specific complications include post-ERCP acute pancreatitis (PEAP, 2–9 %), haemorrhage (1.3–3.7 %), infection (1.9–3.6 %) and duodenal perforation (DP) in descending order of frequency. Specific risk factors for the above-mentioned four main types of complications are listed in Table 9.1. Additionally, a variety of rare complications have been occasionally reported, including pneumothorax, portal venous air embolism, splenic injury and perforation of colonic diverticula. Mostly secondary to operative procedures, the post-ERCP mortality (0.5–1.4 %) is particularly high in elderly patients with comorbidities and in centres with limited caseloads [1–4].

This chapter reviews the imaging appearances of the commonest post-ERCP complications including interstitial oedematous and necrotising PEAP, haemorrhages, retroperitoneal and intraperitoneal DPs, infections and stent-related complications. Most of the emphasis is placed on the pivotal role of multidetector CT, which should be warranted following complex or prolonged ERCP procedures since it represents the most effective modality to detect and grade ERCP-related complications and to monitor nonsurgically treated patients [5].

9.2 Post-ERCP Acute Pancreatitis

9.2.1 Definition, Incidence and Pathogenesis

According to the commonly used consensus definition, the diagnosis of PEAP requires at least two out of the three following criteria:

(a) Consistent new-onset or worsening abdominal pain which is usually persistent, severe, located in the epigastrium and often radiating to the back.

M. Tonolini, MD (✉) • A. Pagani
Radiology Department, "Luigi Sacco" University Hospital, Via G.B. Grassi 74, Milano 20157, Italy
e-mail: mtonolini@sirm.org

© Springer International Publishing Switzerland 2016
M. Tonolini (ed.), *Imaging Complications of Gastrointestinal and Biliopancreatic Endoscopy Procedures*, DOI 10.1007/978-3-319-31211-8_9

Table 9.1 Specific risk factors associated with an increased incidence of the commonest post-ERCP complications

Type of complication	Risk factors
Acute pancreatitis	**Patient specific:**
	Age below 55
	Female gender
	Sphincter of Oddi dysfunction
	Normal bilirubin
	Non-dilated common bile duct
	History of acute pancreatitis
	Non-dilated common bile duct
	Procedure related:
	Difficult or repeated cannulation
	Pancreatic duct CM injection
	Balloon dilatation
	Failure to clear bile duct stone
	Standard or pre-cut sphincterotomy
Haemorrhage	**Primary: sphincterotomy**
	Others:
	Coagulopathy
	Therapeutic anticoagulation
	Haemodialysis
	Acute cholangitis
	Papillary stricture
Duodenal perforation	**Primary: standard or pre-cut sphincterotomy**
	Others:
	Guidewire manipulation
	Previous Billroth II surgery
	Presence of peri-Vaterian diverticula
	Dilated common bile duct
	Guidewire manipulation
	Stricture dilatation
Infection	**Primary: incomplete or failed biliary drainage of obstructed biliary system**
	Others:
	Stenting across tumours
	Combined percutaneous–endoscopic procedures
	Primary sclerosing cholangitis

(b) New or prolongation of hospitalisation for at least 2 days.

(c) Abnormally elevated (at least three times above the upper normal limit) serum lipase or amylase 24 h after the procedure. Notably, a transient asymptomatic increase in serum pancreatic enzymes occurs in the majority (70–75 %) of patients within 4 h after ERCP but resolves within a few days [1, 4, 6].

Generally considered the commonest post-procedural complication, PEAP is probably unavoidable even in the hands of experienced endoscopists and has been reported in literature to occur after 2–9 % of all ERCPs, with a mortality approaching 3 % of cases. A meta-analysis of several prospective studies estimated its incidence at approximately 3.5 % of patients, but PEAP may complicate up to 30 % of high-risk cases. Notably, the incidence of PEAP is much higher in younger patients (below 59 years) following sphincterotomy compared than that in the elderly population [1, 4, 6].

The multifactorial pathogenesis of PEAP involves mechanical factors (such as direct trauma from endoscopy, difficult bile duct cannulation and multiple pancreatic duct injections) along with enzymatic, microbiological and patient-related factors including history of allergy [7–9].

The role of iodinated contrast medium (CM) as one of the cofactors in causing PEAP has been extensively studied. In experimental models of acute pancreatitis, digestive enzyme activation occurs rapidly within acinar cells following an initiating event: secretion blockage leads to accumulation of zymogen granules within cells, their fusion into large vacuoles, enzyme activation and finally cellular injury [7]. Besides the reduced pancreatic blood flow due to CM hyperviscosity, controversy exists on the role of the chemical effect of CM osmolality. Earlier studies reported reduced rates of pancreatic damage and decreased with newer low- or iso-osmolar compared to high-osmolar contrast medium, but other reports including a meta-analysis did not confirm a significantly different risk and outcome of PEAP [8–11].

9.2.2 Imaging Appearances

Albeit not specifically developed for iatrogenic pancreatitis, the revised Atlanta classification differentiates morphologically interstitial oedematous

(IEP) from necrotizing acute pancreatitis (NAP), the latter associated with high probability of infection, subsequent organ failure and increased mortality (12–30 % versus <3 %) [12, 13].

CT findings consistent with IEP include diffuse or localised enlargement of the pancreatic gland with normal homogeneous parenchymal enhancement (reaching attenuation values of 80–150 HU), associated with peripancreatic fat stranding or by fluid-like (measuring 0–30 HU) acute peripancreatic fluid collections (APFC). Containing a mixture of exudates, necrosis and blood, APFCs develop nearby the pancreas, are confined by normal fascial planes but lack a discernible wall and display homogeneous low (0–30 HU) attenuation without contrast enhancement [12–14].

Following ERCP, imaging is generally unnecessary to diagnose PEAP in those patients who meet the above-mentioned clinical and laboratory criteria. Nevertheless, in our experience most clinicians generally request CT within 24–72 h from ERCP in patients with suggestive clinical and laboratory features, to exclude other complications with similar manifestations such as DP. Therefore, a majority of patients with iatrogenic IEP are imaged with near-normal or subtle CT findings such as peripancreatic fat stranding, minimal effusions surrounding the head and neck of the pancreas and extending along the retroperitoneal fascial planes, accompanied by an homogeneously enhancing pancreatic gland (Figs. 9.1 and 9.2) [5].

Borrowing from experience with gallstone AP, "early" contrast-enhanced CT obtained within 2–3 days from the onset of symptoms may underestimate the severity of PEAP and cannot confidently exclude the appearance of necrosis; therefore, repeated scanning is usually needed during the post-ERCP hospitalisation [5, 12–17].

Conversely, NAP is defined by fatty tissue necrosis in either the pancreatic parenchyma or peripancreatic tissue. The usual CT appearance includes variable degrees of pancreatic enlargement and heterogeneity, with single or multiple areas of diminished or absent enhancement consistent with necrosis (Figs. 9.3 and 9.4). In NAP, post-necrotic peripancreatic fluid collections (PNPFCs) are commonly observed in the pancreas, the peripancreatic tissue or both. The differentiation between APFCs and PNPFCs should rely on the presence or absence of glandular necrosis. In a later stage, PNPFCs appear progressively more organised and encapsulated. After 4 weeks from onset, PNPFCs become defined as walled-off pancreatic necrosis after 4 weeks of symptom onset (Fig. 9.4) [5, 12–17].

The severity of AP may be graded according to the modified CT severity index (M-CTSI), which takes into account the presence of pancreatic and/or peripancreatic inflammatory changes, of APFCs, of necrosis (<30 %, 30–50 % and over 50 %) and extrapancreatic complications such as pleural effusion, ascites, vascular or gastrointestinal involvement. Therefore, in PEAP the key issue is the identification of the presence and extent of necrosis [12, 13, 15]. In the only published specific series, PEAP severity was graded according to M-CTSI scores as mild (≤2 points), moderate (4–6) and severe (≤8) in 53.6 %, 42.8 % and 3.6 % of cases, respectively [17].

Furthermore, glandular and peripancreatic changes consistent with PEAP are well demonstrated by MRI (Figs. 9.2 and 9.3). Typical MRI findings of AP include variable degrees of pancreatic enlargement with mildly increased T2-weighted signal intensity from oedema, normal signal on fat-saturated T1-weighted acquisitions, plus peripancreatic inflammatory fat stranding, fluid or collections. Similarly to CT, pancreatic enhancement may appear homogeneous in IEP, diminished or heterogeneous in NAP after intravenous gadolinium CM. In the setting of gallstones, it has been proposed that a limited non-contrast MRI protocol has high correlation with contrast-enhanced CT in the assessment of mild AP. Furthermore, very recently the inclusion of diffusion-weighted sequences in routine MRI protocols before or without CM administration may allow differentiation between normal, inflamed and necrotic pancreas with measurement of apparent diffusion coefficients (ADC) [12, 13, 18, 19].

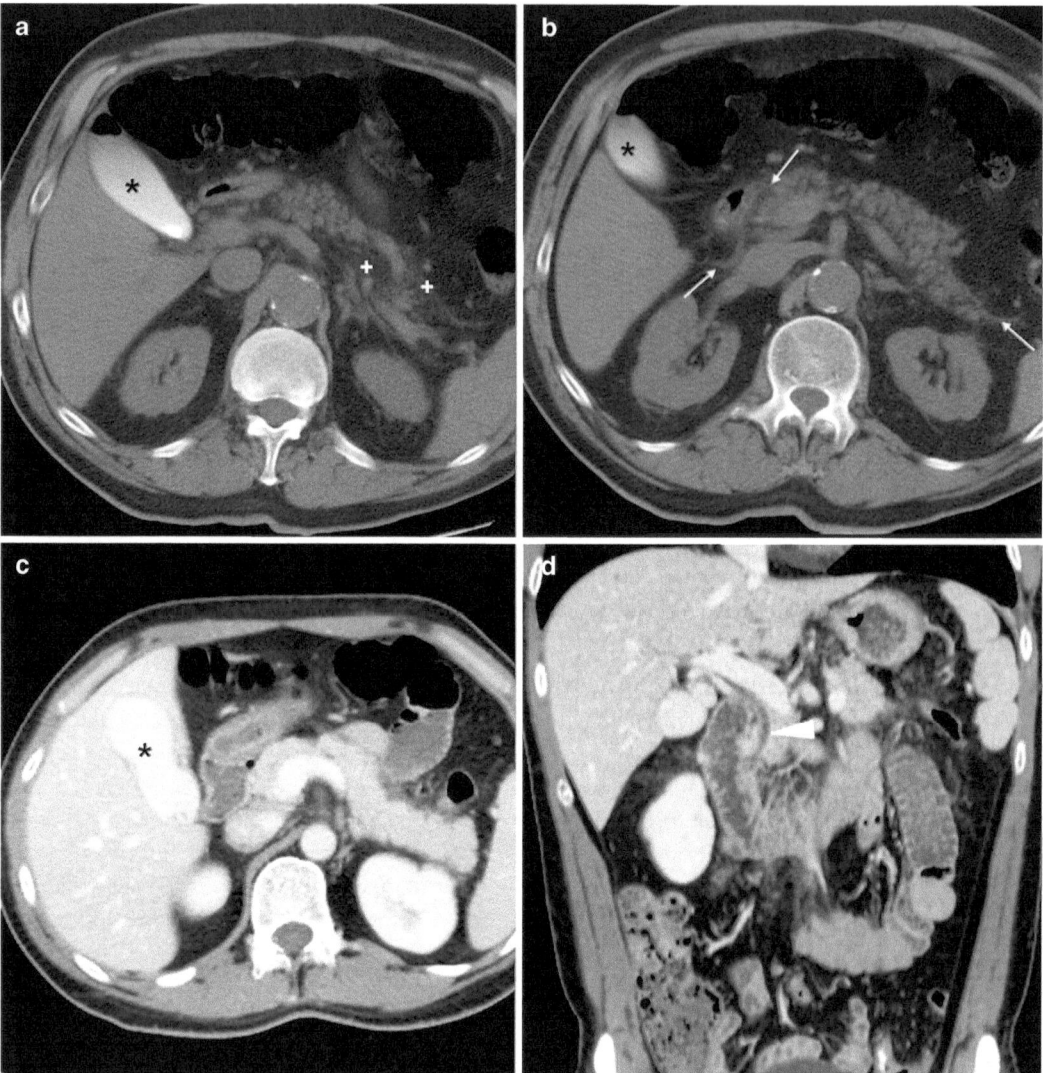

Fig. 9.1 Oedematous post-ERCP acute pancreatitis (PEAP). Two days after ERCP including sphincterotomy and extraction of common bile duct (CBD) stones, a 39-year-old male experienced abdominal pain with increased serum lipase. Unenhanced CT images (**a**, **b**) showed retained contrast medium (CM, *) and some air in the gallbladder, subtle peripancreatic fat stranding (+) and minimal effusion in the pancreatic groove and retroperitoneal fascial planes (*thin arrows*). Post-contrast acquisition showed normal thickness and homogeneous enhancement of the pancreatic gland (**c**), normal calibre of the common bile duct (*arrowhead* in **d**). The patient had an uneventful course with conservative treatment

9.3 Haemorrhage

Generally, bleeding occurs after approximately 1–2 % of ERCPs, most usually after sphincterotomy (see Table 9.1). On the basis of blood loss and transfusion need, haemorrhage is graded as mild in approximately 70 % of cases: conversely clinically significant haemorrhage requiring angiographic, endoscopic or surgical intervention is reported after less than 1/1,000 procedures. Haemorrhage is heralded by haematemesis, melaena or haemoglobin drop and may be delayed up to 2 weeks in up to 50 % of patients [1, 4].

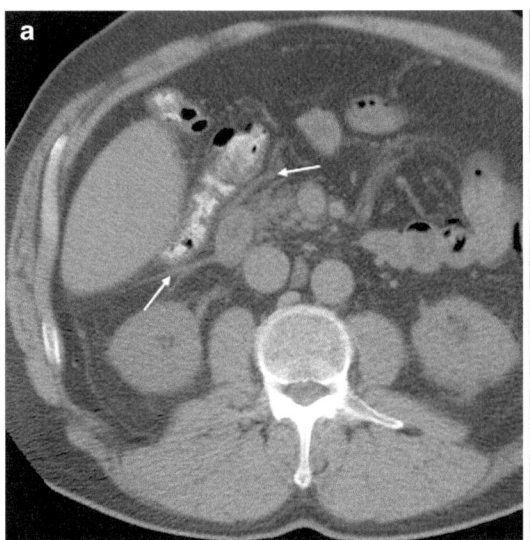 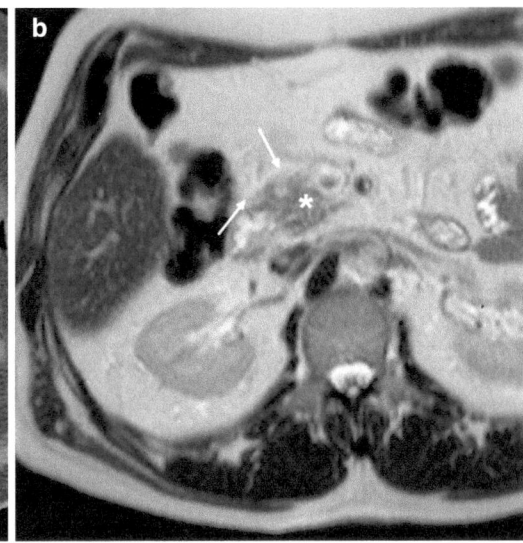

Fig. 9.2 Oedematous PEAP with markedly increased serum amylase 48 h after endoscopic treatment of choledocholithiasis in a 55-year-old male with past history of gallstone acute pancreatitis and laparoscopic cholecystectomy. Unenhanced CT (**a**) and T2-weighted MRI (**b**) images show mild peripancreatic and retroperitoneal fascial fluid (*thin arrows*) without abnormal collections. Clinical symptoms and laboratory changes regressed within 72 h (Reproduced from Open Access Ref. no [5])

Prompt CT imaging may prove helpful to investigate post-ERCP bleeding. Consistent imaging findings include hyperattenuating wall thickening of the duodenum representing intramural haematoma and hyperattenuating blood in the choledochus (Fig. 9.5) or duodenal lumen. In our experience, uncertainty of interpretation may exist between fresh haemorrhage and diluted CM in the duodenal or jejunal lumen. Furthermore, CM-enhanced study including an arterial-phase acquisition may effectively show active contrast extravasation in the duodenum, indicating ongoing bleeding (see case presentation Sect. 9.7.1). Finally, bleeding may occasionally appear as intrahepatic or subcapsular hepatic haematomas with associated haemoperitoneum (see case presentation Sect. 9.7.2) [5, 14, 15, 20, 21].

Repeated endoscopy is the preferred first-line approach to venous bleeding, as it allows to perform several different methods of haemostasis such as local epinephrine flushing, balloon tamponade, haemostatic (fibrin glue) injection, haemoclip placement, electrocoagulation or temporary stent placement. Conversely, failure of endoscopic treatment and CT detection of active bleeding represent indications for endoscopic, interventional (transarterial embolisation) or surgical treatment [22–25].

9.4 Duodenal Perforation

9.4.1 Incidence and Classification

Representing the rarest yet most dreaded occurrence, DP complicates up to 1 % of ERCP procedures and is associated with a non-negligible mortality (9–18 %) [1, 4, 26–34].

In a significant proportion (26–48 %) of cases, DP is identified or at least suspected intraprocedurally during ERCP, by means of CM injection through the endoscope showing extraluminal CM leakage (see case presentation Sect. 9.7.3). Alternatively, presentation occurs hours or days later. Clinical manifestations are often closely similar to those associated with PEAP and not unusually mild compared to the imaging findings [1, 4, 26–34].

The widely employed classification proposed by Stapfer et al. (Table 9.2) categorises DP into four classes in descending order of severity, on the basis of mechanism and anatomical location [33].

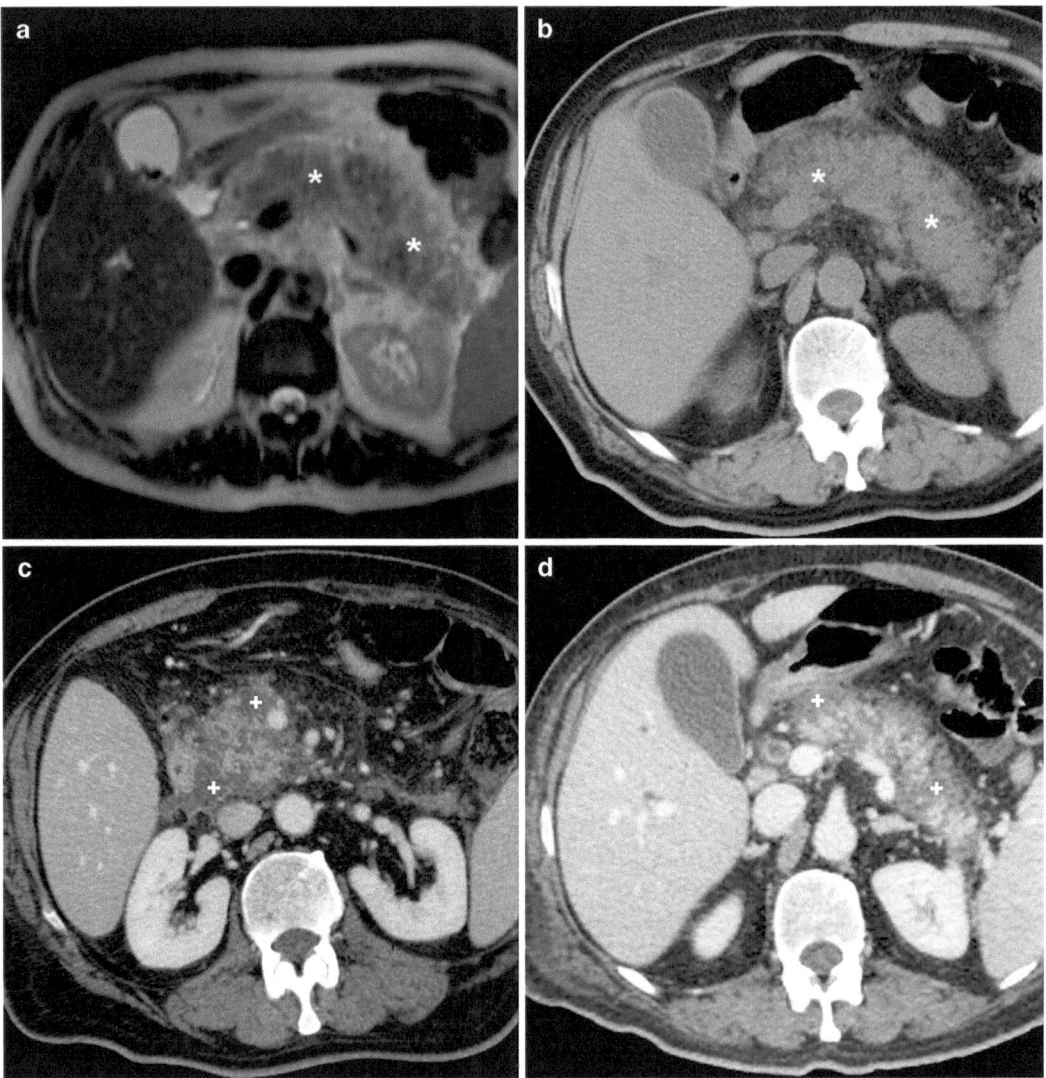

Fig. 9.3 Necrotizing PEAP in a 73-year-old male after ERCP including endoscopic control of mild bleeding from sphincterotomy. Urgent MRI (T2-weighted image in **a**) requested because of abdominal pain with increased C-reactive protein (CRP), leukocyte count and serum lipase showed markedly enlarged pancreatic gland (*) with peripancreatic oedema. Unenhanced (**a**) and contrast-enhanced CT (**c, d**) confirmed severe AP with inhomogeneous enhancement of the enlarged pancreas due to diffuse peripancreatic necrosis (+). The patient finally recovered after 2 weeks of in-hospital conservative treatment (Partly reproduced from Open Access Ref. no [5])

9.4.2 Imaging Appearances and Impact on Management

The imaging hallmark of DP is represented by extraluminal air, which may be sometimes recognised within the duodenal wall, but most commonly dissects through the retroperitoneum.

In our experience, the typical appearance of a type II DP includes air collecting posteriorly to the duodenum and pancreatic head, in the right anterior pararenal and perirenal spaces. Air is often seen surrounding the inferior vena cava, portal vein and splanchnic vessels, sometimes crosses the midline along the retroperitoneal

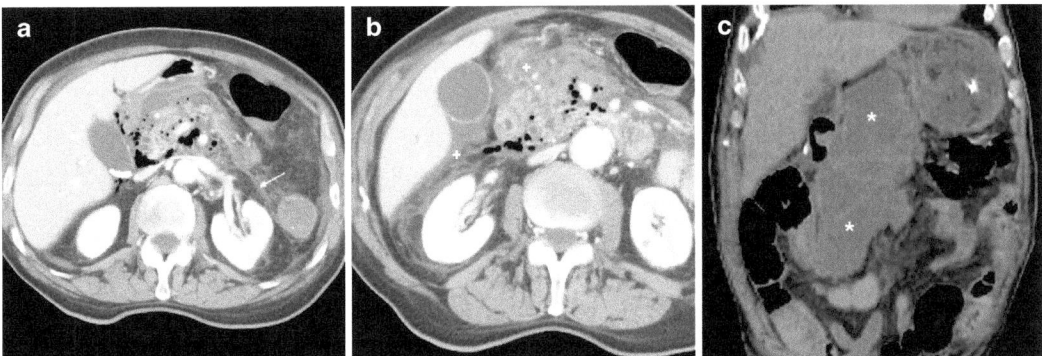

Fig. 9.4 Necrotizing PEAP plus retroperitoneal air in a 79-year-old male occurring 48 h after endoscopic sphincterotomy and removal of choledocholithiasis. Contrast-enhanced multidetector CT (**a**, **b**) showed enlarged, markedly inhomogeneous, poorly enhancing pancreas with fascial (*thin arrow* in **a**), peripancreatic and infrahepatic (+ in **b**) fluid, gas bubbles along the superior mesenteric vessels and in the periduodenal region. Pleural effusion was present bilaterally. Urgent laparotomic surgery confirmed severe necrotic–haemorrhagic pancreatitis. During a prolonged intensive care unit stay, follow-up unenhanced CT (**c**) showed appearance of a vast walled-off post-necrotic collection (*) (Reproduced from Open Access Ref. no [5])

fascial planes and occasionally tracks upwards to reach the posterior mediastinum (Figs. 9.6 and 9.7 and case presentation Sect. 9.7.3) [4, 5, 15, 16, 29].

However, the presence and amount of retroperitoneal air at imaging does not linearly correlate with the severity of the injury or with the need for invasive treatment, since it rather reflects the degree of continuous endoscopic air insufflation and manipulation after an undetected injury occurred. Therefore, successful nonoperative management of type II DP with extensive retroperitoneal air is possible, provided that the patient does not develop peritonitis, fever or impending shock. However, negative physical findings do not reliably exclude surgery since severe DP may be masked clinically by the retroperitoneal site especially in elderly or chronically ill patients [5, 14–16, 35].

Although controversy exists about the optimal approach, this practical system in the management of ERCP-related DP should be individualised according to its type, clinical picture and imaging findings. Type I (endoscope-related) duodenal wall perforations invariably require early surgery. Conversely, nowadays, the majority (approximately 70 %) of patients with peri-Vaterian (type II) DP are considered amenable to endoclipping (see Fig. 8.1) or conservative treatment with nasogastric drainage, parenteral nutrition, intravenous hydration and antibiotics. The approach to management of stable patients with DP is increasingly nonsurgical and proves successful in almost 90 % of cases with a correct patient selection. Unfortunately, delayed recognition of type I perforations and failure of conservative treatment are still associated with a high (50 %) mortality rate from sepsis. According to the ESGE guidelines, the indications for surgical treatment include:

(a) Clinical features are symptoms, signs and laboratory changes indicating:
   - Sepsis
   - Peritonitis
(b) Imaging features:
   - Pneumoperitoneum (Fig. 9.8)
   - Periduodenal or retroperitoneal fluid collections
   - Major contrast extravasation at ERCP, CT or upper gastrointestinal study with water-soluble CM (see case presentation Sect. 9.7.3)
   - Massive subcutaneous emphysema
(c) Retained stones or basket/wire endoscopic instruments.
(d) Failure of conservative management.

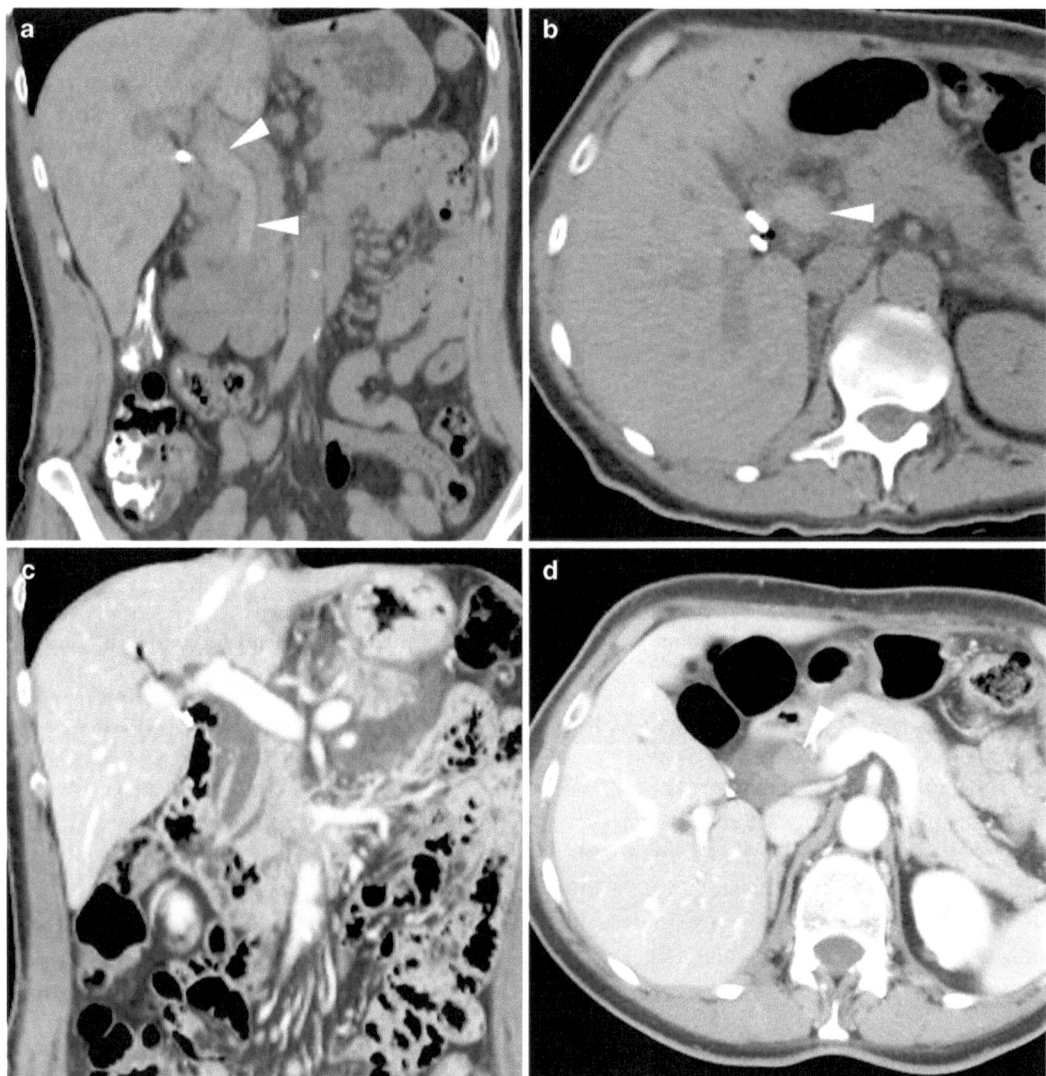

Fig. 9.5 Haemobilia following ERCP in a 57-year-old female with benign papillary stenosis and previous cholecystectomy, manifesting with abdominal pain and mild haemoglobin drop. Unenhanced (**a, b**) and post-contrast (**c, d**) multidetector CT images showed moderate dilatation and hyperattenuating (45 HU) content of the CBD (*arrowheads*) which was initially misinterpreted as retained CM injected during the procedure. Conversely, repeated endoscopy disclosed intraluminal haemorrhage in the CBD without signs of active bleeding. This self-limiting complication resolved on conservative treatment (Partly reproduced from Open Access Ref. no [5])

Table 9.2 Classification of duodenal perforations according to Stapfer et al.

Type	Description	Comment
I	Endoscope-related lateral or medial duodenal wall perforations	Often large and distant from the ampulla, requires surgical intervention in most cases
II	Retroperitoneal peri-Vaterian perforations resulting from (pre-cut) sphincterotomy	Of variable severity but most often discrete and amenable to conservative management
III	Distal common bile duct injuries secondary to guidewire insertion or instrumentation for stone extraction	Amenable to conservative management
IV	Isolated retroperitoneal air from excessive insufflation	Does not require specific treatment

Adapted from Ref. no. [33]

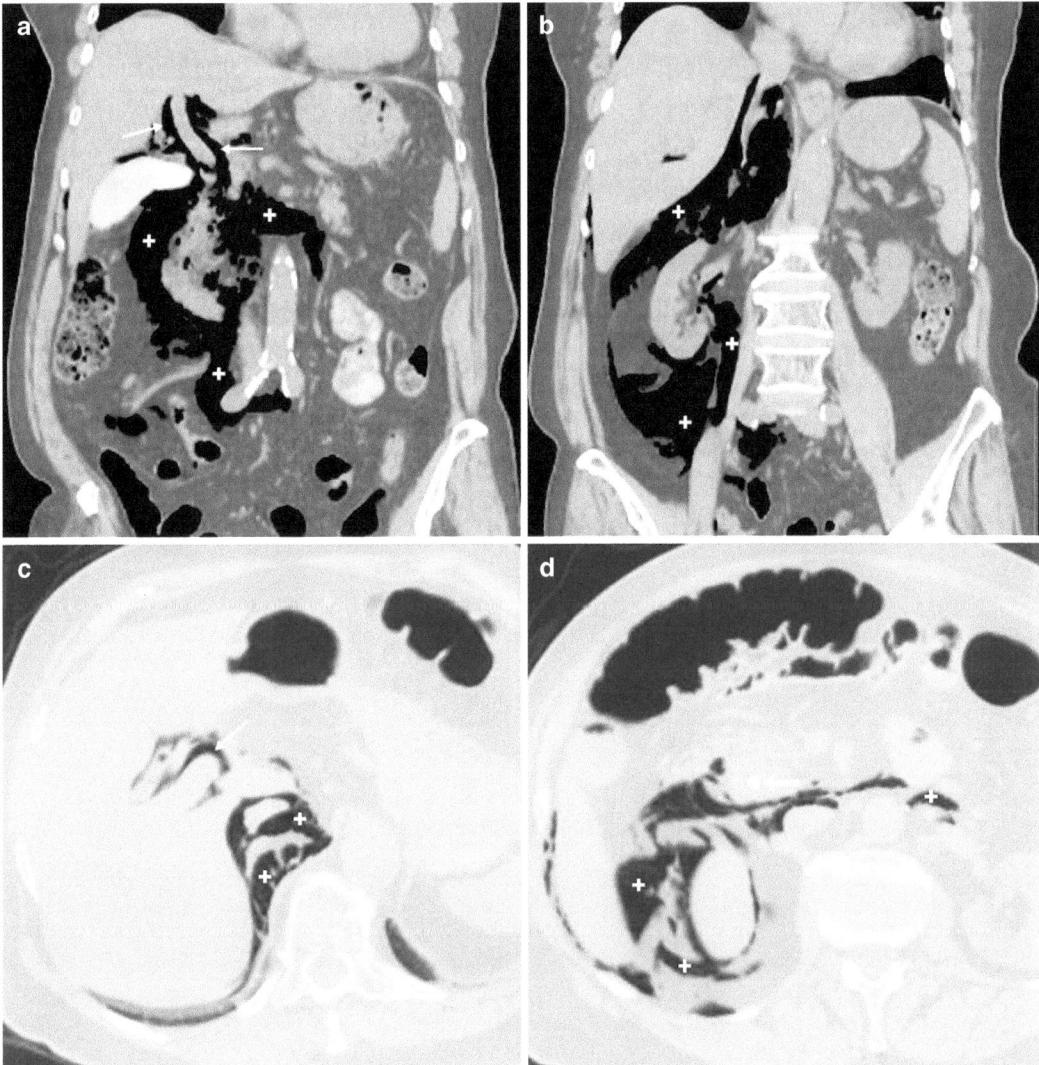

Fig. 9.6 Severe retroperitoneal (Type II) duodenal perforation (DP) in an 80-year-old woman following ERCP with sphincterotomy, incomplete retrieval of choledocholithiasis and positioning of plastic CBD stent (*arrow* in **d**). Post-procedural unenhanced CT viewed at both soft tissue (**a**, **b**) and bone (**c**, **d**) window settings showed extensive retroperitoneal air (+) predominantly located in the right peri- and pararenal spaces, around the descending duodenum and tracking along the inferior vena cava and portal vein (*thin arrows*). Surgical exploration dictated by sepsis failed to detect a perforation site, and the patient finally recovered (Reproduced from Open Access Ref. no [5])

Therefore, the interpreting radiologist should carefully report the presence of extraluminal CM leakage, pneumoperitoneum and fluid collections which represent the key imaging findings which usually contraindicate a conservative approach. Surgery may include perforation closure or duodenal exclusion, retroperitoneal drainage, CBD exploration and T-tube insertion [4, 14, 26–34].

During conservative treatment, repeat CT may be warranted after 48–72 h interval to confirm sealed leaks and absent fluid collections and

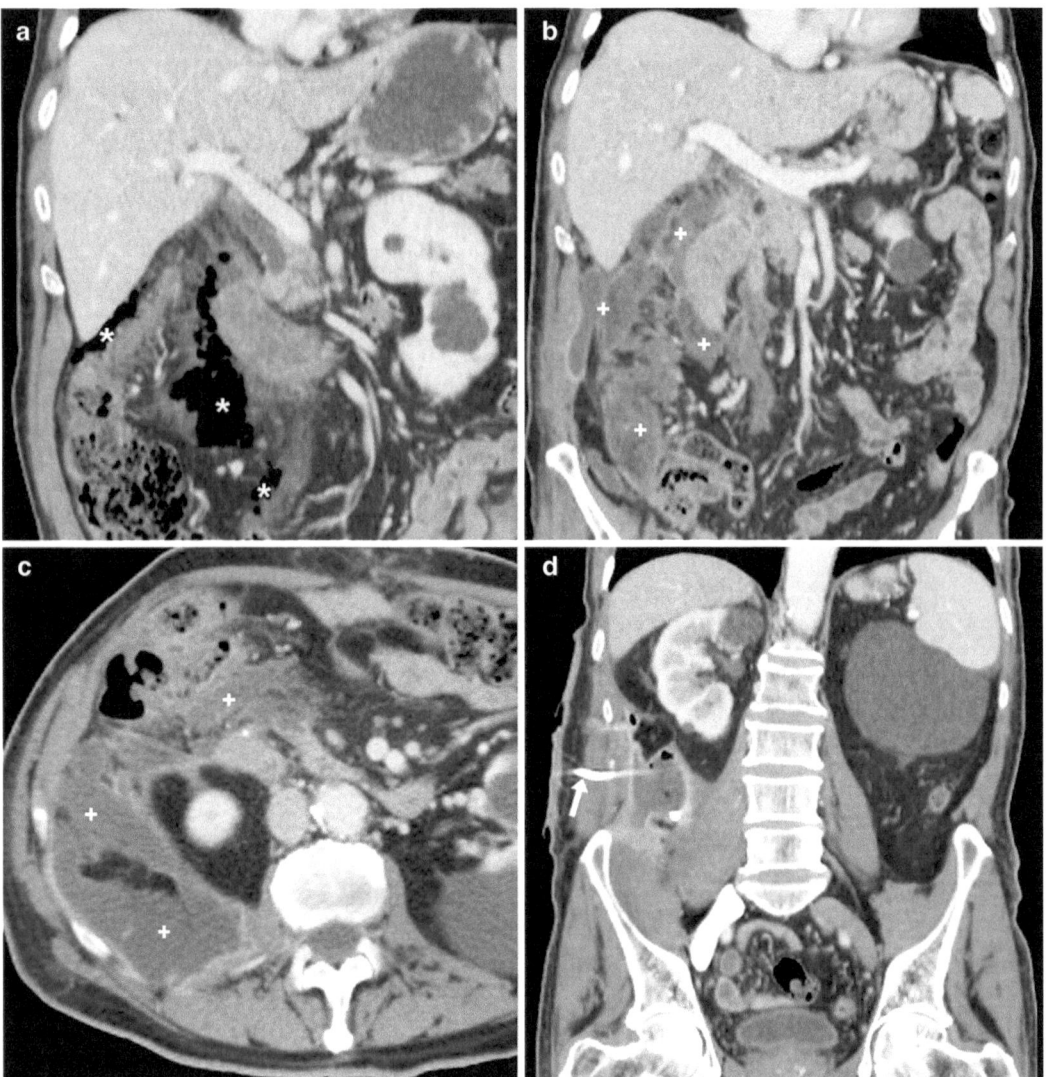

Fig. 9.7 Failed conservative management of DP in an 83-year-old male with a chronic duodenal stricture who underwent ERCP to prevent further episodes of infectious cholangitis. The next day, contrast-enhanced CT (**a**) showed moderate right-sided retroperitoneal air (*). Follow-up CT (**b, c**) 4 days later showed formation of multiple confluent periduodenal and right parieto-colic fluid-like infected collections (+), with extensive occupation of ipsilateral posterior pararenal space, which required percutaneous drainage (*arrow* in **d**) to relieve sepsis (Partly reproduced from Open Access Ref. no [5])

to monitor the patient until recovery. Whenever a fluid collection develops, percutaneous drainage should be considered [5, 14–16, 30, 35].

9.5 Post-ERCP Infections

The current clinical guidelines recommend antibiotic prophylaxis in known or suspected biliary obstruction. However, the development of bacteraemia is a common event (15–27%) after diagnostic or therapeutic ERCP. Whereas the reported incidence of clinically significant iatrogenic infections is limited (1–3%), sepsis represents a common cause of death [1, 4].

The spectrum of post-ERCP infectious complications encompasses cholecystitis, acute cholangitis, liver abscesses and systemic sepsis. Occurring in approximately 0.2–0.5% of patients, cholecystitis has been correlated to

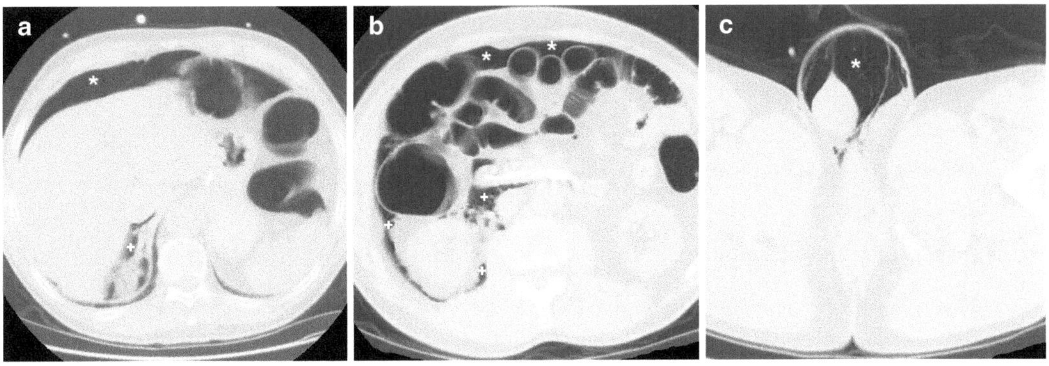

Fig. 9.8 Stapfer type I DP with moderate retroperitoneal air (+) plus pneumoperitoneum extending to the scrotum (*) shown by emergency unenhanced CT (**a–c**) in a 62-year-old male undergoing ERCP treatment of choledo-cholithiasis. Laparotomic surgery allowed duodenotomy and suture of posterior duodenal wall discontinuity, toilette and drainage of peritoneal cavity. Subsequent course was uneventful and repeated CT with oral CM at discharge (not shown) excluded extraluminal contrast leak (Reproduced from Open Access Ref. no [5])

cholelithiasis and intraprocedural filling of the gallbladder with CM, is heralded by appearance of luminal overdistension and circumferential mural thickening and may sometimes be complicated by perforation (Fig. 9.9) [5, 15, 16].

Acute cholangitis represents a potentially life-threatening condition if not promptly and appropriately treated, which typically develops in an obstructed biliary system and after biliary instrumentation. Its pathogenesis involves microbial colonisation and overgrowth in stagnant bile: the resulting increased intraductal pressure causes cholangiovenous reflux of bacteria and toxins into the bloodstream and represents the key factor associated with clinical severity, risk of sepsis and mortality [36, 37]. Infectious cholangitis clinically manifests with fever, jaundice, abdominal pain and abnormal liver function tests. Multidetector CT and MRCP generally depict variable degrees of central, diffuse or segmental bile duct dilatation, with pneumobilia, increased attenuation or signal layering from purulent bile, and filling defects from intraluminal stones or sludge. The most characteristic imaging appearance is represented by mural thickening and enhancement of CBD and intrahepatic duct walls (Fig. 9.10) [5, 14–16].

More recently, other imaging appearances have been described, which allow supporting the clinical diagnosis of acute cholangitis and monitoring changes during treatment: these changes include showing patchy or wedge-shaped parenchymal areas of increased MRI signal intensity, and markedly inhomogeneous arterial-phase parenchymal enhancement with hyperenhancing "geographic" regions representing transient attenuation differences from increased arterial blood supply [38–40].

Finally, CT or MRI allows identification of septic complications, particularly the development of liver abscesses, which display the typical appearance of fluid-like hypoattenuating collections with enhancing periphery (Fig. 9.11, case presentation Sect. 9.7.2). Accessory signs of sepsis such as atelectasis/pneumonia and splenic or renal infarcts may be observed (Fig. 9.10). Alternatively, sepsis may develop from superinfection of PNPFCs or abnormal collections from DP (Fig. 9.7) [5, 14–16].

9.6 Stent-Related Complications

The endoscopic positioning of plastic or metallic self-expanding metal stents (SEMS) represents the ideal minimally invasive treatment for biliary strictures, with very high technical (98–99%) and clinical (80%) success rates. However, biliary stenting is associated with a significant risk of complications, which are estimated to occur in up to 40% of patients overall [41–44].

Early complications following biliary stenting are relatively rare and include haemorrhage (see case presentation Sect. 9.7.2), PEAP, stent

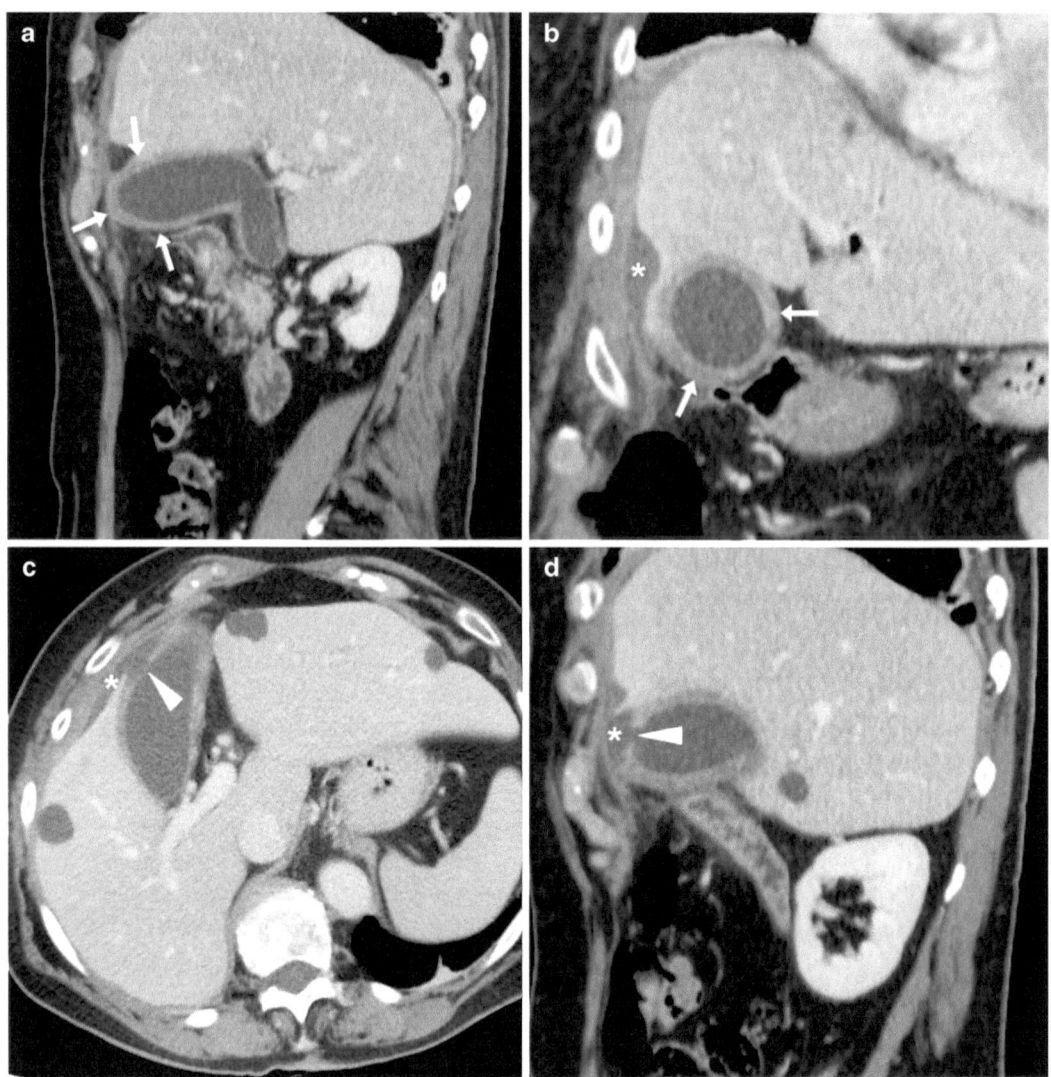

Fig. 9.9 Acute cholecystitis in a 66-year-old female manifesting with fever and transverse upper abdominal pain 3 days after ERCP with sphincterotomy and biopsy of ampullary adenoma, despite antibiotic prophylaxis. Multiplanar contrast-enhanced CT images (**a–d**) show thickened gallbladder wall (*arrows*) with focal perforation (*arrowhead* in **c**) and localised collection (*) which required emergency laparotomic cholecystectomy (Reproduced from Open Access Ref. no [5])

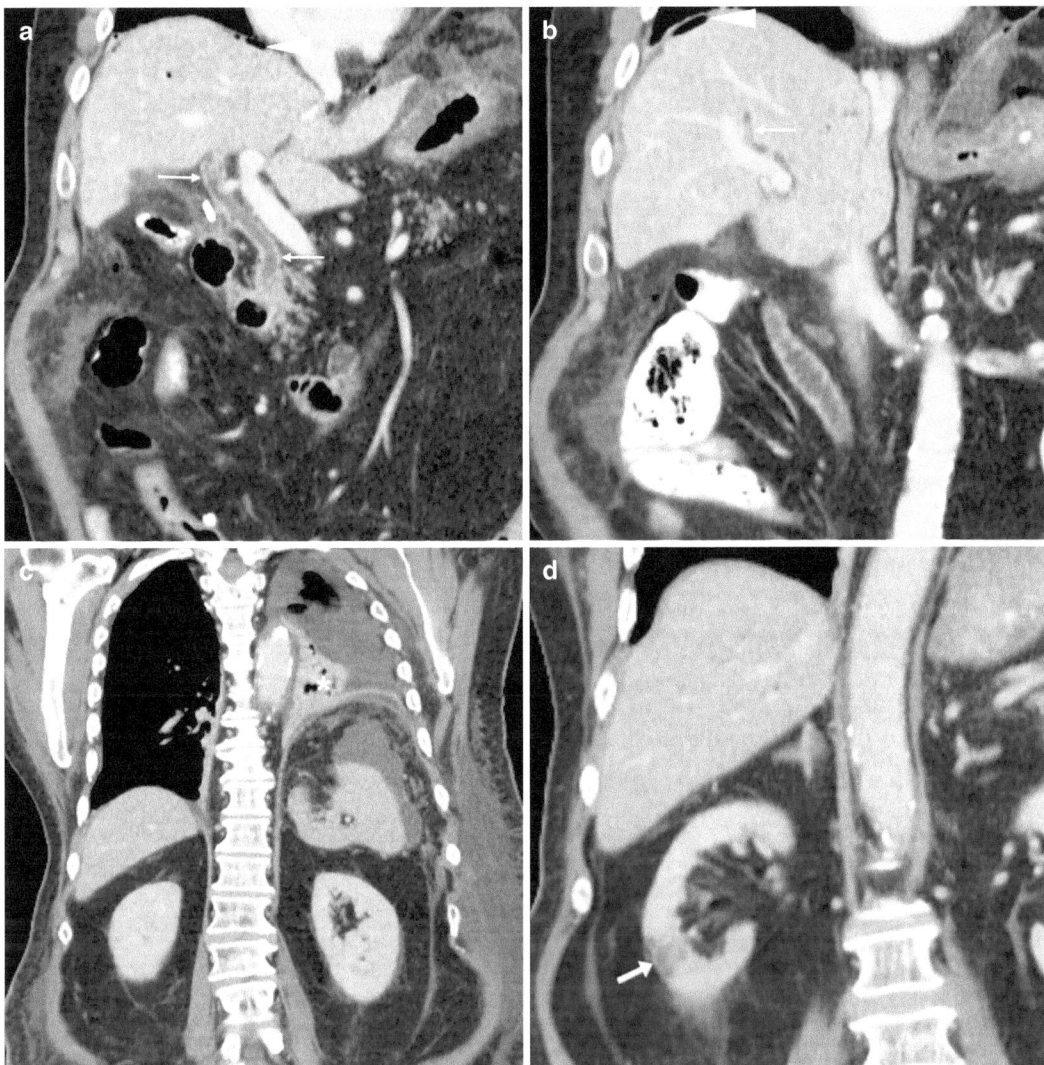

Fig. 9.10 (Cholangitis and sepsis in an 81-year-old female following endoscopic stone retrieval. Multiplanar contrast-enhanced CT images (**a–d**) showed minimal pneumoperitoneum (*arrowheads*) and peritoneal effusion, thickened enhancing walls of CBD and main intrahepatic ducts (*thin arrows*). Additionally, left-sided pneumonia (* in **c**) and a limited renal infarct (*arrow* in **d**) were seen. Worsening clinical conditions dictated surgery, which revealed biliary peritonitis from contained cystic duct injury. The patient recovered after a long intensive care unit stay (Reproduced from Open Access Ref. no [5])

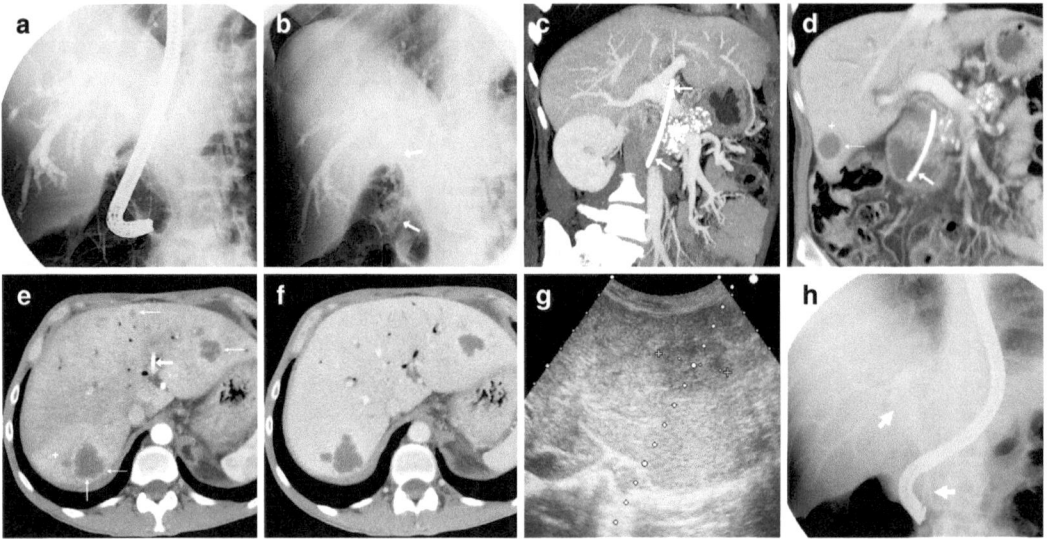

Fig. 9.11 A 43-year-old male had inoperable CBD carcinoma with liver and nodal metastases. After confirmation of severe cholestasis during endoscopic cholangiography (**a**), the CBD stricture was trespassed using a guidewire and a plastic stent (*arrows* in **b**) was positioned. Effective relief (decrease of serum bilirubin from 23 to 5) was obtained. After chemotherapy, the patient suffered from abdominal pain and malaise. Multidetector CT (**c–f**) including MIP reconstruction (**c**) documented the correct position of the stent (*arrows*) with its distal end in the duodenal lumen (**d**). Note severe pancreatic calcifications (in c) corresponding to known chronic alcohol-related pancreatitis. Furthermore, some variable-sized liver lesions with fluid-like content, enhancing periphery (*thin arrows*) and transient hyperenhancement of the surrounding parenchyma in the arterial phase (**e**) were noted, suggesting abscesses. Differentiation from metastases required ultrasound-guided percutaneous aspiration biopsy (**g**), and the plastic stent was replaced with two SEMS (**h**)

misplacement, perforation (Fig. 9.12) and injury to the CBD or main pancreatic duct [5, 15, 44, 45].

Chronic stent-related complications are more commonly observed. By far, the most frequent event is stent obstruction (Fig. 9.13), which is reported to occur in 25–35 % of patients. Stents may be occasionally collapse or become fractured, a situation which is exquisitely depicted by CT. Infections such as cholangitis, liver abscesses (Fig. 9.11) and sepsis are often observed in patients with biliary stents. Finally, biliary stents may migrate after a variable time lapse. Stent dislodgement occurs in up to 6 % of patients, is more frequent with plastic stents compared to SEMS and may occur proximally, such as in patients with malignancies, or distally. Migrated stents in the bowel may be expelled with stools or remain asymptomatic: the use of imaging allows detecting their presence before endoscopic removal [5, 14, 41–45].

9.7   Clinical Cases Presentations

9.7.1   Post-ERCP Acute Duodenal Haemorrhage

A 77-year-old woman with obstructive jaundice had CT (Fig. 9.14a, b) diagnosis of gallbladder carcinoma with direct liver invasion. Operative ERCP, performed to relieve the intrahepatic biliary obstruction, was interrupted after sphincterotomy because of duodenal bleeding, which was treated with epinephrine injection and endoscopic clipping. Hours after the unsuccessful procedure, she suffered from acute abdominal pain with impending haemodynamic shock. Performed to investigate possible complications, emergency multidetector CT (Fig. 9.14c–e) excluded signs of duodenal perforation and of acute pancreatitis. Active CM extravasation was seen in the duodenal lumen, consistent with persistent arterial haemorrhage [46].

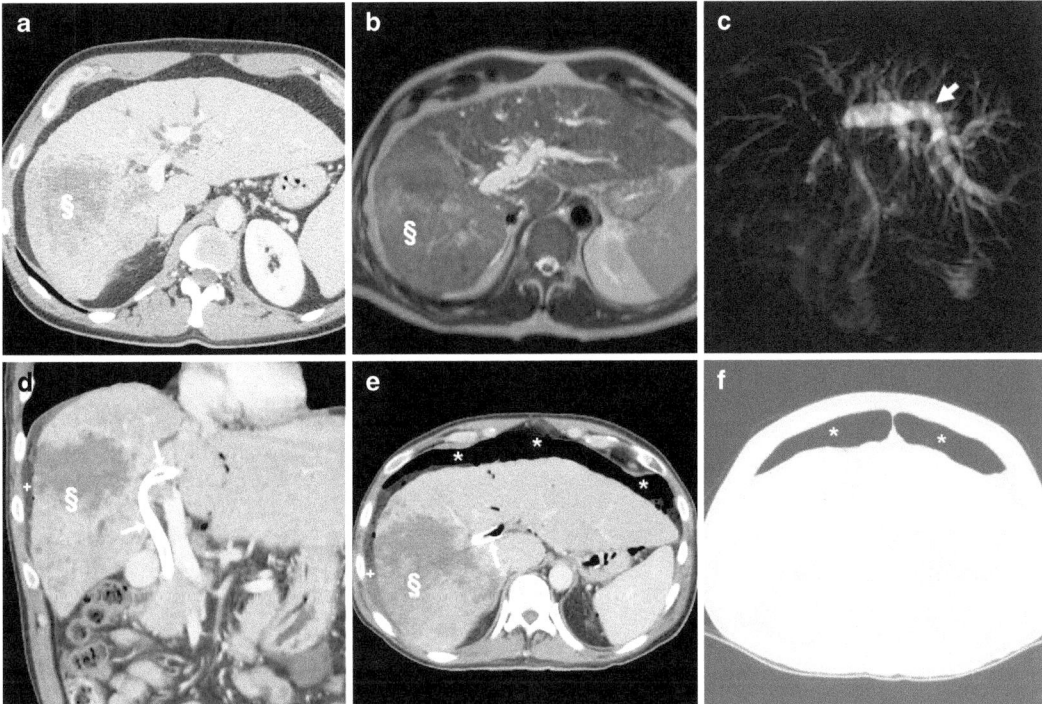

Fig. 9.12 A 63-year-old male had a large intrahepatic cholangiocarcinoma (§) as documented by initial contrast-enhanced CT (**a**) and MRI (T2-weighted image in **b**). MRCP (**c**) showed left-sided intrahepatic biliary obstruction (short arrow) which was treated with positioning of a SEMS to decrease jaundice and allow chemotherapy. Post-procedural CT showed distension of the left intrahepatic biliary system from the correctly positioned SEMS (*arrows* in **d**, **e**), and development of pneumoperitoneum (*), best seen and quantified by viewing at lung window settings (**f**). The patient recovered with conservative treatment

Endovascular therapeutic embolisation of the gastroduodenal artery achieved stopping bleeding. Afterwards percutaneous transhepatic biliary drainage (Fig. 9.14f) with placement of two internal–external biliary drainage catheters was performed to relieve intrahepatic biliary obstruction [46].

9.7.2 Various Complications After ERCP and Biliary Stenting: Liver Haematoma, Followed by Superinfection with Abscess Formation, and Ultimate Stent Displacement

Following laparoscopic cholecystectomy, a 39-year-old male developed a Bismuth type II iatrogenic bile duct injury (Fig. 9.15a, b) which required immediate reintervention to remove the surgical clips. Ten months later, 24 h after endoscopic positioning of a covered metallic biliary stent (Fig. 9.15c), he experienced sudden abdominal pain, vomiting and hypotension [47].

Emergency multidetector CT (Fig. 9.15d) showed the development of a massive subcapsular haematoma compressing the liver which was attributed to guidewire manipulation, plus abundant peritoneal effusion. The next day, progressive blood loss and increasing hepatic haematoma at repeated MDCT (Fig. 9.15e) dictated immediate surgical evacuation (Fig. 9.15f) [47]. One month after hospital discharge, the patient was rushed to the emergency department with worsening right-sided thoracic–abdominal pain and fever over a week. Urgent MDCT (Fig. 9.16) showed pleural effusion, lung atelectasis and a huge liver

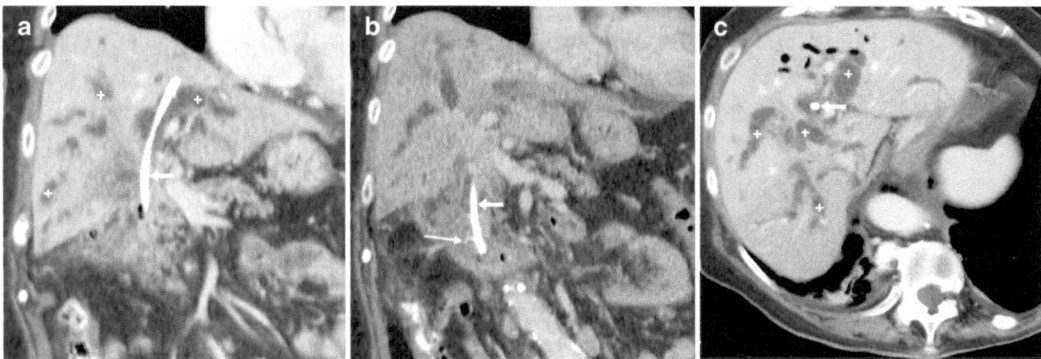

Fig. 9.13 An elderly female with from hilar (Klatskin-type) cholangiocarcinoma (same patient of Fig. 8.4) underwent endoscopic positioning of plastic stent to palliate high-grade jaundice. After some weeks, follow-up CT (a–c) showed reappearance of severe intrahepatic biliary obstruction (+) with correctly placed stent (*arrows*) which was consistent with stent obstruction. Note small anchoring "claw" (*thin arrow*) at the lower extremity of the stent

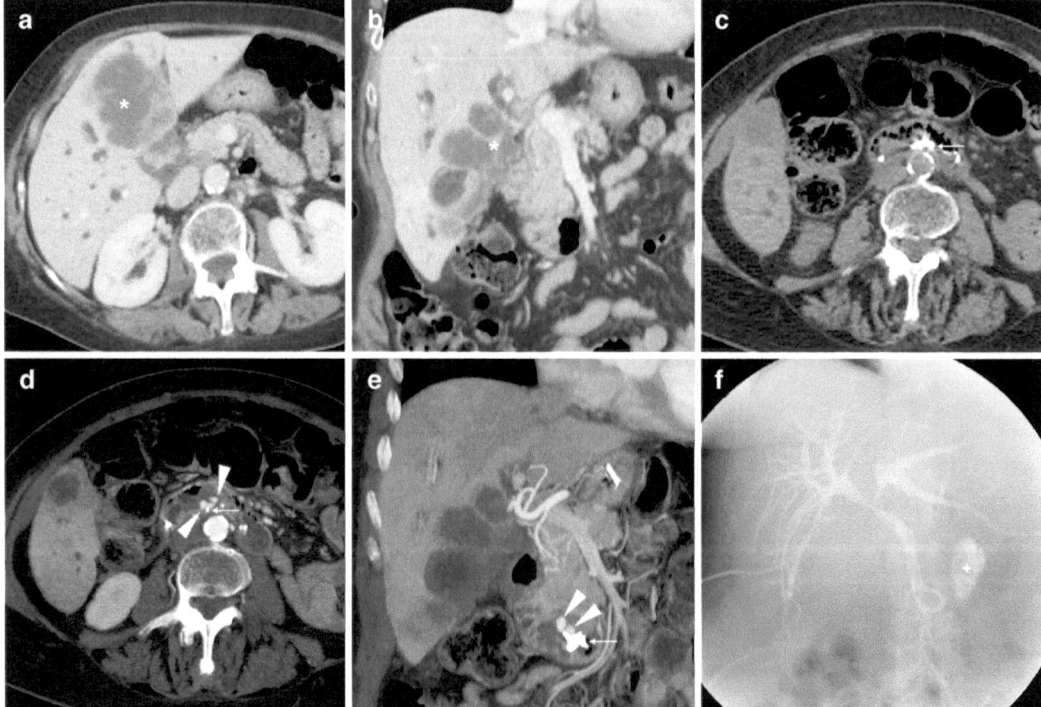

Fig. 9.14 At admission, axial (**a**) and coronal (**b**) contrast-enhanced multidetector CT images showed a large infiltrating polylobulated neoplastic mass (*) arising from the gallbladder's fundus with dilated intrahepatic bile ducts. Post-ERCP emergency CT (**c–e**) showed endoscopic metallic clips (*arrow* in unenhanced image **c**), thickening of duodenal wall with intraluminal contrast extravasation (*arrowheads*) consistent with active haemorrhage, which was effectively documented with maximum-intensity projection (MIP) reconstruction viewed at vascular window settings (**d**). After therapeutic angiographic embolisation and percutaneous transhepatic biliary drainage, fluoroscopic image (**f**) showed distension of intrahepatic bile ducts after placement of two internal–external biliary drainage catheters with iodinated contrast medium flowing into the duodenum (+) (Partly reproduced from Ref. [46] and Open Access Ref. [5])

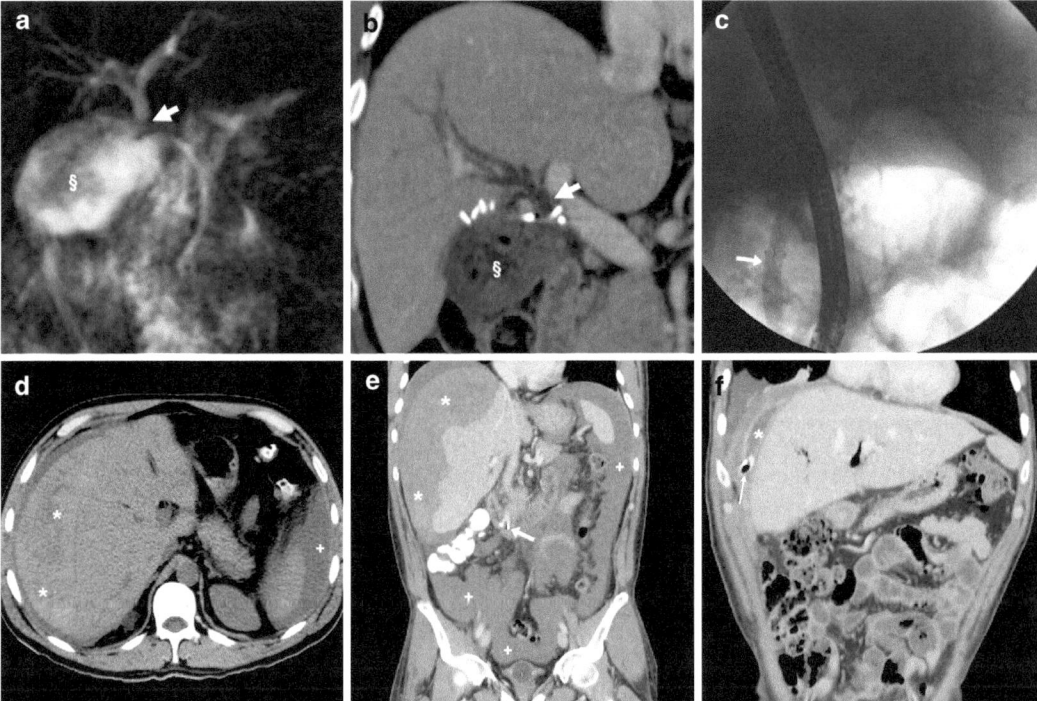

Fig. 9.15 Coronal thick-slab MRCP image (**a**) and maximum-intensity projection CT (MIP, **b**) images showed postoperative haematoma in the gallbladder fossa (§), moderately dilated intrahepatic ducts, a 7-mm wide, 1.5-cm long common hepatic duct stump with an abrupt termination consistent with Bismuth type II injury (*short arrows*) and normal-calibre choledochus caudally to the ductal discontinuity. To achieve long-term stricture treatment, an 8-cm long covered metallic stent with characteristic radiopaque reticular "mesh" appearance (*arrow* in **c**) was positioned endoscopically. Twenty-four hours later, multidetector CT (**d**) detected a massive hyperattenuating subcapsular liver haematoma (*) and haemoperitoneum (+), which progressed at repeated contrast-enhancement CT 24 h later (**e**) causing compression of the liver. Note biliary stent in place (*arrow* in **e**). Postoperative CT (**f**) showed effective surgical evacuation of haemoperitoneum and haematoma (*) with drainage (*thin arrow*) in place (Partially reproduced from Ref. [47] and Open Access Ref. [5])

abscess. Percutaneous drainage evacuated 3 liters of stinking pus. Clinical, laboratory and imaging (Fig. 9.16c, d) resolution was obtained [47].

During endoscopic replacement, the biliary stent was not found anymore (Fig. 9.16e), displaced and probably lost with stools [47].

9.7.3 Post-ERCP Perforation

An elderly male with choledocholithiasis and several multiple comorbidities underwent therapeutic ERCP including pre-cut sphincterotomy and stone retrieval using a basket device. During ERCP, fluoroscopy (Fig. 9.17a) showed a sizeable extraluminal collection of iodinated CM, indicating periampullary perforation (type II according to the Stapfer's classification system) [48].

Hours after the procedure, the patient suffered from acute abdominal pain. Multidetector CT (Fig. 9.17b–f) showed posterior pneumomediastinum, perihepatic and right parietocolic pneumoperitoneum and development of extensive retroperitoneal emphysema. The intrahepatic ducts and CBD appeared persistently distended and opacified, with a few residual lithiasis

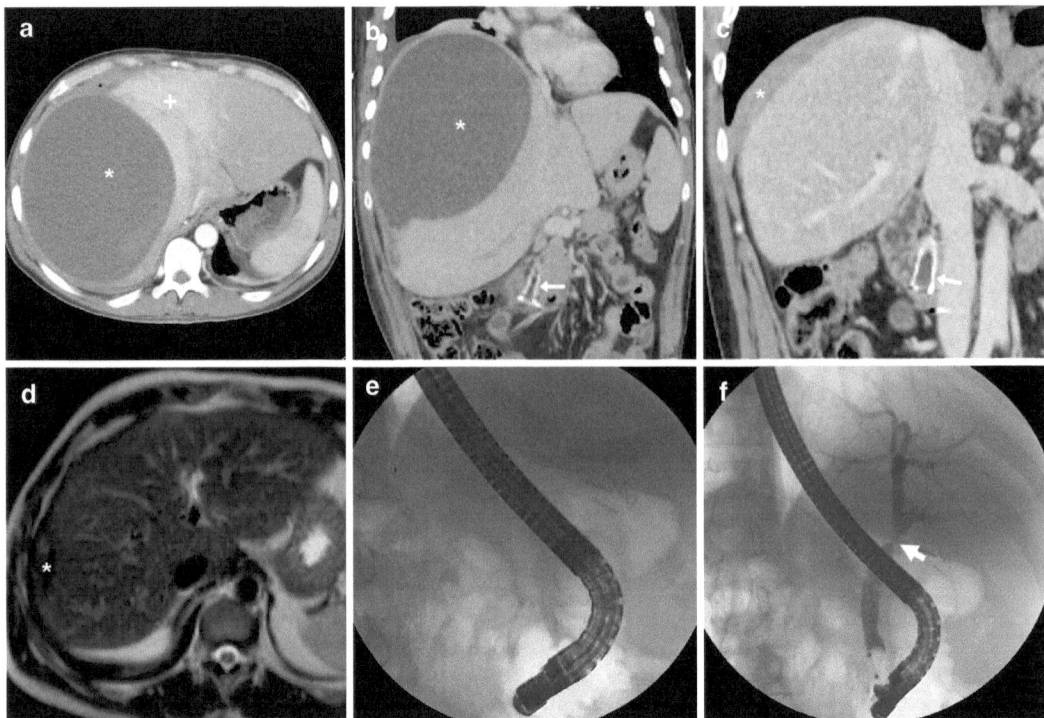

Fig. 9.16 A month after evacuation of subcapsular hepatic haematoma in Fig. 9.15, arterial (**a**) and venous-phase (**b**) images from emergency CT showed the development of a huge, predominantly fluid-attenuating (15 Hounsfield Units) subphrenic collection (*) with inflammatory enhancement of the surrounding, compressed liver parenchyma (+) and thin rim-like enhancement, consistent with an abscess which was percutaneously evacuated. Note ipsilateral pleural effusion and basal lung atelectasis, correctly positioned metallic CBD stent (*arrows*). Follow-up CT (**c**) and long-term MRI (T2-weighted image in **d**) showed resolved subphrenic abscess with development of low signal intensity consistent with fibrosis (*). Subsequently, during endoscopic replacement, the biliary stent was not found anymore (**e**), displaced and probably lost with stools. Endoscopic cholangiography (**f**) confirmed persistent iatrogenic biliary stricture (*short arrow*) with reduced upstream dilatation (Partially reproduced from Ref. [47] and Open Access Ref. [5])

fragments [48].Considering the worsening clinical conditions with development of peritonitis, and the imaging findings including periampullary perforation and pneumoperitoneum, the attending surgeon chose to perform urgent laparotomy.

After confirmation of intra-abdominal free air, surgery included opening and toilet of common bile duct and positioning of Kehr T-tube. Ten days later, the patient finally recovered and was discharged from the hospital [48].

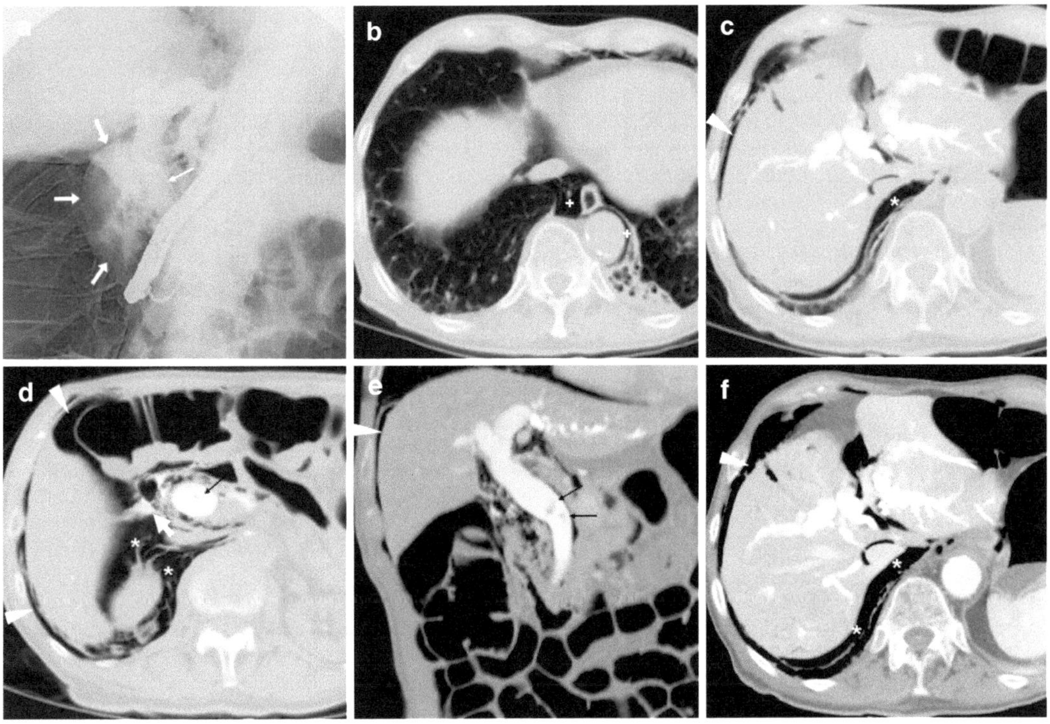

Fig. 9.17 Fluoroscopic image during ERCP (**a**) showed opacification of dilated intrahepatic ducts and CBD (note guidewire indicated by *thin arrow*) and of a sizeable extraluminal collection of iodinated CM (demarcated by *arrows*) consistent with periampullary perforation. Urgent multidetector CT including image review at bone window settings detected posterior pneumomediastinum (+ in **b**) surrounding the distal oesophagus and descending aorta, mild perihepatic and right parietocolic pneumoperitoneum (*arrowheads* in **c–f**), persistently extravasated CM (*short arrow* in **d**), extensive retroperitoneal emphysema (*) with air surrounding the inferior vena cava and portal vein, persistent dilatation and opacification by CM injected during ERCP of the intrahepatic system and CBD with small residual lithiasis fragments (*thin arrows* in **d**, **e**). Note gaseous bowel distension (**e**) from insufflation during endoscopy (Partially reproduced from Ref. [48] and Open Access Ref. [5])

References

1. Anderson MA, Fisher L, Jain R et al (2012) Complications of ERCP. Gastrointest Endosc 75: 467–473
2. Glomsaker T, Hoff G, Kvaloy JT et al (2013) Patterns and predictive factors of complications after endoscopic retrograde cholangiopancreatography. Br J Surg 100:373–380
3. Kapral C, Duller C, Wewalka F et al (2008) Case volume and outcome of endoscopic retrograde cholangiopancreatography: results of a nationwide Austrian benchmarking project. Endoscopy 40:625–630
4. Silviera ML, Seamon MJ, Porshinsky B et al (2009) Complications related to endoscopic retrograde cholangiopancreatography: a comprehensive clinical review. J Gastrointest Liver Dis 18:73–82
5. Tonolini M, Pagani A, Bianco R (2015) Cross-sectional imaging of common and unusual complications after endoscopic retrograde cholangiopancreatography. Insights Imag 6:323–338
6. Dumonceau JM, Andriulli A, Elmunzer BJ et al (2014) Prophylaxis of post-ERCP pancreatitis: European Society of Gastrointestinal Endoscopy (ESGE) Guideline - updated June 2014. Endoscopy 46:799–815
7. Pezzilli R, Romboli E, Campana D et al (2002) Mechanisms involved in the onset of post-ERCP pancreatitis. JOP 3:162–168
8. Pfau PR, Mosley RG, Said A et al (2006) Comparison of the effect of non-ionic and ionic contrast agents on pancreatic histology in a canine model. JOP 7:27–33
9. Johnson GK, Geenen JE, Johanson JF et al (1997) Evaluation of post-ERCP pancreatitis: potential causes noted during controlled study of differing contrast media. Midwest Pancreaticobiliary Study Group. Gastrointest Endosc 46:217–222
10. Goebel C, Hardt P, Doppl W et al (2000) Frequency of pancreatitis after endoscopic retrograde cholangiopancreatography with iopromid or iotrolan: a randomized trial. Eur Radiol 10:677–680
11. George S, Kulkarni AA, Stevens G et al (2004) Role of osmolality of contrast media in the development of

post-ERCP pancreatitis: a metanalysis. Dig Dis Sci 49:503–508

12. Sheu Y, Furlan A, Almusa O et al (2012) The revised Atlanta classification for acute pancreatitis: a CT imaging guide for radiologists. Emerg Radiol 19:237–243

13. Zaheer A, Singh VK, Qureshi RO et al (2013) The revised Atlanta classification for acute pancreatitis: updates in imaging terminology and guidelines. Abdom Imaging 38:125–136

14. Saddala P, Ramanathan S, Tirumani SH et al (2015) Complications of minimally invasive procedures of the abdomen and pelvis: a comprehensive update on the clinical and imaging features. Emerg Radiol 22:283–294

15. Pannu HK, Fishman EK (2001) Complications of endoscopic retrograde cholangiopancreatography: spectrum of abnormalities demonstrated with CT. Radiographics 21:1441–1453

16. Wax BN, Katz DS, Badler RL et al (2006) Complications of abdominal and pelvic procedures: computed tomographic diagnosis. Curr Probl Diagn Radiol 35:171–187

17. Woods RW, Akshintala VS, Singh VK et al (2014) CT severity of post-ERCP pancreatitis: results from a single tertiary medical center. Abdom Imaging 39:1162–1168

18. Miller FH, Keppke AL, Dalal K et al (2004) MRI of pancreatitis and its complications: part 1, acute pancreatitis. AJR Am J Roentgenol 183:1637–1644

19. de Freitas TF, Schraibman V, Ardengh JC et al (2014) Diffusion-weighted magnetic resonance imaging indicates the severity of acute pancreatitis. Abdom Imaging 40:265–271

20. Horton KM, Jeffrey RB Jr, Federle MP et al (2009) Acute gastrointestinal bleeding: the potential role of 64 MDCT and 3D imaging in the diagnosis. Emerg Radiol 16:349–356

21. Jaeckle T, Stuber G, Hoffmann MH et al (2008) Acute gastrointestinal bleeding: value of MDCT. Abdom Imaging 33:285–293

22. So YH, Choi YH, Chung JW (2012) Selective embolization for post-endoscopic sphincterotomy bleeding: technical aspects and clinical efficacy. Korean J Radiol 13:73–81

23. Katsinelos P, Kountouras J, Chatzimavroudis G (2010) Endoscopic hemostasis using monopolar coagulation for postendoscopic sphincterotomy bleeding refractory to injection treatment. Surg Laparosc Endosc Percutan Tech 20:84–88

24. Tsou YK, Lin CH, Liu NJ (2009) Treating delayed endoscopic sphincterotomy-induced bleeding: epinephrine injection with or without thermotherapy. World J Gastroenterol 15:4823–4828

25. Maleux G, Bieden J, Laenen A et al (2014) Embolization of post-biliary sphincterotomy bleeding refractory to medical and endoscopic therapy: technical results, clinical efficacy and predictors of outcome. Eur Radiol 24:2779–2786

26. Avgerinos DV, Llaguna OH, Lo AY et al (2009) Management of endoscopic retrograde cholangiopancreatography: related duodenal perforations. Surg Endosc 23:833–838

27. Kim J, Lee SH, Paik WH et al (2012) Clinical outcomes of patients who experienced perforation associated with endoscopic retrograde cholangiopancreatography. Surg Endosc 26:3293–3300

28. Machado NO (2012) Management of duodenal perforation post-endoscopic retrograde cholangiopancreatography. When and whom to operate and what factors determine the outcome? A review article. JOP 13:18–25

29. Miller R, Zbar A, Klein Y et al (2013) Perforations following endoscopic retrograde cholangiopancreatography: a single institution experience and surgical recommendations. Am J Surg 206:180–186

30. Paspatis GA, Dumonceau JM, Barthet M et al (2014) Diagnosis and management of iatrogenic endoscopic perforations: European Society of Gastrointestinal Endoscopy (ESGE) Position Statement. Endoscopy 46:693–711

31. Polydorou A, Vezakis A, Fragulidis G et al (2011) A tailored approach to the management of perforations following endoscopic retrograde cholangiopancreatography and sphincterotomy. J Gastrointest Surg 15:2211–2217

32. Rabie ME, Mir NH, Al Skaini MS et al (2013) Operative and non-operative management of endoscopic retrograde cholangiopancreatography-associated duodenal injuries. Ann R Coll Surg Engl 95:285–290

33. Stapfer M, Selby RR, Stain SC et al (2000) Management of duodenal perforation after endoscopic retrograde cholangiopancreatography and sphincterotomy. Ann Surg 232:191–198

34. Kodali S, Monkemuller K, Kim H et al (2015) ERCP-related perforations in the new millennium: a large tertiary referral center 10-year experience. United Eur Gastroenterol J 3:25–30

35. Sartelli M, Viale P, Catena F et al (2013) 2013 WSES guidelines for management of intra-abdominal infections. World J Emerg Surg 8:3

36. Mosler P (2011) Diagnosis and management of acute cholangitis. Curr Gastroenterol Rep 13:166–172

37. Hong MJ, Kim WS, Kin HC et al (2012) Comparison of the clinical characteristics and imaging findings of acute cholangitis with and without biliary dilatation. Br J Radiol 85:e1219–e1225

38. Catalano OA, Sahani DV, Forcione DG et al (2009) Biliary infections: spectrum of imaging findings and management. Radiographics 29:2059–2080

39. Menu Y, Vuillerme MP (2002) Non-traumatic abdominal emergencies: imaging and intervention in acute biliary conditions. Eur Radiol 12:2397–2406

40. Watanabe Y, Nagayama M, Okumura A et al (2007) MR imaging of acute biliary disorders. Radiographics 27:477–495

41. van Boeckel PG, Vleggaar FP, Siersema PD (2009) Plastic or metal stents for benign extrahepatic biliary strictures: a systematic review. BMC Gastroenterol 9:96

42. Matlock J, Freeman ML (2005) Endoscopic therapy of benign biliary strictures. Rev Gastroenterol Disord 5:206–214

43. Judah JR, Draganov PV (2007) Endoscopic therapy of benign biliary strictures. World J Gastroenterol 13: 3531–3539

44. Siriwardana HP, Siriwardena AK (2005) Systematic appraisal of the role of metallic endobiliary stents in the treatment of benign bile duct stricture. Ann Surg 242:10–19

45. Catalano O, De Bellis M, Sandomenico F et al (2012) Complications of biliary and gastrointestinal stents: MDCT of the cancer patient. AJR Am J Roentgenol 199:W187–W196

46. Pagani A, Tonolini M (2014) EuroRAD Case 11665. Post-ERCP acute duodenal haemorrhage. doi:10.1594/EURORAD/CASE.11665:Available at: URL: http://www.eurorad.org/case.php?id=11665

47. Tonolini M (2012) EuroRAD Case 10384. Spectrum of complications following biliary stent positioning. doi:10.1594/EURORAD/CASE.10384:Available at: URL: http://www.eurorad.org/case.php?id=10384

48. Rigiroli F, Tonolini M, Pagani A (2014) EuroRAD Case 11409. Imaging diagnosis and surgical triage of post-therapeutic ERCP perforation. doi:10.1594/EURORAD/CASE.11409:Available at: URL: http://www.eurorad.org/case.php?id=11409

Part IV

Complications of Colonoscopy and Colorectal Interventional Procedures

10

Emilia Bareggi and Alessandra Dell'Era

10.1 Lower Gastrointestinal Endoscopy: An Overview

Lower gastrointestinal endoscopy (LGIE) or colonoscopy is an endoscopic procedure that evaluates the colon and the distal ileum. It is an invasive procedure that should be performed with caution and in the appropriate setting due to its intrinsic risks. LGIE is commonly used to evaluate different disorders of the lower digestive tract, including screening and surveillance of colorectal neoplasia, and to perform therapeutic interventions such as removal of colonic polyps and dilatation of benign or malign strictures with eventual placement of stent.

10.1.1 The Procedure

Colonoscopy consists of the endoscopic examination of the rectum and colon and may be extended to visualise the distal ileum. A flexible tube is passed through the anus and pushed up to the caecum, while gently inflating the colon to allow vision and injecting water to allow better evaluation of the colonic walls. During colonoscopy mucosal biopsies can be taken, and polyps can be removed with

E. Bareggi (✉) • A. Dell'era
Gastroenterology Unit, "Luigi Sacco" University Hospital, Via G.B. Grassi 74, Milan 20157, Italy
e-mail: bareggi.emilia@gmail.com

different devices according to their size. The patient is generally positioned in the left lateral decubitus position and sometimes is moved to the supine position to ease the colonoscope progression. Sedation can be performed simply by using sedative drugs, adding an opioid if necessary depending on the duration of the procedure and patient tolerance.

10.1.2 Patient- and Procedure-Related Risk Factors and Contraindications

The risk of complications must be considered before performing a colonoscopy. If the benefit–risk ratio is against colonoscopy, other techniques should be considered such as double-contrast barium enema, water enema CT or CT colonography. The risk of complications is highest in the elderly, in patients with significant comorbidities, fulminant colitis, diverticular disease, personal history of abdominal surgery or radiation that may cause the presence of adherences, anticoagulant or antiplatelet therapy.

10.2 Complications of Diagnostic Colonoscopy

Complications related to colonoscopy may be due to the bowel preparation and the sedation for the procedure (not treated in this chapter), procedure itself or to therapeutic techniques employed during the procedure. They can manifest during the procedure itself, immediately after the procedure or in the following days. After colonoscopy, the most common symptom reported by patients is pain, which can be due to gaseous distension but also to perforation or post-polypectomy syndrome. The patient reporting pain should be carefully evaluated for signs of peritonitis.

The most common serious complications of colonoscopy are perforation (up to 0.2 %) and bleeding (up to 0.11 %) [1–6]; other very rare complications include colonoscope incarceration in an hernia, splenic haematoma or rupture, volvulus of the colon, glutaraldehyde-induced colitis, pneumomediastinum and pneumothorax. In diagnostic colonoscopy, reported mortality rates range from 0.02 % to 0.06 %, with morbidity rates of 0.14–0.25 %.

10.2.1 Colonic Perforation

Perforation during a diagnostic colonoscopy may occur in approximately 0–0.19 % of cases [7]. *Risk factors* for perforation include severe diverticular disease, previous abdominal and pelvic surgery and severe active colitis.

Perforation can be distinguished into pneumatic perforation and mechanical perforation. The former (*pneumatic perforation*) occurs when the increase in the intraluminal pressure may cause the rupture of the colon wall. This is more likely to happen when the wall is thinner (e.g. transmural ulcers, right colon) or where the wall tension is higher (e.g. in the caecum where the radius is greater). Conversely, the latter (*mechanical perforation*) usually occurs when the colonoscope is forcefully inserted causing laceration of the colon wall due to the shaft or the tip of the endoscope. This is more likely to occur in presence of inflamed colon (e.g. inflammatory bowel disease, ischaemic colitis or diverticulitis).

Clinical manifestations: in some cases perforation may be recognised during endoscopy because peritoneal structures (e.g. vessels, fatty tissue) may be visualised or because adequate distension of the colon may not be maintained. The patient may present abdominal pain, and there may be haemodynamic changes (e.g. in heart rate, blood pressure and O2 saturation). In the majority of cases, perforation becomes evident in the hours after colonoscopy: the patient presents increasing pain, failure to pass gas and, eventually, signs of peritonitis.

Prevention: careful examination of the colon, avoiding overinflation or hard pushing and avoiding excessive looping may reduce the risk of perforation. If possible, the use of CO_2 could reduce the risk, because it is rapidly absorbed from the lumen instead of air. There is evidence that colonoscopies performed by endoscopists with low procedure volume are more frequently associated with high risk of perforation and bleeding. Particular care should be taken in patients with severe colitis, but normally it is better to avoid complete colonoscopy in these patients.

Diagnosis: the diagnosis can be made by visualisation of the perforation site during endoscopy.

In this case, perforation can be recognised with visualisation during the examination of extraintestinal/peritoneal structures such as mesenteric fat, vessels or surrounding serous. If the site of perforation is not suddenly visualised, clinical suspicion of perforation during the examination must be in the case of sudden onset of pain, difficulty maintaining insufflation or in case of rapid change in the patient's clinical status.

In the majority of patients, the diagnosis of perforation is delayed, variably from 1 to 42 days: in these cases the commonest symptom is the persistent or worsening abdominal pain, sometimes associated by abdominal distension. Suspicion is further increased in presence of tachycardia, fever, general abdominal tenderness, rigidity, leucocytosis and failure to pass flatus.

When physical findings indicate peritonitis, abdominal X-ray is warranted to detect pneumoperitoneum. As discussed in the following imaging chapters, with high clinical suspicion but negative X-ray, performing CT is suggested since it is more sensitive for detection of perforation [8].

Treatment options: in all patients in whom a perforation is diagnosed, antibiotic therapy, intravenous hydration, fasting patient and nasogastric suction should be instituted. Surgical consultation must be obtained in all cases. If the perforation is recognised during endoscopy, the perforation site may be closed placing clips. If the perforation is small, conservative treatment is the best option; in all other cases, surgical intervention is needed [9].

10.3 Complications of Operative Colonoscopy

The two major complications of operative colonoscopy are perforation during polypectomy, endoscopic mucosal resection (EMR) or endoscopic submucosal dissection (ESD), and haemorrhage.

10.3.1 Colonic Perforation During Polypectomy, Endoscopic Mucosal Resection (EMR) or Endoscopic Submucosal Dissection (ESD)

The perforation rates for polypectomy, EMR or ESD are listed in Table 10.1 [1, 2, 4, 6, 10–14].

Besides the causes seen in diagnostic endoscopy, colonic perforation during therapeutic endoscopy may be due to thermal injury caused by the use of hot biopsy forceps or polypectomy snare or can be due to excessive removal of tissue during polypectomy. *Risk factors* are an excessive application of electrocoagulation and contact of the head of polyp with the opposite colonic wall during the application of the electrocoagulation.

It is described that using submucosal saline "lift" at the base of large polyps, especially localised in the right column, so to separate mucous

from submucosal layer, may reduce the risk of perforation post-polypectomy.

Normally clinical manifestations, diagnosis and treatment are the same of perforations which occur in diagnostic colonoscopy.

Sometimes in patients with a small bowel perforation, called microperforations, the pain and tenderness remain localised, but radiological studies can confirm the presence of free gas in the abdominal cavity under the diaphragm.

In 0.003–0.1 % of cases, a transmural burn without perforation may mimic perforation from the clinical point of view, but no air is observed on abdominal radiographs or CT. This will be discussed in depth in the appropriate imaging chapter. In the majority of cases, this **post-polypectomy syndrome** resolves with conservative treatment. It is the result of electrocoagulation injury to the bowel wall that induces a localised peritonitis, and typically the clinical manifestations are fever, localised pain, localised peritoneal signs and leucocytosis, 1 or 5 days after a colonoscopy.

10.3.2 Haemorrhage

Colonic bleeding almost exclusively results from operative colonoscopy, but can occasionally occur also during diagnostic colonoscopy. Multiple studies have reported a risk of haemorrhage of 0.1–0.6 % [9]. Bleeding rates for polypectomy, EMR and ESD are reported in Table 10.1 [7, 12, 15].

Risk factors may be the use of antiplatelets or anticoagulant drugs, polyp size, number of polyps removed, poor technique in which the polyp is cut before achieving adequate electrocoagulation of the vessels and inadequate haemostasis after polypectomy. Patient comorbidities, like cardiovascular, respiratory or renal diseases or elderly age, may increase the risk of bleeding [2, 16–21].

Prevention: adequate management of antiplatelets and anticoagulant drugs [16] and good technique may help prevent bleeding (e.g. cautious use of electrocoagulation, adrenaline injection before polypectomy). Although data are

Table 10.1 Perforation and bleeding rate of polypectomy, endoscopic mucosal resection and endoscopic submucosal dissection

	Perforation	Bleeding
Polypectomy	0.004–0.5 %	0.01–3.3 %
Endoscopic mucosal resection	0–5 %	10 %
Endoscopic submucosal dissection	5–10 %	10 %

contrasting, clips may be placed in the polypectomy site after polypectomy to prevent delayed bleeding [22, 23].

Clinical manifestation: bleeding may be observed during endoscopy but sometimes delayed bleeding may occur. In the first case, bleeding may present as oozing but, especially in pedunculated polyps, arterial spurt is possible. Delayed bleeding occurs usually after 1–14 days and the patient may present with proctorrhagia or melaena.

Treatment options: in case of evidence of bleeding during the procedure, haemostatic therapy, with adrenaline injection, argon plasma coagulation and clip or endoloop placement, should be instituted. Delayed bleeding is usually self-limiting, if the patient is not on anticoagulant therapy. If the bleeding does not stop, a repeated colonoscopy should be performed to identify and treat the site of bleeding. The site of bleeding can be identified endoscopically or angiographically. Normally acute post-polypectomy haemorrhage is soon recognised and treated endoscopically. Only in the minority of cases, bleeding persists and so the gastrointestinal surgeon and the radiology team should be alerted. In fact, if endoscopy is unsuccessful, treatment modality includes angiographic embolisation and surgery.

It must be kept in mind that selective arterial catheterisation and embolisation are associated to ischaemic colonic necrosis, and elective surgery should be performed after bleeding has stopped.

10.3.3 Complications During Colonic Dilatation

Patients with surgical anastomoses or with Crohn's disease may present benign strictures of the anastomosis or of the colon. Colonic dilatation may be employed to treat these strictures [24]. The reported complication rate after this procedure in patients without Crohn's disease is 0 % [25, 26], while in patients with Crohn's disease ranged between 0 % and 18 % [27]. Almost all complications were perforations.

For *clinical manifestations*, *diagnosis* and *treatment options*, see above.

10.3.4 Complications During Colonic Stent Placement

Patients with malignant obstruction of the colon may be treated with self-expandable metal stents (SEMS) [28]. Complications associated with this procedure are perforation (3.7–4.5 %), stent migration (9.8–11.8 %) and stent occlusion (7.3–12 %).

Clinical manifestations: for perforation see above. In case of stent migration or occlusion, the patient may present with clinical signs of colon obstruction (pain, progressive failure to pass faeces and gas, faecal vomiting).

Diagnosis is made by abdominal radiographs which shows a dilated colon and the position of the migrated stent.

Treatment options: the migrated stent should be removed and a new one should be placed. In case of an occluded stent, a coaxial one can be placed.

References

1. Kahn K (1986) Indications for selected medical and surgical procedures – a literature review and ratings of appropriateness. Diagnostic upper gastrointestinal endoscopy. The Rand Corporation, Santa Monica
2. Reiertsen O, Skjoto J, Jacobsen CD et al (1987) Complications of fiberoptic gastrointestinal endoscopy – five years' experience in a central hospital. Endoscopy 19:1–6
3. Gilbert DA, Hallstrom AP, Shaneyfelt SL et al (1984) The National ASGE survey – complications of colonoscopy. Gastrointest Endosc 30:156
4. Habr-Gama A, Waye JD (1989) Complications and hazards of gastrointestinal endoscopy. World J Surg 13:193–201
5. Macrae FA, Tan KG, Williams CB (1983) Towards safer colonoscopy: a report on the complications of 5000 diagnostic or therapeutic colonoscopies. Gut 24:376–383
6. Waye JD, Lewis BS, Yessayan S (1992) Colonoscopy: a prospective report of complications. J Clin Gastroenterol 15:347–351
7. Bowles CJA, Leicester R, Romaya C et al (2004) A prospective study of colonoscopy practice in the Uk today: are we adequately prepared for national colorectal cancer screening for tomorrow? Gut 53:277–283
8. Stapakis JC, Thickman D (1992) Diagnosis of pneumoperitoneum: abdominal CT vs. upright chest film. J Comput Assist Tomogr 16:713–716

9. ASGE (2011) Complications of colonoscopy. Gastrointest Endosc 74(4):745–752

10. Shinya H (1982) Complications: prevention and management. In: Colonoscopy: diagnostic and treatment of colonic diseases. Igaku-Shoin, New York, pp 199–208

11. Nivatvonga S (1986) Complications in colonoscopic polypectomy. An experience with 1555 polypectomies. Dis Colon Rectum 29:825–830

12. Saito Y, Uraoka T, Yamaguchi Y et al (2010) A prospective, multicenter study of 1111 colorectal endoscopic submucosal dissections (with video). Gastrointest Endosc 72:1217–1225

13. Tanaka S, Oka S, Kaneko I et al (2007) Endoscopic submucosal dissection for colorectal neoplasia: possibility of standardization. Gastrointest Endosc 66: 100–107

14. Repici A, Pellicano R, Strangio G et al (2009) Endoscopic mucosal resection for early colorectal neoplasia: pathologic basis, procedures, and outcomes. Dis Colon Rectum 52:1502–1515

15. Kantsevoy SV, Adler DG, Conway JD et al (2008) Endoscopic mucosal resection and endoscopic submucosal dissection. Gastrointest Endosc 68:11–18

16. Eisen GM, Baron TH, Dominitz JA et al (2002) Guideline on the management of anticoagulation and antiplatelet therapy for endoscopic procedures. Gastrointest Endosc 55:775–779

17. Kim HS, Kim TI, Kim WH et al (2006) Risk factors for immediate postpolypectomy bleeding of the colon: a multicenter study. Am J Gastroenterol 101:1333–1341

18. Hui AJ, Wong RM, Ching JY et al (2004) Risk of colonoscopic polypectomy bleeding with anticoagulants and antiplatelet agents: analysis of 1657 cases. Gastrointest Endosc 59:44–48

19. Sawhney MS, Salfiti N, Nelson DB et al (2008) Risk factors for severe delayed postpolypectomy bleeding. Endoscopy 40:115–119

20. Singh M, Mehta N, Murthy UK et al (2010) Postpolypectomy bleeding in patients undergoing colonoscopy on uninterrupted clopidogrel therapy. Gastrointest Endosc 71:998–1005

21. Witt DM, Delate T, McCool KH et al (2009) Incidence and predictors of bleeding or thrombosis after polypectomy in patients receiving and not receiving anticoagulation therapy. J Thromb Haemost 7:1982–1989

22. Luigiano C, Ferrara F, Ghersi S et al (2010) Endoclip-assisted resection of large pedunculated colorectal polyps: technical aspects and outcome. Dig Dis Sci 55:1726–1731

23. Shioji K, Suzuki Y, Kobayashi M et al (2003) Prophylactic clip application does not decrease delayed bleeding after colonoscopic polypectomy. Gastrointest Endosc 57:691–694

24. Harrison ME, Anderson MA, Appalaneni V et al (2010) The role of endoscopy in the management of patients with known and suspected colonic obstruction and pseudo-obstruction. Gastrointest Endosc 71:669–679

25. Di Giorgio P, De Luca L, Rivellini G et al (2004) Endoscopic dilation of benign colorectal anastomotic stricture after low anterior resection: a prospective comparison study of two balloon types. Gastrointest Endosc 60:347–350

26. Ambrosetti P, Francis K, De Peyer R et al (2008) Colorectal anastomotic stenosis after elective laparoscopic sigmoidectomy for diverticular disease: a prospective evaluation of 68 patients. Dis Colon Rectum 51:1345–1349

27. Hassan C, Zullo A, De Francesco V et al (2007) Systematic review: endoscopic dilatation in Crohn's disease. Aliment Pharmacol Ther 26:1457–1464

28. Watt AM, Faragher IG, Griffin TT et al (2007) Self-expanding metallic stents for relieving malignant colorectal obstruction: a systematic review. Ann Surg 246:24–30

11 Imaging Techniques and Expected Post-colonoscopy Appearances

Anna Ravelli, Alessandro Campari,
and Massimo Tonolini

11.1 Introduction

Optical colonoscopy (OC) represents the cornerstone for diagnosis of most large bowel disorders. In recent years new techniques have been developed in order to improve patient tolerance to colonoscopy, such as insufflation of carbon dioxide (CO_2) instead of room air, warm water colonoscopy, cap colonoscopy and use of spasmolytics such as glucagon or hyoscine butylbromide. However, OC still remains associated with post-procedural pain and discomfort and has a potential risk for morbidity and occasional mortality. Albeit rare, haemorrhage and perforation are the two commonest and most feared colonoscopy-related complications, particularly following therapeutic procedures such as polypectomy, mucosal resection, submucosal dissection and argon plasma coagulation. A significant proportion (up to 33 %) of patients complained of minor intestinal symptoms such as abdominal fullness, bloating, discomfort or pain after OC, even without therapeutic procedures. Severe complications

occur in about 0.3 % of patients, the vast majority (almost 85 % of cases) after polypectomy [1–6]. Leffler et al. reported an incidence of emergency room visits within 2 weeks from the procedure of 0.84 % for all OCs and 0.95 % for screening OCs. Generally, no imaging is necessary if the patient's clinical conditions evolve favourably. Conversely, further investigations are warranted if the patient fails to improve or routine laboratory assays reveal abnormalities such as leucocytosis, elevated acute phase reactants or blood loss [7].

11.2 Post-colonoscopy Findings: Imaging Assessment

Since imaging is not required following OC in asymptomatic patients, no specific colonic or extra-colonic findings related to uncomplicated diagnostic endoscopy have been described in the English literature. When cross-sectional imaging is performed for whatever reason within a few hours after an ordinary diagnostic OC, radiologists can reasonably expect to observe distension of the colon and almost complete absence of faeces in the lumen. Segmental residual gaseous distension of the colon may be found, secondary to gas insufflation during endoscopy. Whereas colonic distension decreases and disappears within hours when ambient air is inflated, the colon collapses even faster when CO_2 is employed

A. Ravelli (✉) • A. Campari
School of Radiology, S. Paolo University Hospital, via di Rudinì, Milan 20142, Italy
e-mail: ellian@alice.it; alessandro.campari@unimi.it

M. Tonolini
Radiology Department, "Luigi Sacco" University Hospital, Via G.B. Grassi 74, Milan 20157, Italy
e-mail: mtonolini@sirm.org

© Springer International Publishing Switzerland 2016
M. Tonolini (ed.), *Imaging Complications of Gastrointestinal and Biliopancreatic Endoscopy Procedures*, DOI 10.1007/978-3-319-31211-8_11

[4]. Absence of faeces in the colonic lumen after colonoscopy is also an expected finding, since the goal of preoperative bowel preparation with low-residue diet and purgatives is to empty the colon of all faecal material to achieve high diagnostic accuracy and therapeutic safety. Intraluminal fluid and some air–fluid levels can be seen at postoperative imaging because fluid flushing is usually performed during the procedure, e.g. to clear luminal residues [8].

11.3 Post-polypectomy Findings: Clips and Coils

Bleeding is one of the commonest complications that may occur during operative OC, especially (up to 1 % of procedures) after therapeutic procedures such as polypectomy. In most cases the site of the haemorrhage is identified during endoscopy, and different techniques are used to obtain haemostasis: simple strangulation of the residual polyp stalk, repeated electrocoagulation, local adrenaline injection, argon plasma photocoagulation, endoloop ligature or endoscopic clips placement [1, 4, 9, 10]. Metal clips placed endoscopically to control bleeding remain visible on plain radiographs and CT scans as a marker of complicated OC (Fig. 11.1). Furthermore, contrast-enhanced CT including arterial and venous phase acquisition is required to assess or exclude persistent active bleeding. When bleeding cannot be stopped endoscopically, such as in the case of arterial vessel damage, prompt endovascular arterial embolisation or surgical ligation is mandatory. As for endoscopic or surgical clips, endovascular coils are visible at imaging, and they also indicate a previous haemorrhagic complication. Colonic ischaemic injury may result from bleeding or therapeutic arterial occlusion, leading to necrosis of a colonic segment. Contrast-enhanced CT is the modality of choice to assess this pathologic condition. The characteristic imaging findings of colonic ischaemia include absence or reduced enhancement of the injured intestinal wall, bowel wall thickening, abnormal distension or stricture of the bowel lumen,

pneumatosis intestinalis with or without portal venous gas, extraluminal fluid collection in close proximity to the ischaemic colonic tract and, in severe cases, free perforation and ascites indicating peritonitis [11].

11.4 Post-polypectomy Findings: Post-polypectomy Electrocoagulation Syndrome (PPES)

11.4.1 Definition, Incidence and Risk Factors

Post-polypectomy electrocoagulation syndrome (PPES), also termed post-polypectomy syndrome or transmural burn syndrome, is characterised by focal colonic wall thickening and adjacent peritoneal inflammation (serositis) in absence of perforation, demonstrated with imaging after polypectomy with electrocautery. This uncommon entity has been reported in a variable proportion (0.14–2 %) of patients who underwent endoscopic polypectomy. Some authors have identified risk factors for developing PPES such as hypertension, resection of polyps larger than 2 cm or without polypoid shape. Furthermore, the right colon is probably more prone to develop PPES because of its relatively thinner wall [4, 12–16].

11.4.2 Pathogenesis

During polypectomy, the electrical current is applied to the polyp stalk by means of a snare and may extend through the colonic layers, crossing the muscularis propria and the serosa and resulting in a localised transmural burn. Three parameters are related to the level of the thermal tissue injury: intensity, duration and diameter of application of the current, partly dependent on the size of the polyp and its morphology. In the majority of cases, the thermal damage occurs at the site of polypectomy; conversely the lesion can develop at the opposite aspect of the colonic wall when the head of the polyp abuts the latter [1, 3–5, 14].

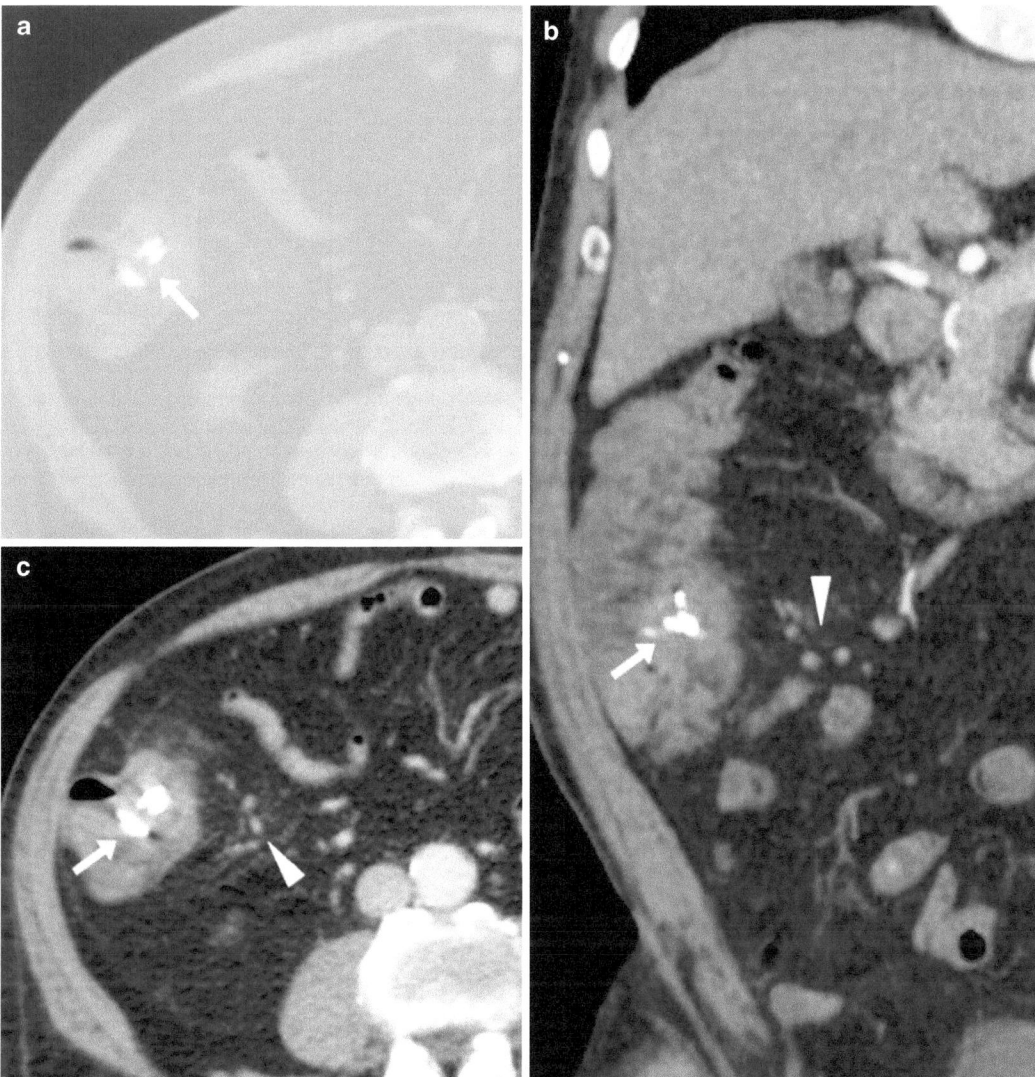

Fig. 11.1 Contrast-enhanced multidetector CT performed shortly after polypectomy complicated by intraoperative bleeding. Axial unenhanced image viewed at lung window settings (**a**) depicted the metallic clips as linear high-attenuation structures (*arrows*) positioned at the inner aspect of the caecal wall and excluded the presence of intramural or extraluminal gas. Post-contrast study including arterial (**b**) and venous (**c**) phases showed mild inflammatory-type pericolonic fat stranding (*arrowheads*). The absence of contrast extravasation confirmed stopped bleeding

11.4.3 Clinical Features

Patients with PPES typically present with abdominal pain and localised or diffuse tenderness, fever, tachycardia and leucocytosis. Symptoms develop in the first few days, often within 12 h after the procedure [3–5, 12, 14, 17]. Symptoms of PPES often mimic those of perforation with localised peritonitis; therefore the onset of acute or progressive abdominal pain should raise concern for possible post-polypectomy injury and appropriately investigated [18].

11.4.4 Imaging Appearance: Plain Radiographs and CT

In most patients presenting to the emergency department, plain radiographs of the thorax and abdomen are generally requested as the initial

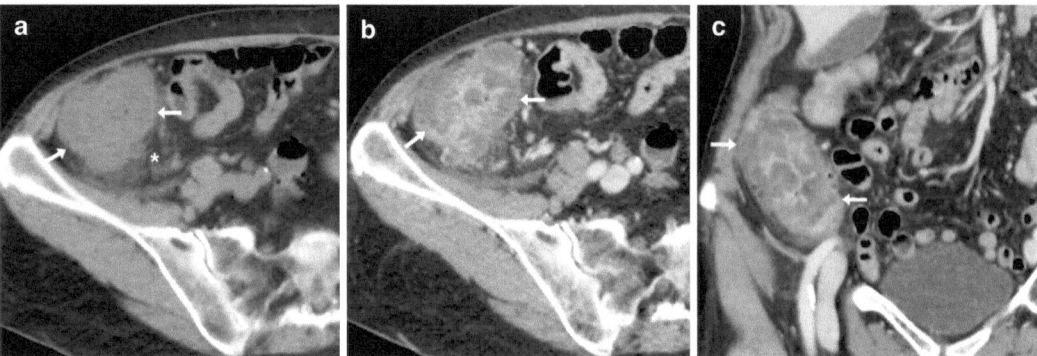

Fig. 11.2 Unenhanced (**a**) and post-contrast (**b, c**) CT study depicted characteristic imaging appearance of PPES in a 64-year-old woman who suffered from right-sided abdominal pain after endoscopic polypectomy. Corresponding to the site of recent polypectomy, the caecum showed an 8-cm long segment involved by marked circumferential wall thickening (*arrows*). The stratified appearance corresponds to enhancing serosa and mucosa separated by thickened oedematous hypoattenuating submucosa. Inflammatory perivisceral fat stranding (* in **a**) is associated. Extraluminal gas and abnormal collections were excluded. The patient had an uneventful course with conservative treatment

investigation, particularly in order to immediately rule out free extravisceral air. Radiographs are preferably obtained in the upright or at least sitting position, to detect air as increased lucency under the diaphragm which is the hallmark of free perforation. Following unremarkable plain radiographs without pneumoperitoneum, in patients with consistent symptoms and laboratory changes, multidetector CT represents a useful second-line investigation. In patients with PPES, CT reviewed with bone or lung window settings confirms the absence of extraintestinal gas (Fig. 11.1). Furthermore, CT typically reveals the characteristic appearance of circumferential segmental thickening of the colonic wall, associated with pericolic fluid and inflammatory-type fat stranding at the site of recent polypectomy (Figs. 11.2 and 11.3). Coronal and sagittal reconstructions allow a panoramic view of the bowel, thus increasing the radiologist's confidence in the interpretation of colonic injuries. These findings, in absence of free air or haematoma, are strongly consistent with a clinical–radiologic diagnosis of PPES. In literature there are no reports about confirmation of PPES through biopsy at site of the colonic wall thickening [3, 4, 14]. Some authors [3, 4] suggested that a contrast enema with water-soluble-iodinated contrast could be performed to distinguish between free and localised perforation. However, in our experience multidetector CT is sufficient to appropriately decide between conservative or surgical treatment, since extraluminal air is confidently detected or excluded on unenhanced scans, and post-contrast imaging at least in the portal venous phase better depicts inflammatory changes in colonic wall and perivisceritis, together with the presence of bleeding or haematomas [1, 3, 9, 12, 19].

11.4.5 Treatment and Follow-Up

Since symptoms of PPES are usually self-limiting within a few days and progression to perforation is rare, the therapeutic approach is typically conservative, sometimes without hospitalisation. Supportive care generally includes bed rest, clinical observation, analgesia, intravenous fluids, bowel rest and antibiotics if clinically necessary [1, 3, 5, 12, 14, 16]. In the literature we could not find any published reports concerning the evolution of cross-sectional imaging findings in patients with PPES during clinical follow-up. In our experience, plain radiographs are of limited value in the follow-up of PPES. In some patients (Figs. 11.3 and 11.4) we have performed serial CT follow-up which documented partial or progressive decrease of the characteristic mural and perivisceral changes [18].

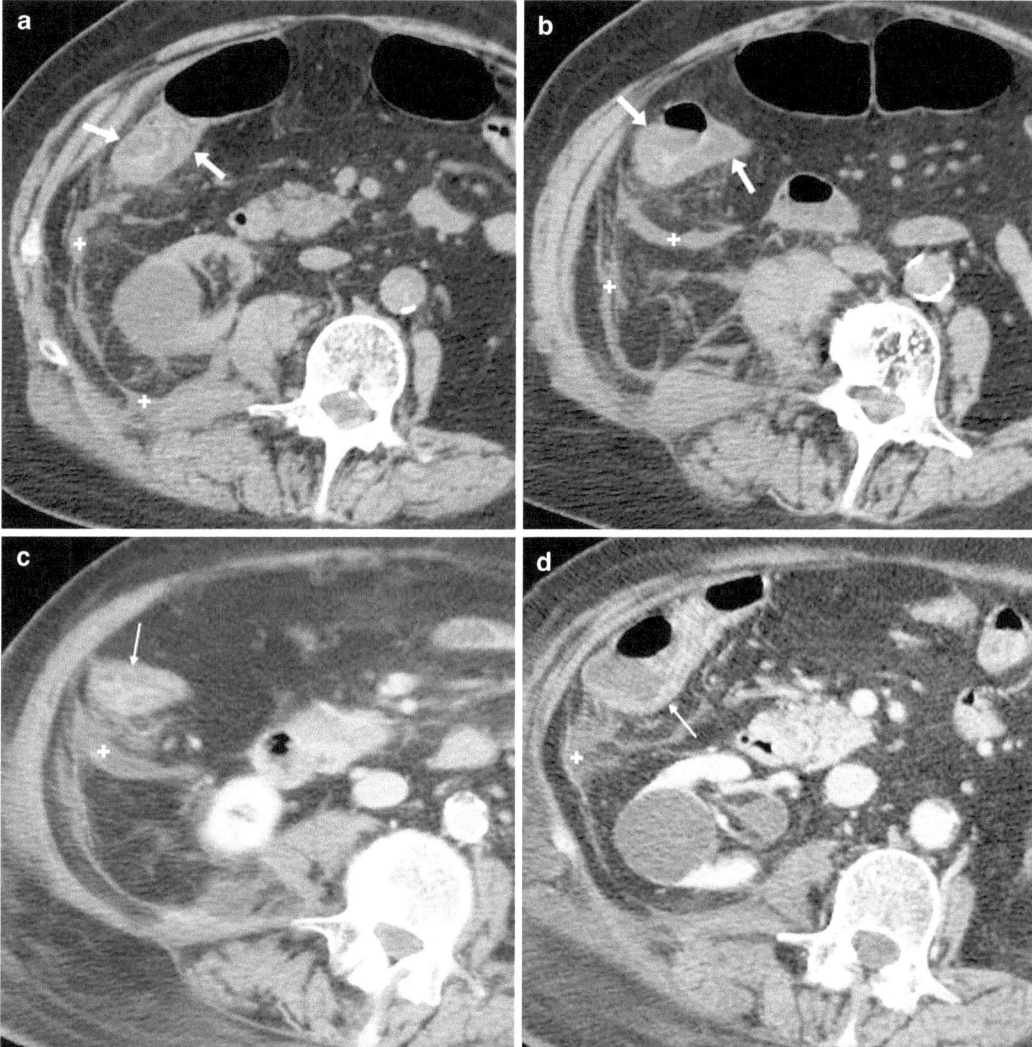

Fig. 11.3 A 38-year-old woman experienced abdominal pain and distension following endoscopic polypectomy at the proximal transverse colon. Unenhanced axial CT images (**a**, **b**) showed findings consistent with PPES, including circumferential mural thickening (*arrows*), inflammatory-type stranding of pericolonic fat and moderate ipsilateral fascial effusion (+). During conservative treatment, 3 days later follow-up contrast-enhanced CT (**c**, **d**) demonstrated decreased thickening of the colonic abnormality (*thin arrows*) with hypoenhancing oedematous submucosa and partial persistence of retroperitoneal fluid (+)

Conclusion

Since clinical signs and symptoms of PPES closely mimic those of colonic perforation, awareness of this pathologic condition is very important for the radiologist because differentiation of PPES from perforation by means of CT can prevent the patient surgical exploration or other unnecessary invasive treatments [5, 18].

11.5 Case Presentation: Post-polypectomy Electrocoagulation Syndrome

A 54-year-old woman with unremarkable past medical history presented to the emergency department complaining of abdominal pain 48 h after operative colonoscopy including

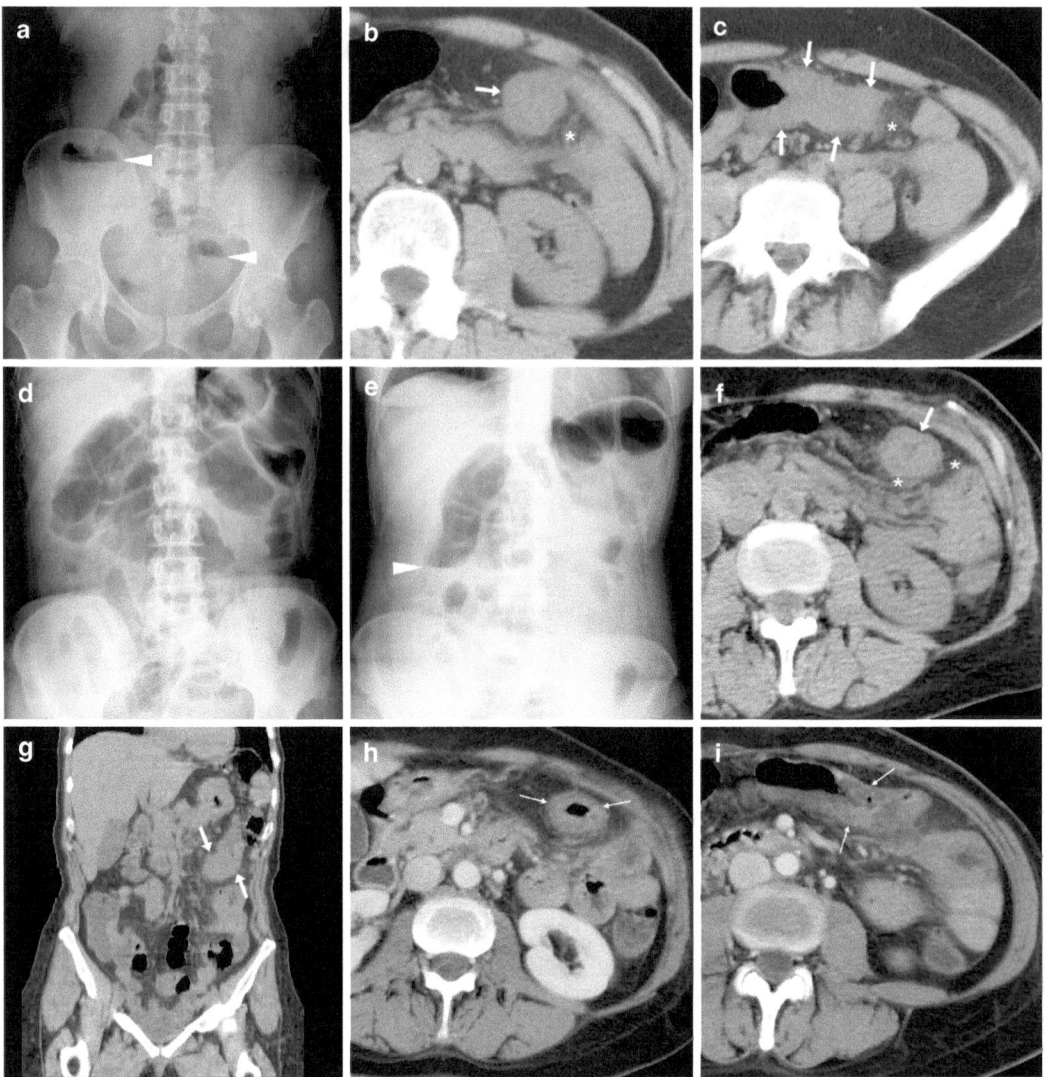

Fig. 11.4 Upright plain abdominal radiograph (**a**) showed moderate gaseous bowel content with some ileo-caecal air–fluid levels (*arrowheads*), excluded sub-phrenic and abnormal extraluminal air collections. Immediate unenhanced CT (**b, c**) detected a 9-cm long segment with marked circumferential mural thickening (*arrows*) without stratification at the distal transverse colon, associated with inflammatory-type stranding of perivisceral fat (*) and minimal peritoneal effusion. Two days later, repeat supine (**d**) and upright (**e**) plain radio-graphs did not detect appearance of extraluminal air. Increased gaseous distension was noted in the transverse and right-sided colon with a prominent caecal air–fluid level (*arrowhead* in **e**). 72 h after admission repeated unenhanced CT (**f, g**) showed persistence of marked cir-cumferential thickening (*arrows*) involving a segment of the distal transverse colon, still associated with inflam-matory-type stranding of perivisceral fat (*). Eight days after admission, follow-up contrast-enhanced CT (**h, i**) showed moderate decrease of both segmental colonic thickening (*thin arrows*) and perivisceral fat stranding and disappearance of peritoneal fluid

biopsies and polypectomy performed. Physical examination revealed a distended, tender abdomen with poor peristalsis and question-able Blumberg's sign. Laboratory assays reveal leucocytosis and markedly increased C-reactive protein. At admission, plain radio-graphs (Fig. 11.4a) showed only moderate gas-eous bowel content with some air–fluid levels.

Fig. 11.5 Same patient as Fig. 11.4; graphs show trends of laboratory parameters including C-reactive protein, neutrophil count and haemoglobin over 11 days of hospitalisation

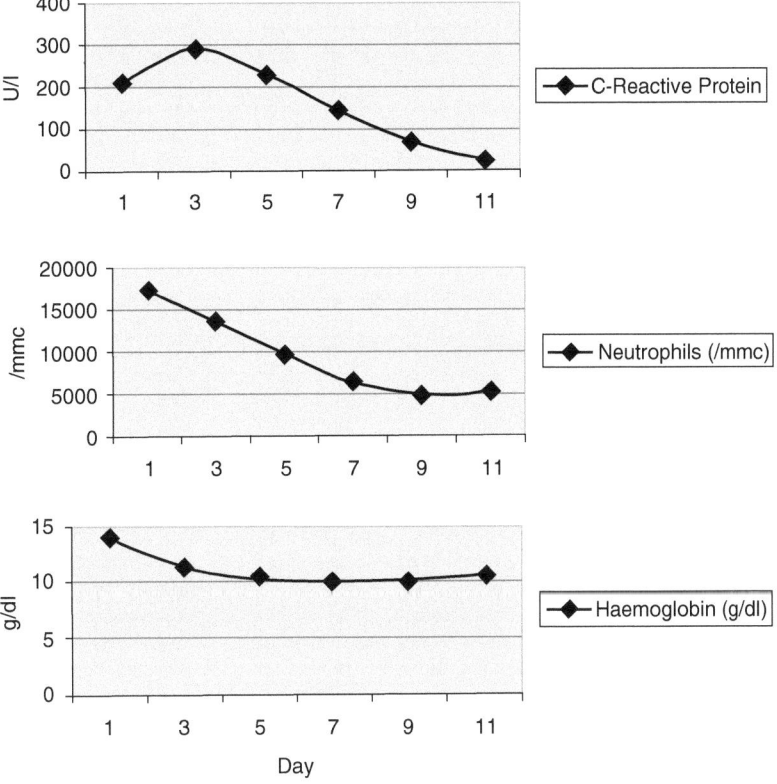

Early unenhanced CT (Fig. 11.4b, c) detected a segmental thickening of the distal transverse colon with associated inflammatory-type stranding of perivisceral fat. In absence of signs of perforation, conservative treatment (intravenous fluids and antibiotics) of PPES was started. 48 h after admission, repeated radiographs (Fig. 11.4d, e) revealed increasing gaseous distension of the transverse and right-sided colon. Repeated CT 72 h after admission (Fig. 11.4f, g) showed stable findings. During 11 days of hospitalisation, C-reactive protein and neutrophil count progressively decreased, whereas haemoglobin levels initially decreased to 10 g/dl and then stabilised within 5 days (Fig. 11.5). Finally, contrast-enhanced CT performed 8 days after admission (Fig. 11.4h, i) showed partial improvement with decreased colonic thickening and perivisceral fat stranding [Partly reproduced with permission from Ref. no 18].

References

1. Kim DH, Pickhardt PJ, Taylor AJ et al (2008) Imaging evaluation of complications at optical colonoscopy. Curr Probl Diagn Radiol 37:165–177
2. Blotiere PO, Weill A, Ricordeau P et al (2014) Perforations and haemorrhages after colonoscopy in 2010: a study based on comprehensive French health insurance data (SNIIRAM). Clin Res Hepatol Gastroenterol 38(1):112–117
3. Lohsiriwat V (2010) Colonoscopic perforation: incidence, risk factors, management and outcome. World J Gastroenterol 16:425–430
4. Green J (2006) BSG guidelines in gastroenterology – complications of gastrointestinal endoscopy http://www.bsg.org.uk/clinical-guidelines/endoscopy/guidelines-on-complications-of-gastrointestinal--endoscopyhtml
5. ASGE Standards of Practice Committee, Fisher DA, Maple JT, Ben-Menachem T et al (2011) Complications of colonoscopy. Gastrointest Endosc 74(4):745–752
6. Schmidt-Tänzer W, Eickhoff A (2014) What influences the quality of prevention colonoscopy? Viszeralmedizin 30(1):26–31

7. Leffler DA, Kheraj R, Garud S et al (2010) The incidence and cost of unexpected hospital use after scheduled outpatient endoscopy. Arch Intern Med 170(19):1752–1757

8. Wexner SD, Beck DE, Baron TH et al (2006) A consensus document on bowel preparation before colonoscopy: prepared by a Task Force from the American Society of Colon and Rectal Surgeons (ASCRS), the American Society for Gastrointestinal Endoscopy (ASGE), and the Society of American Gastrointestinal and Endoscopic Surgeons (SAGES). American Society of Colon and Rectal Surgeons (ASCRS); American Society for Gastrointestinal Endoscopy (ASGE); Society of American Gastrointestinal and Endoscopic Surgeons (SAGES). Surg Endosc 20(7):1147–1160

9. Wax BN, Katz DS, Badler RL et al (2006) Complications of abdominal and pelvic procedures: computed tomographic diagnosis. Curr Probl Diagn Radiol 35:171–187

10. Shaish H, Gilet A, Gerard P (2015) 'It's all foreign to me': how to decipher gastrointestinal intraluminal foreign bodies. Abdom Imaging 40(7):2173–2192

11. Moschetta M, Telegrafo M, Rella L et al (2014) Multi-detector CT features of acute intestinal ischemia and their prognostic correlations. World J Radiol 6(5):130–138

12. Benson BC, Myers JJ, Laczek JT (2013) Postpolypectomy electrocoagulation syndrome: a

mimicker of colonic perforation. Case Rep Emerg Med 2013:687931

13. Choo WK, Subhani J (2012) Complication rates of colonic polypectomy in relation to polyp characteristics and techniques: a district hospital experience. J Interv Gastroenterol 2(1):8–11

14. Hirasawa K, Sato C, Makazu M et al (2015) Coagulation syndrome: delayed perforation after colorectal endoscopic treatments. World J Gastrointest Endosc 7(12):1055–1061

15. Lee SH, Kim KJ, Yang DH et al (2014) Postpolypectomy fever, a rare adverse event of polypectomy: nested case-control study. Clin Endosc 47:236–241

16. Cha JM, Lim KS, Lee SH et al (2013) Clinical outcomes and risk factors of post-polypectomy coagulation syndrome: a multicenter, retrospective, case-control study. Endoscopy 45:202–207

17. Ko CW, Riffle S, Shapiro JA et al (2007) Incidence of minor complications and time lost from normal activities after screening or surveillance colonoscopy. Gastrointest Endosc 65(4):648–656

18. Tonolini M (2014) Post-polypectomy electrocoagulation syndrome {Online} URL: http://www.eurorad.org/case.php?id=11612

19. Maniatis V, Chryssikopoulos H, Roussakis A et al (2000) Perforation of the alimentary tract: evaluation with computed tomography. Abdom Imaging 25:373–379

Imaging Appearances of Post-colonoscopy Complications

12

Alessandro Campari, Anna Ravelli, and Massimo Tonolini

12.1 Introduction

Optical colonoscopy (OC) is an irreplaceable tool for diagnosis and treatment of a wide range of colonic conditions, including screening and surveillance of colorectal cancer. Since OC requires intubation of the length of the colon and manipulation of the instrument, this procedure carries a low but real risk for morbidity and mortality, which increases as endoscopy assumes a more therapeutic role. Post-endoscopy complications are presently declining due to improved technology and greater operator experience, but continue to occur with a not negligible frequency because of the increasing number and complexity of procedures. After OC up to 33 % of patients report at least one minor gastrointestinal symptom, and serious adverse events occur in about 0.3 % of cases in the vast majority (over 85 %) after polypectomy. Adverse events may be caused by the pre-colonoscopy bowel preparation, by the sedation or by the procedure itself [1, 2]. Perforation is the commonest procedure-specific complications and will be further discussed in this chapter.

Haemorrhage is the second most common complication, which occurs in 0.1–0.6 % of all colonoscopies [1] and in up to 1 % of interventive procedures [3]. Risk factors for bleeding include coagulation disorders and removal of large polyps. Significant bleeding can be immediately detected and treated during the procedure, but delayed (secondary) haemorrhage may also occur after 1–14 days [4]. Treatment options for secondary haemorrhage are either endoscopic, surgical or endovascular. In haemodynamically stable patients, accurate preoperative planning can be obtained with contrast-enhanced multidetector CT. CT may suggest the site of bleeding depicting high-attenuation blood within the bowel lumen on precontrast scans and/or detect contrast extravasation indicating active bleeding, a finding which directs endoscopic, surgical or interventional treatment [5]. Furthermore, CT can depict intramural haematoma, extracolonic haemorrhage and haemoperitoneum and give information on vascular supply, because anatomic variants are commonly encountered [6, 7]. Very rare complications of OC include colitis, splenic lesions, volvulus and acute diverticulitis [1, 2, 8]. Not unusually, post-colonoscopy injuries may be unrecognised by the endoscopist, and clinical symptoms or laboratory signs might develop later: up to 0.95 % of patients who underwent OC visit the emergency room within 14 days from the procedure [9]. Early detection has a direct impact on patient's outcome, as most complications require prompt

A. Campari (✉) • A. Ravelli
School of Radiology, S. Paolo University Hospital, via di Rudinì, Milano 20142, Italy
e-mail: alessandro.campari@unimi.it; ellian@alice.it

M. Tonolini
Radiology Department, "Luigi Sacco" University Hospital, Via G.B. Grassi 74, Milano 20157, Italy
e-mail: mtonolini@sirm.org

© Springer International Publishing Switzerland 2016
M. Tonolini (ed.), *Imaging Complications of Gastrointestinal and Biliopancreatic Endoscopy Procedures*, DOI 10.1007/978-3-319-31211-8_12

management. Therefore, cross-sectional imaging with CT plays a key role in detection of OC complications, providing precise information about site, mechanism and severity of the damage, together with associate conditions.

12.2 Colonoscopic Perforation

12.2.1 Incidence, Risk Factors and Pathogenesis

Albeit uncommon, bowel perforation represents one of the most feared complications of colonoscopy, associated with significant morbidity and even mortality. Estimated perforation rate ranges between 0.03% and 0.8% for diagnostic colonoscopies in both the symptomatic and screening settings. Risk factors associated with an increased risk of perforation can be divided in patient-related and procedure-related. The former include advanced age (>80 years), female gender, high body mass index (BMI), haemodialysis, hospitalisation (especially in intensive care), diverticulosis and other colonic diseases such as colitis and inflammatory bowel diseases (IBD). Procedure-related risk factors include interventional procedure, resection of polyps larger than 1 cm or more than four polyps, emergency conditions and limited operator experience. The risk of perforation is four times superior (up to 5%) for polypectomy compared to diagnostic endoscopic procedures. Among therapeutic interventions, endoscopic mucosal resection (EMR), endoscopic submucosal dissection (ESD), argon plasma coagulation (APC) and dilatation have higher rates of perforation (11%) than simple polypectomy [1, 4, 10–13]. Although death after OC is rare (1/3,500 procedures), post-colonoscopy perforation is associated with a significant (8–15%) mortality rate, mostly related to the underlying disease and comorbidities [10, 11, 14]. Mechanisms of perforation include mechanical force on the colonic wall from the endoscope, especially in a pathological area, barotrauma from air insufflation and direct damage from interventions. Mechanical trauma is more frequent in the sigmoid colon and the rectosigmoid junction; it can either be direct at the apex of the endoscope or abrasive from its side. Pneumatic distension may lead to wall tears that cause perforation when extended to the serosa; this kind of damage usually occurs in the caecum because the wall of the right colon is thinner than the left and colonic wall tension is highest in the caecum. Therapeutic OC may cause perforation because of passage of instruments through the colon wall or by means of thermal injury. The sigmoid colon and rectosigmoid junction are the most common sites of perforation (70–80% of cases), due to the sharp angulation at the junction and the mobility of the sigmoid, together with the common presence of diverticulosis [2].

12.2.2 Clinical Features and Treatment

Approximately 30% of iatrogenic colon perforation are detected during endoscopy and may be successfully treated with endoluminal clipping. Conversely the commonest presentation includes symptoms and signs of peritonitis manifesting hours to 3 days after the procedure. The vast majority (90%) of patients present within 48 h and never more than 5 days after the procedure [10, 11, 15]. Colonoscopy-related perforation can progress to peritonitis and sepsis, resulting in serious morbidity with a mean 1–3 weeks hospital stay. Recognition and treatment within 24 h are associated with better outcome, fewer intestinal resections and reduced morbidity and hospital stays. A better outcome is also observed in patients who received bowel preparation prior to colonoscopy [11, 14–16]. The clinical manifestations of postcolonoscopy perforation depend on the site and size of the perforation, the amount of faecal spillage into the peritoneum and the premorbid condition of the patient. Practically, iatrogenic colonic perforation should be suspected when a patient complains of abdominal pain, distention and fever after OC. Tachycardia, fever, abdominal tenderness and leucocytosis should raise a strong suspicion. Failure to pass flatus despite obvious distension also suggests the diagnosis of perforation [2]. The choice between surgery and nonoperative management should consider the type of injury, previous bowel preparation, underlying colonic disease and clinical conditions. Laparoscopic or laparotomic surgical management is often needed, with either primary suture (70%) or bowel resection with colonic anastomosis or stoma creation. Endoluminal clipping is successful in up to 81% of cases and may obviate the need for surgery in patients with endoscopy-related perforations [10, 14, 17]. Since early recognition and treatment are associated with reduced morbidity, high level of suspicion and prompt investigation are recommended. Conservative treatment including intravenous fluids, bowel rest and broad-spectrum antibiotics is feasible in patients in good conditions, perforations unnoticed during endoscopy, early diagnosis, no signs of peritonitis and proper colonic preparation [11, 15, 16].

12.2.3 Role of Imaging

Colonic perforation causes extraluminal leakage of gas, which may collect in the peritoneal cavity, retroperitoneal spaces, mesentery or ligaments, depending on the affected site. Furthermore, bowel wall damage results in perivisceral inflammation and possible formation of phlegmon, abscess collections and peritonitis. The role of imaging includes demonstration of the perforation, localisation of the injury site and detection of further complications [18]. When perforation is suspected, plain radiographs of the thorax and abdomen are generally performed as initial investigation, preferably in the upright position. If the patient is unable to stand, sitting position or left lateral decubitus is an acceptable alternative. Radiographs may detect pneumoperitoneum as convex radiolucency beneath the domes of the diaphragm in erect position or outlining the liver in the lateral decubitus. Unfortunately, even when acquired with an optimal technique, plain radiographs have moderate (50–70%) sensitivity for pneumoperitoneum, even lower for retroperitoneal gas. In the supine position, only large gas collections can be appreciated as increased lucency over the liver projection. Additionally, conventional radiographs are insensitive to the presence of extraluminal fluid [3]. Conversely, multidetector CT readily detects small amount of free intra- or extraperitoneal gas and fluid with absolute sensitivity. The European Society of Gastrointestinal Endoscopy (ESGE) position statement recommends that symptoms or signs suggestive of iatrogenic perforation after an endoscopic procedure should be carefully evaluated and documented, possibly with a CT scan, in order to prevent any diagnostic delay. When CT findings are inconclusive, close monitoring with repeated CT scan may be indicated [13].

12.2.4 Computed Tomography (CT) Technique and Findings

Whereas unenhanced CT is sufficient for confident detection or exclusion of extraluminal gas, contrast-enhanced CT enables a better depiction of the perforation site and of associated complications. In our experience, the oral or rectal administration of water-soluble contrast medium does not result in substantial added benefit for detecting iatrogenic perforation, is often cumbersome and may lead to diagnostic delay. The entire abdomen from the dome of the diaphragm to the pelvic floor should always be included in the scanned volume. The use of thin slices, multiplanar reconstruction (MPR) and image review at the bone or lung window settings are recommended to enhance sensitivity for detection of intramural and extraluminal air, mural pathology and perivisceral inflammation. The CT diagnosis of perforation is based on direct and indirect findings. Direct findings are represented by extraluminal gas and discontinuation of the visceral wall. Visualisation of the discontinuity of the wall is possible in less than 50% of cases, probably due to the small size of most injuries. However small foci of extraluminal gas may congregate near the perforation site, hinting at its location [3, 19]. Free gas distribution following iatrogenic colonic perforation depends on the site of injury: perforation of intraperitoneal colonic segments on a mesentery, including the transverse, sigmoid and caecum, commonly occurs on the mobile antimesenteric aspect, causing free intraperitoneal gas, whereas injury to the ascending, descending colon and rectum usually results in extraperitoneal collections [3, 11, 14]. However, perforation of intraperitoneal segments can also result in extraperitoneal collections when the injury affects the mesenteric aspect of the colon. In extraperitoneal perforations, gas can occasionally track through the visceral space that forms an anatomic connection between the retroperitoneum, the mediastinum and the neck, causing pneumomediastinum and/or subcutaneous emphysema [3, 20]. Indirect findings of perforation include perivisceral inflammatory fat stranding, segmental wall thickening and abnormal wall enhancement consistent with mural ischaemia. Although iatrogenic perforation usually occurs in a prepared bowel, the incidence of extraluminal bacteric contamination is high, leading to phlegmon, abscess formation or peritonitis. In the latter complication, abdominal free fluid collects in the most dependent portions of the peritoneum, such as the hepatorenal fossa (Morrison's pouch), the paracolic gutters, the mesenteric root and the pelvis [3] (Figs. 12.1, 12.2, 12.3, and 12.4).

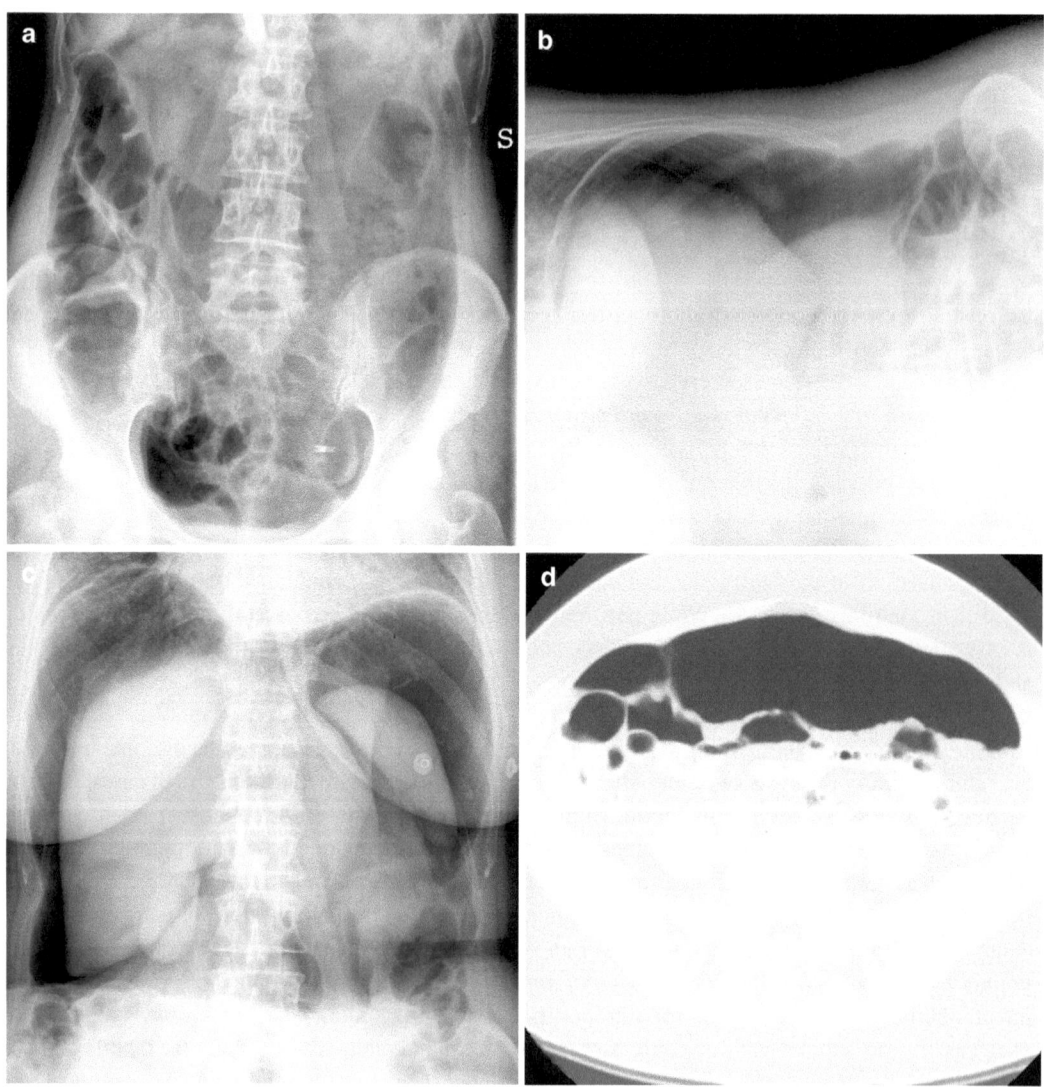

Fig. 12.1 Severe pneumoperitoneum as a result of iatrogenic perforation. Anteroposterior plain radiograph acquired in supine patient (**a**) shows slightly increased lucency of all abdominal quadrants, compatible with gas collection, but cannot assess gas site and extension. Radiograph obtained with patient in lateral decubitus (**b**) demonstrates significant lucency under the lateral abdominal wall and the left diaphragm, consistent with pneumoperitoneum. Radiograph obtained with patient seated (**c**) better depicts the pneumoperitoneum as an obvious lucency between the domes of the diaphragm and the abdominal organs. Axial CT image viewed at soft tissue window settings (**d**) confirms the pneumoperitoneum and excludes retroperitoneal gas collections

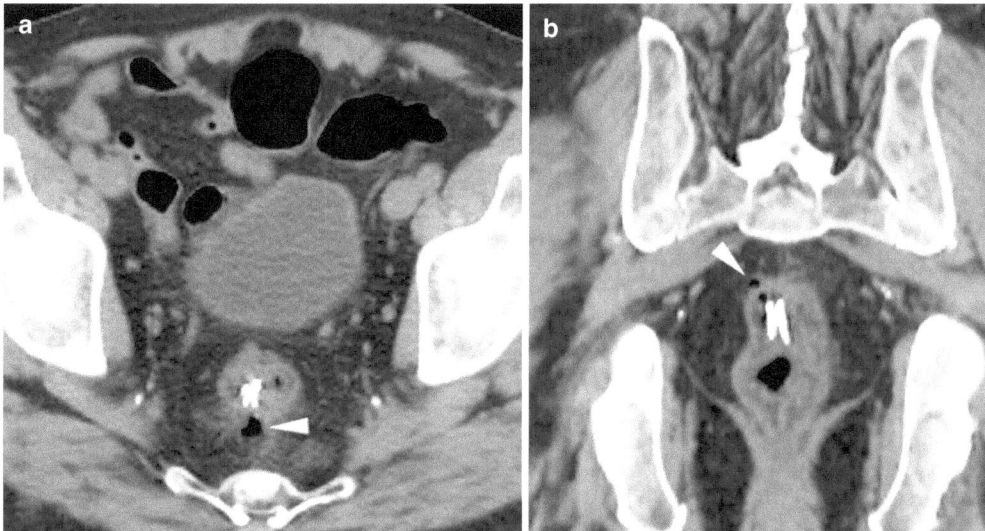

Fig. 12.2 Iatrogenic rectal perforation successfully treated with intraoperative endoscopic clipping. Axial (**a**) and coronal (**b**) unenhanced CT images show small amount of perivisceral gas (*arrowhead*) in close proximity to intraluminal metallic clips, surrounded by inflammatory mesorectal fat stranding

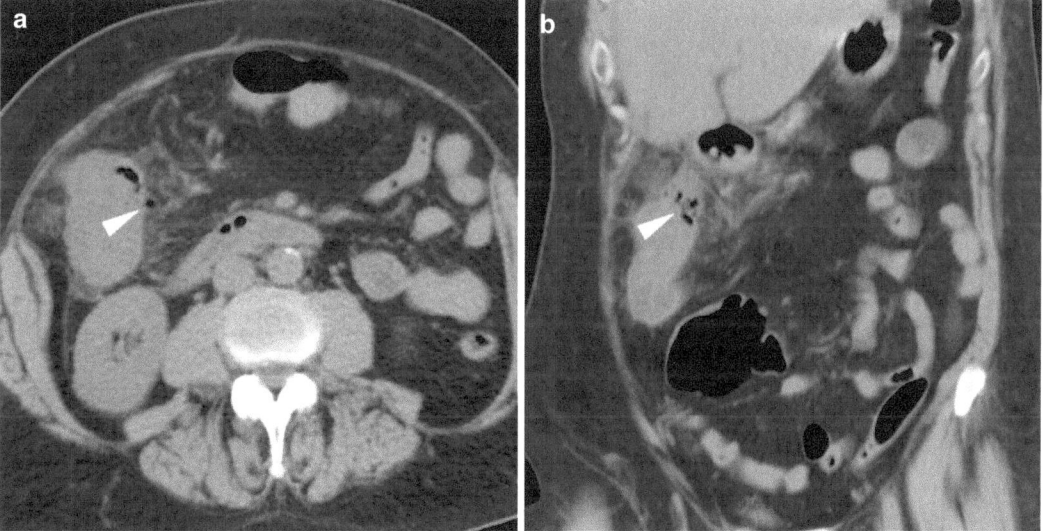

Fig. 12.3 Evolution of small iatrogenic perforation. Axial (**a**) and coronal (**b**) unenhanced CT images depict small amount of intraperitoneal free gas (*arrowhead*) adjacent to the right colon, together with diffuse peritoneal fat stranding and thickening of the renal fascia. After clinical worsening during hospitalisation, axial (**c**) and coronal (**d**) unenhanced CT images demonstrate increase of the free fluid volume and the fat stranding

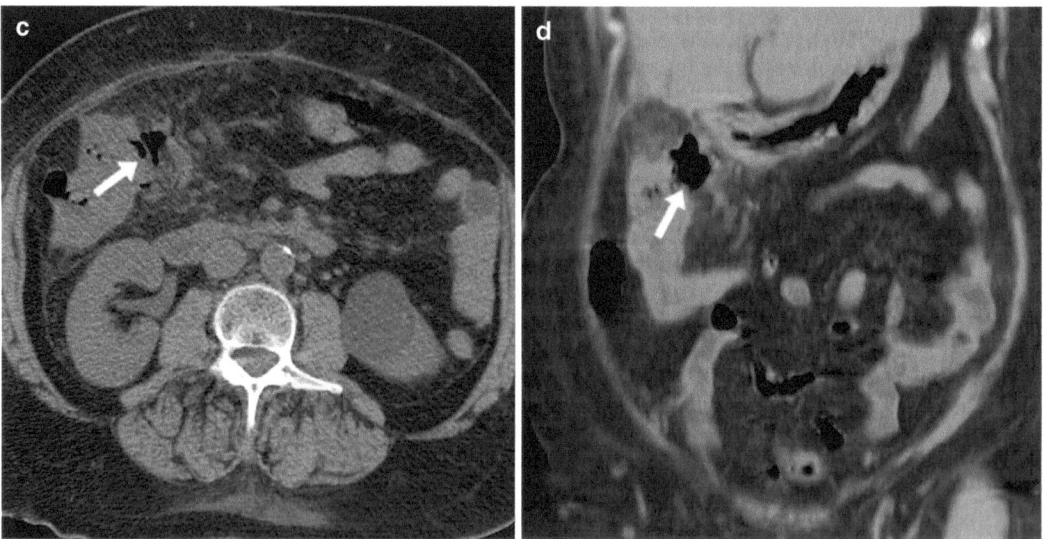

Fig. 12.3 Continued

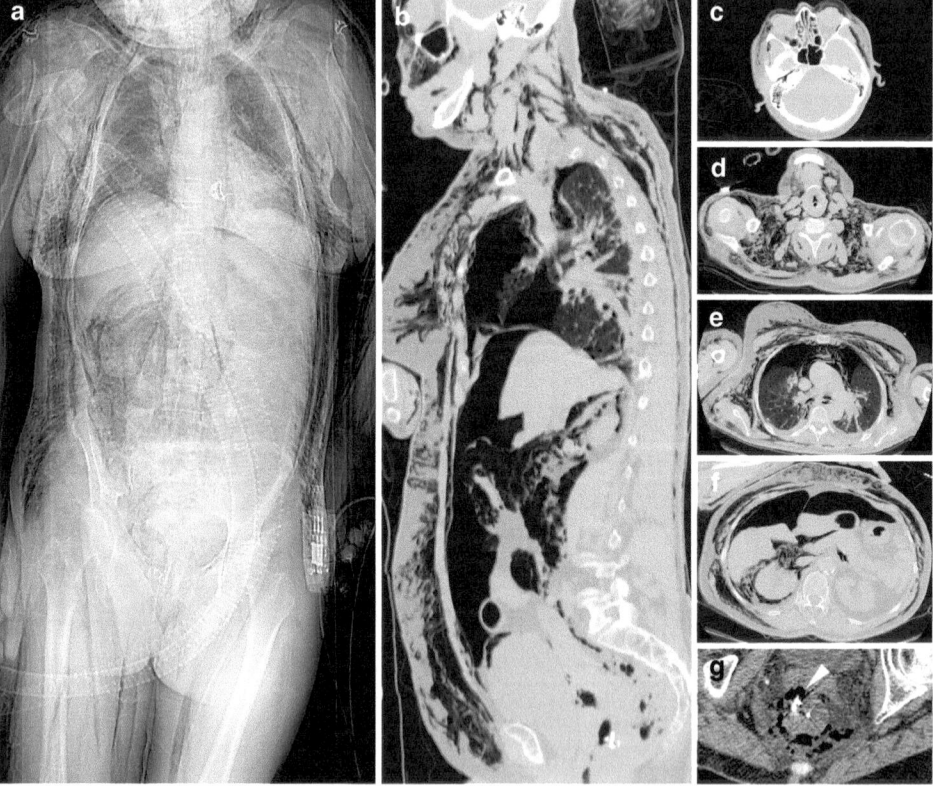

Fig. 12.4 Unsuccessful endoluminal clipping after rectal perforation during optical colonoscopy assessed with unenhanced CT. Scout view (**a**) demonstrates extensive subcutaneous emphysema. Sagittal reconstruction and axial images viewed at lung window settings (**b**) demonstrate retro-pneumoperitoneum, pneumoperitoneum, pneumothorax and pneumomediastinum, together with massive emphysema in the deep subfascial and subcutaneous spaces of the abdomen, thorax, neck and head (**c–f**). Axial image viewed at soft tissue window settings (**g**) demonstrates extraluminal gas (*arrowhead*) at the leakage site in close proximity to metallic clips in the rectum

12.3 Case Presentation: Iatrogenic Colon Perforation During Operative Colonoscopy

A 69-year-old female patient affected with primary biliary cirrhosis, pulmonary fibrosis, diabetes and sigmoid colon diverticulosis complained of abdominal pain 24 h after operative colonoscopy including resection of a 7-mm sessile polyp of the sigmoid colon and argon plasma coagulation of ascending colon angiodysplasias. Physical examination revealed bilateral pelvic tenderness without frank peritonism. Laboratory assays demonstrated anaemia (10.5 g/dl), increased lactate dehydrogenase (300 U/l) and C-reactive protein (90 mg/l). Chest and abdominal radiographs (Fig. 12.5a) excluded

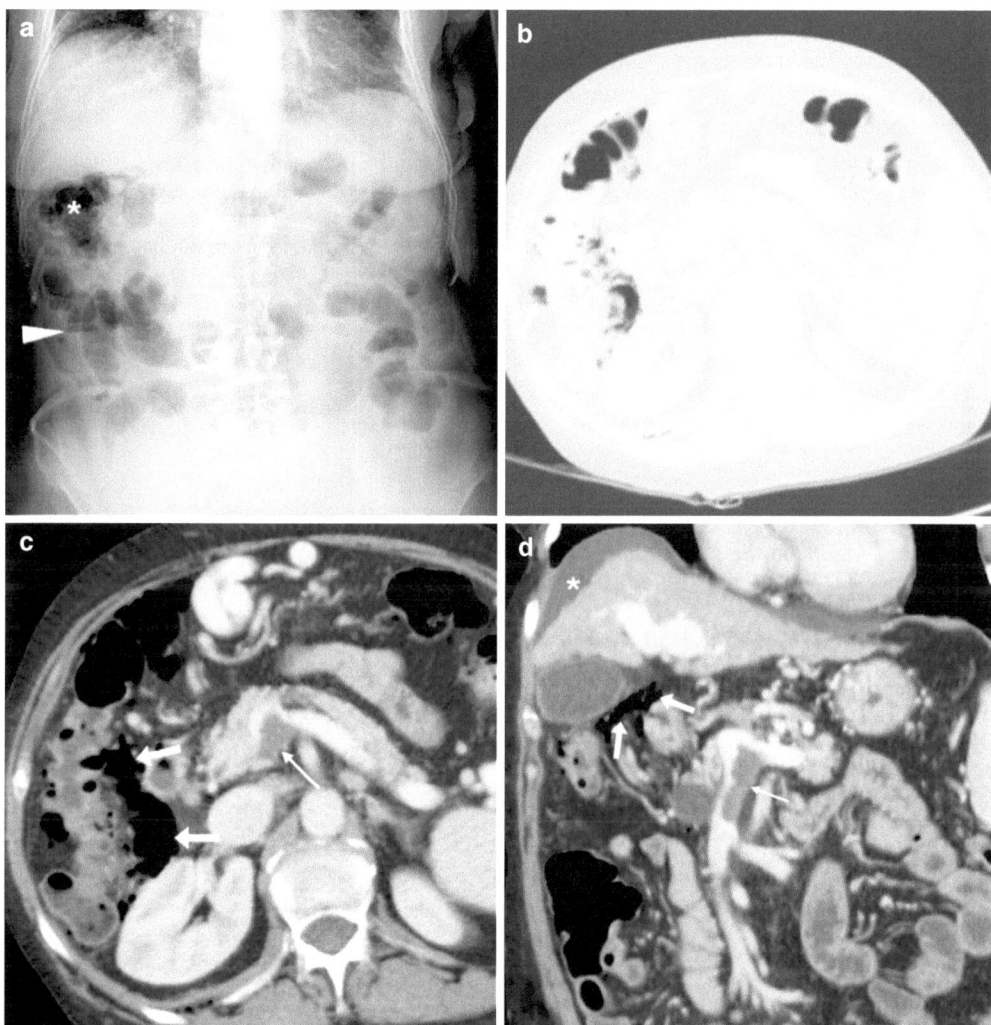

Fig. 12.5 Upright plain abdominal radiograph (**a**) does not disclose subphrenic air collections consistent with pneumoperitoneum and reveals some ileal air–fluid levels in the right hemiabdomen (*arrowheads*), a bubbly gaseous infrahepatic radiolucency (*) partly superimposed to the right colonic flexure projection. Preliminary unenhanced CT image viewed at lung window settings (**b**) reveals extraluminal gas (*arrows*) surrounding the right hepatic flexure and the ascending colon, without pneumoperitoneum. Contrast-enhanced axial (**c**) and coronal (**d**) CT images show sizeable extraperitoneal gas collection (*arrows*) surrounding the right flexure and ascending colon. Additionally, moderate perihepatic peritoneal effusion (* in c), recanalised paraumbilical vein and partial portomesenteric venous thrombosis (*thin arrows*) are noted

subphrenic pneumoperitoneum and revealed some ileal air–fluid levels in the right hemiabdomen together with a circumscribed "bubbly" gaseous infrahepatic radiolucency, which was partly superimposed to the right colonic flexure. Immediate multidetector CT investigation (Fig. 12.5b–d) confirmed absence of free pneumoperitoneum and depicted a sizeable extraperitoneal gas surrounding the right hepatic flexure and ascending colon, consistent with iatrogenic perforation of the right colon from argon plasma coagulation. No abnormalities were seen nearby the polypectomy site at the sigmoid. Additionally, moderate perihepatic peritoneal effusion, recanalised paraumbilical vein and partial portomesenteric venous thrombosis were noted. Considering the absent clinical and imaging signs of peritonitis, the attending surgeon opted for nonsurgical treatment including bowel rest, intravenous fluids and broad-spectrum antibiotics, allowing clinical, imaging and laboratory improvement within a few days [Partly reproduced with permission from Ref. no 18].

References

1. Committee ASoP, Fisher DA, Maple JT, Ben-Menachem T (2011) Complications of colonoscopy. Gastrointest Endosc 74:745–752
2. Green J (2006) BSG guidelines in gastroenterology – complications of gastrointestinal endoscopy. http://www.bsg.org.uk/clinical-guidelines/endoscopy/guidelines-on-complications-of-gastrointestinal--endoscopyhtml
3. Kim DH, Pickhardt PJ, Taylor AJ et al (2008) Imaging evaluation of complications at optical colonoscopy. Curr Probl Diagn Radiol 37:165–177
4. Blotiere PO, Weill A, Ricordeau P et al (2013) Perforations and haemorrhages after colonoscopy in 2010: a study based on comprehensive French health insurance data (SNIIRAM). Clin Res Hepatol Gastroenterol 38(1):112–117
5. Laing CJ, Tobias T, Rosenblum DI et al (2007) Acute gastrointestinal bleeding: emerging role of multidetector CT angiography and review of current imaging techniques. Radiograph: Rev Publ Radiol Soc N Am 27:1055–1070
6. Wax BN, Katz DS, Badler RL et al (2006) Complications of abdominal and pelvic procedures: computed tomographic diagnosis. Curr Probl Diagn Radiol 35:171–187
7. Geffroy Y, Rodallec MH, Boulay-Coletta I et al (2011) Multidetector CT angiography in acute gastrointestinal bleeding: why, when, and how. Radiograph: Rev Publ Radiol Soc N Am 31:E35–E46
8. Ishii N, Fujita Y (2015) Colonic diverticulitis after endoscopic band ligation performed for colonic diverticular hemorrhage. ACG Case Rep J 2:218–220
9. Leffler DA, Kheraj R, Garud S et al (2010) The incidence and cost of unexpected hospital use after scheduled outpatient endoscopy. Arch Intern Med 170:1752–1757
10. Hagel AF, Boxberger F, Dauth W et al (2012) Colonoscopy-associated perforation: a 7-year survey of in-hospital frequency, treatment and outcome in a German university hospital. Colorectal Dis 14:1121–1125
11. Lohsiriwat V (2010) Colonoscopic perforation: incidence, risk factors, management and outcome. World J Gastroenterol 16:425–430
12. Hamdani U, Naeem R, Haider F et al (2013) Risk factors for colonoscopic perforation: a population-based study of 80118 cases. World J Gastroenterol 19:3596–3601
13. Paspatis GA, Dumonceau JM, Barthet M et al (2014) Diagnosis and management of iatrogenic endoscopic perforations: European Society of Gastrointestinal Endoscopy (ESGE) Position Statement. Endoscopy 46:693–711
14. Samalavicius NE, Kazanavicius D, Lunevicius R et al (2013) Incidence, risk, management, and outcomes of iatrogenic full-thickness large bowel injury associated with 56,882 colonoscopies in 14 Lithuanian hospitals. Surg Endosc 27:1628–1635
15. Castellvi J, Pi F, Sueiras A et al (2011) Colonoscopic perforation: useful parameters for early diagnosis and conservative treatment. Int J Colorectal Dis 26:1183–1190
16. Won DY, Lee IK, Lee YS et al (2012) The indications for nonsurgical management in patients with colorectal perforation after colonoscopy. Am Surg 78:550–554
17. Kim JS, Kim BW, Kim JI et al (2013) Endoscopic clip closure versus surgery for the treatment of iatrogenic colon perforations developed during diagnostic colonoscopy: a review of 115,285 patients. Surg Endosc 27:501–504
18. Tonolini M, Rigiroli F (2014) Iatrogenic colon perforation during operative colonoscopy: imaging triage {Online}. URL: http://www.eurorad.org/casephp?id=11594
19. Kim HC, Yang DM, Kim SW et al (2014) Gastrointestinal tract perforation: evaluation of MDCT according to perforation site and elapsed time. Eur Radiol 24:1386–1393
20. Falidas E, Anyfantakis G, Vlachos K et al (2012) Pneumoperitoneum, retropneumoperitoneum, pneumomediastinum, and diffuse subcutaneous emphysema following diagnostic colonoscopy. Case Rep Surg 2012:108791

Massimo Tonolini

13.1 Colonoscopic Perforation in Inflammatory Bowel Diseases: Incidence and Risk Factors

In patients with chronic inflammatory bowel diseases (IBD), ileocolonoscopy with biopsies represents the cornerstone for diagnosis, assessment of disease extent and activity, prediction of prognosis, monitoring of therapeutic effects and neoplastic surveillance and may allow therapeutic procedures such as stricture dilatation [1, 2].

In the general population, the reported incidence of colonoscopic perforation (CP) is greatly variable (in the range 0.03–0.3 %) and substantially higher when interventional procedures are performed. Although data on iatrogenic perforations in Crohn's disease (CD) and ulcerative colitis (UC) are scarce and conflicting, there is significant concern that the thickened, non-compliant inflamed colonic wall and the presence of strictures increase the risk of CP up to 0.52–1 % in IBD populations. A recent study published in Journal of Crohn's and Colitis reported CP to occur after endoscopy in 1 % of IBD inpatients, a figure which is significantly higher (1.83 adjusted odds ratio; 95 % confidence interval 1.40–2.38)

compared to control inpatients without IBD, without differences between CD and UC. IBD resulted in an independent risk factor for CP even after adjusting for age, sex, comorbidities and endoscopic interventions such as polypectomy and dilatation. Advanced age, female gender, operator experience and therapeutic dilatation were independent risk factors for CP. Conversely biopsy, polypectomy and comorbidities were not associated with an increased risk [2].

However, whether IBD patients are at increased risk of CP compared to the general population remains debated. A large cohort including all consecutive patients seen over 13 years at a tertiary referral centre revealed a much lower incidence (0.168 %) rate of CP, including two occurrences in stricturing CD and two in UC patients, which was attributed to the higher expertise in performing IBD endoscopy procedures. The same study emphasised the role of steroids as a key risk factor and the frequent need (three out of four patients) for surgical repair with or without stoma [1, 2].

13.2 Colonoscopic Perforation in Inflammatory Bowel Disease: Imaging Assessment

Similarly to the general population, in patients with IBD, the hallmark of CP includes new-onset or worsening abdominal pain, distention and

M. Tonolini
Radiology Department, "Luigi Sacco" University
Hospital, Via G.B. Grassi 74, Milan 20157, Italy
e-mail: mtonolini@sirm.org

© Springer International Publishing Switzerland 2016
M. Tonolini (ed.), *Imaging Complications of Gastrointestinal and Biliopancreatic Endoscopy Procedures*, DOI 10.1007/978-3-319-31211-8_13

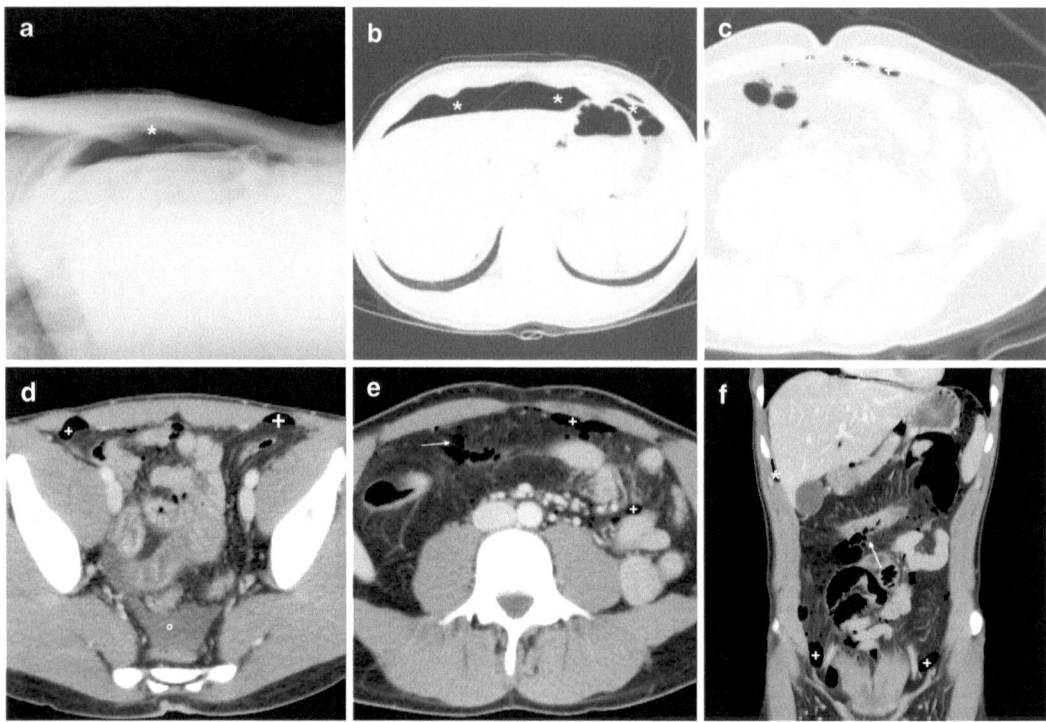

Fig. 13.1 Iatrogenic perforation in a 28-year-old male with ileocolonic Crohn's disease (CD), who suffered from acute abdominal pain and peritonitis immediately after colonoscopy, interrupted because of an impassable stricture of the descending colon. Tangential abdominal radiograph (**a**) showing nondependent air crescent (*) consistent with significant pneumoperitoneum. Immediate multidetector CT (**b–f**) confirmed 3-cm thick supramesocolic pneumoperitoneum (*) best visible with lung window settings (**b, c**) associated with minimal inframesocolic free air (+) and fluid in the peritoneal cul-de-sac (*o* in **d**). The perforation site in the transverse colon was identified as a focal mural discontinuity (*thin arrows* in **e**, **f**) from which air is directly seen flowing outside the lumen. The patient underwent urgent laparoscopy with creation of ileostomy, followed by elective recanalisation and segmental resection of the colonic stricture

fever after colonoscopy. When CP is clinically suspected, urgent chest and abdominal (preferably upright) radiographs are usually requested in most patients. However, borrowing from experience with spontaneous perforations, plain films have only moderate (below 50–70 %) sensitivity for free air. In patients unable to stand, significant pneumoperitoneum may be appreciated radiographically as increased lucency over the liver in the supine projection and nondependent air crescent in tangential or lateral decubitus views (Fig. 13.1) [3, 4].

Conversely, due to its excellent sensitivity for detection of extraluminal air and free fluid, CT represents the preferred modality for investigation of suspected CP. Including visualisation at lung or bone window settings, careful interpretation of CT studies may effectively show the perforation site, most usually indicated by coalescent foci of extraluminal gas and/or fluid and sometimes directly identifiable as a focal bowel wall discontinuity (Figs. 13.1 and 13.2). Additionally, peritoneal effusion (Fig. 13.1) and serosal thickening or hyperenhancement support a diagnosis of peritonitis [3–6]. Alternatively, similarly to the general population characteristic, CT findings consistent with post-polypectomy electrocoagulation syndrome (PPES) may be observed including segmental circumferential thickening of the colonic wall at the site of recent polypectomy, associated

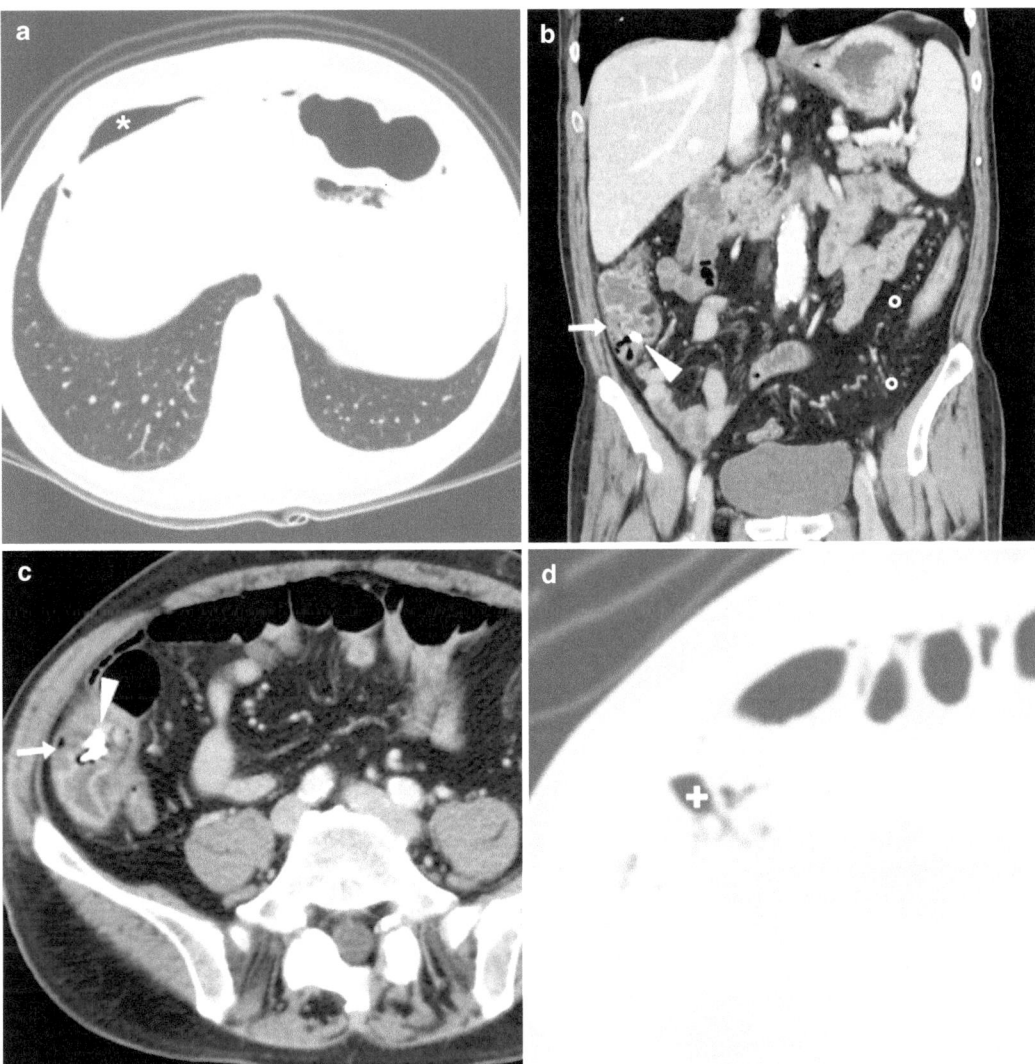

Fig. 13.2 Iatrogenic caecal perforation during endo-scopic submucosal dissection in a 71-year-old male with ulcerative colitis (UC) and a 2-cm flat granular lesion with central ulceration, treated endoscopically with four clips. Unenhanced (**a**) and post-contrast (**b**, **c**) images from urgent multidetector CT showed minimal subphrenic pneumoperitoneum (* in **a**), focal oedematous-type mural thickening of the caecum (*arrows* in **b**, **c**) and presence of metallic clips (*arrowheads*). Detailed CT image at lung window settings (**d**) showing the perforation site identi-fied by minimal extraluminal air (+) flowing outside (*thin arrow*) the ventral aspect of the caecum. The patient then underwent total proctocolectomy with J-pouch creation and protective ileostomy

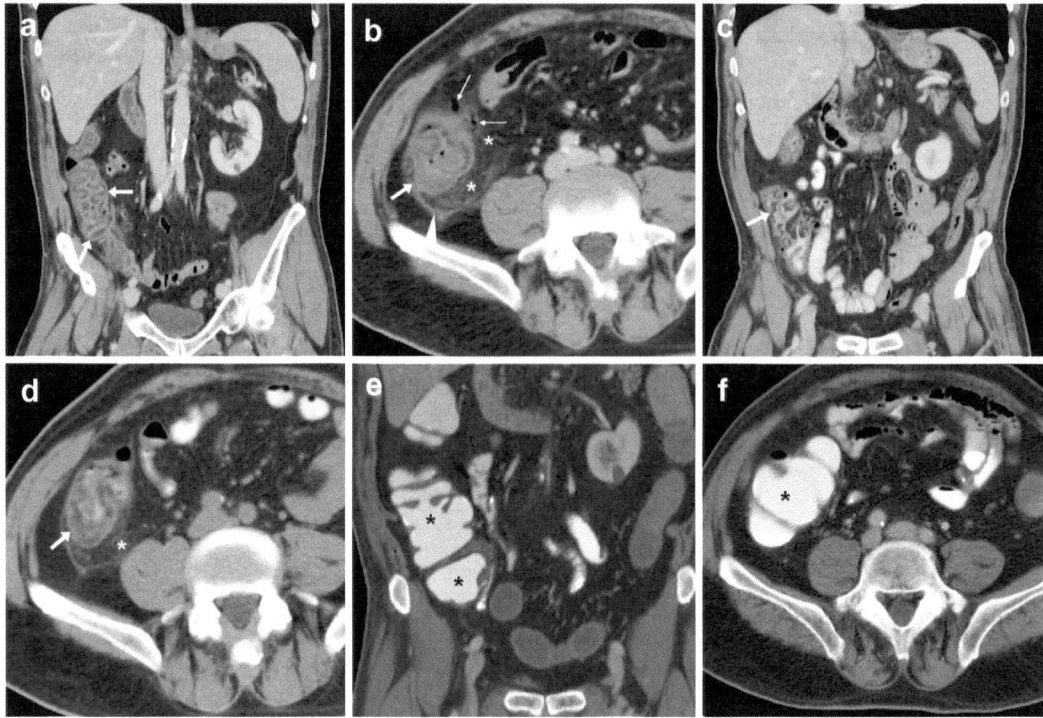

Fig. 13.3 One day after endoscopic polypectomy with diathermic loop and peripheral coagulation with argon plasma probe of a sessile polyp of the ascending colon, a 61-year-old patient with UC suffered from fever and right-sided abdominal pain without peritonism, with laboratory findings of elevated C-reactive protein (67 mg/L) and leucocytosis (11,510 cells/mmc). Urgent contrast-enhanced multidetector CT (**a**, **b**) showed stratified mural thickening of the caecum and ascending colon (*arrows*) with oedematous submucosa, inflammatory stranding of the pericaecal fat (*), two millimetric gas bubbles (*thin arrows*) and minimal fascial fluid (*arrowhead* in **b**) consistent with post-polypectomy electrocoagulation syndrome (PPES). Conservative treatment allowed resolution of symptoms and laboratory changes over a few days. Repeated CT a week later (**c**, **d**) showed decreasing oedematous mural thickening of the caecum (*arrows*) and near-complete regression of iatrogenic perivisceral (*) and fascial changes. Follow-up CT with positive intraluminal contrast (**e**, **f**) showed well-distended right hemicolon (*) with normal mural thickness and normalised perivisceral structures

with pericolonic fluid and inflammatory-type fat stranding (Fig. 13.3) [5–7].

13.3 Case Presentation: Colonoscopic Perforation in Crohn's Disease

A 26-year-old woman had a long-standing history of stricturing-type ileocolonic CD refractory to medical therapies and previous ileocolonic resection 9 years earlier. Two years earlier an excluding loop ileostomy was created to obviate obstruction due to anal and rectosigmoid stenosis. Currently hospitalised to undergo elective anal dilatation, she underwent colonoscopy which confirmed severe stiffness of the sigmoid and descending colon and impassable ileocolonic anastomosis because of stricturing relapse with inflamed friable mucosal surface. The planned anal dilatation was ultimately not performed.

Hours after endoscopy, she complained of progressively worsening abdominal pain. Plain radiographs (Fig. 13.4a, b) and CT (Fig. 13.4c–f) showed abundant intraperitoneal free air and identified the site of perforation at the descending colon [8].

Whereas in the general population early diagnosis and treatment of CP are crucial to limit morbidity and mortality, in IBD patients the treatment decision between surgery and

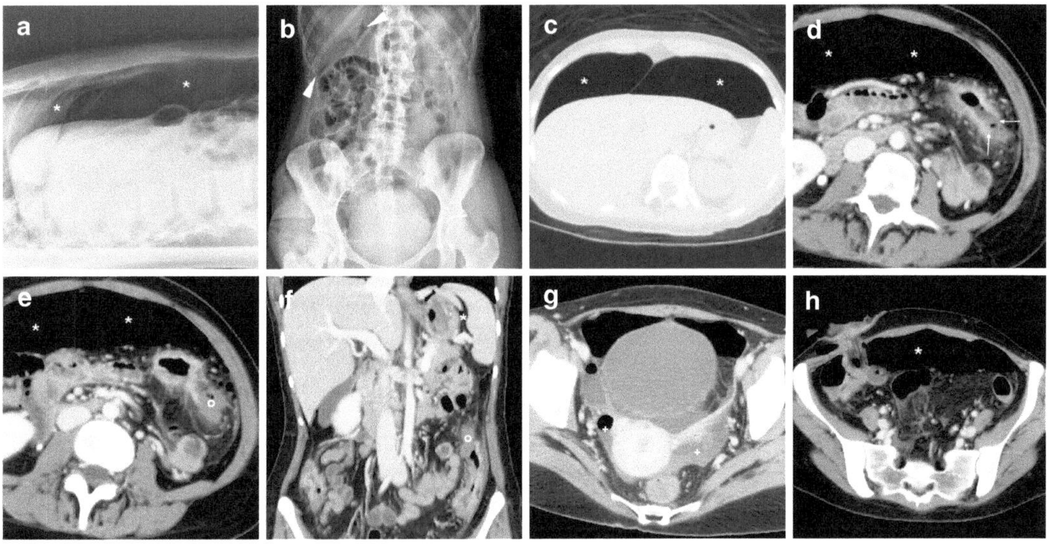

Fig. 13.4 Post-procedural tangential abdominal radiograph showed massive pneumoperitoneum (*), poorly appreciable in the supine projection as increased lucency outlining the liver (*arrowheads* in **b**). Urgent multidetector CT (**c–f**) confirmed free pneumoperitoneum (*) and showed the descending colon with enhancing wall thickening and hypervascularity of the mesentery with prominent vasa recta ("comb sign") consistent with active CD. Additionally, a mural discontinuity (*thin arrows*) consistent with perforation was clearly visible, from which enteral material and gas flowed in a collection (o) abutting the large bowel. Repeated contrast-enhanced CT 72 h later (**g, h**) showed persistent pneumoperitoneum (*) and moderate peritoneal effusion (+) with enhancing peritoneal serosa (Partly reproduced with permission from Ref. no [8])

nonoperative strategy should ultimately be based upon a combination of factors, particularly regarding underlying colonic disease, presence or absence of peritonitis and postoperative bowel anatomy. In this patient conservative treatment including bowel rest, hydration and intravenous antibiotic allowed progressive resolution of symptoms and of physical abnormalities. Follow-up CT 3 days later showed stable findings concerning perforation and appearance of mild pelvic peritonitis (Fig. 13.4g, h). The attending surgeon chose to delay elective recanalisation after clinical improvement [1, 8–10].

References

1. Buisson A, Chevaux JB, Hudziak H et al (2013) Colonoscopic perforations in inflammatory bowel disease: a retrospective study in a French referral centre. Dig Liver Dis 45:569–572
2. Navaneethan U, Parasa S, Venkatesh PG et al (2011) Prevalence and risk factors for colonic perforation during colonoscopy in hospitalized inflammatory bowel disease patients. J Crohns Colitis 5:189–195
3. Borofsky S, Taffel M, Khati N et al (2014) The emergency room diagnosis of gastrointestinal tract perforation: the role of CT. Emerg Radiol 22:315–327
4. Maniatis V, Chryssikopoulos H, Roussakis A et al (2000) Perforation of the alimentary tract: evaluation with computed tomography. Abdom Imaging 25:373–379
5. Kim DH, Pickhardt PJ, Taylor AJ et al (2008) Imaging evaluation of complications at optical colonoscopy. Curr Probl Diagn Radiol 37:165–177
6. Wax BN, Katz DS, Badler RL et al (2006) Complications of abdominal and pelvic procedures: computed tomographic diagnosis. Curr Probl Diagn Radiol 35:171–187
7. Benson BC, Myers JJ, Laczek JT (2013) Postpolypectomy electrocoagulation syndrome: a mimicker of colonic perforation. Case Rep Emerg Med 2013:687931
8. Pagani A, Tonolini M, Bareggi E (2014) EuroRAD Case 11741. Colonoscopic perforation in Crohn's disease {Online}. URL: http://www.eurorad.org/case.php?id=11741. doi:10.1594/EURORAD/CASE.11741
9. Castellvi J, Pi F, Sueiras A et al (2011) Colonoscopic perforation: useful parameters for early diagnosis and conservative treatment. Int J Colorectal Dis 26:1183–1190
10. Samalavicius NE, Kazanavicius D, Lunevicius R et al (2013) Incidence, risk, management, and outcomes of iatrogenic full-thickness large bowel injury associated with 56,882 colonoscopies in 14 Lithuanian hospitals. Surg Endosc 27:1628–1635

Imaging of Complications of Colonic Stents

Brice Malgras, Athur Berger, Paul Bazeries,
Christophe Aubé, Mourad Boudiaf,
and Philippe Soyer

14.1 Introduction

Intestinal obstruction may be the revealing symptom of colorectal cancer in up to 30 % of patients. Previous studies have reported poor outcome and substantial postoperative mortality for patients with obstructive colorectal cancers [1–3]. Emergency surgery, although controversial, is an option in this situation but conveys high morbidity (40–60 %) and mortality (8–20 %) [4, 5]. Moreover, for patients with left colonic obstruction, up to 40–60 % of them ultimately have permanent stoma after emergency surgery [3]. In order to improve these results, self-expandable metallic stents (SEMS) have been proposed since the 1990s, first as a palliative treatment and then as a bridge to surgery [6, 7].

14.2 Indications

14.2.1 Palliative Treatment in Malignant Stenosis

Two different clinical situations must be distinguished. For patients with very poor lifetime expectancy, stent insertion is associated with a better quality of life and less unnecessary surgery. For patients with longer lifetime expectancy who will receive chemotherapy, SEMS can avoid stoma, which is generally permanent, and is associated with lower morbidity rate, shorter time to first chemotherapy, better quality of life and similar survival compared to surgery [8–11]. Two randomised controlled trials reported a lower rate of stoma performance, a better quality of life [12]

B. Malgras, MD (✉)
Department of Surgical Oncology, Hôpital
Lariboisière, AP-HP, 2, rue Ambroise-Paré,
Paris cedex 10 75475, France

Sorbonne Paris Cité, Université Diderot-Paris 7,
10, avenue de Verdun, Paris 75010, France

UMR Inserm 965, Hôpital Lariboisière,
2, rue Ambroise-Paré, Paris 75010, France
e-mail: bricemalgras@hotmail.com

A. Berger, MD
Department of Gastroenterology and Hepatology,
CHU d'Angers, Angers 49933, France

P. Bazeries, MD • C. Aubé, MD, PhD
Department of Radiology, CHU d'Angers,
Angers 49933, France

M. Boudiaf, MD
Department of Abdominal and Interventional
Imaging, Hôpital Lariboisière,
AP-HP, 2, rue Ambroise-Paré, Paris cedex 10 75475,
France

P. Soyer, MD, PhD
Sorbonne Paris Cité, Université Diderot-Paris 7,
10, avenue de Verdun, Paris 75010, France

UMR Inserm 965, Hôpital Lariboisière,
2, rue Ambroise-Paré, Paris 75010, France

Department of Abdominal and Interventional
Imaging, Hôpital Lariboisière, AP-HP, 2, rue
Ambroise-Paré, Paris cedex 10 75475, France

© Springer International Publishing Switzerland 2016
M. Tonolini (ed.), *Imaging Complications of Gastrointestinal and Biliopancreatic Endoscopy
Procedures*, DOI 10.1007/978-3-319-31211-8_14

and a shorter hospital stay for patients who received SEMS placement in comparison with those who were treated by surgery. A third randomised controlled trial was terminated prematurely because of safety considerations related to a high colonic perforation rate in the SEMS group [13], especially delayed perforations in patients who were treated by systemic chemotherapy and antiangiogenic drug (bevacizumab) [10]. Some authors reported that adjuvant bevacizumab therapy nearly tripled the risk of colonic perforation in the case of stent placement [14]. Authors claimed that surgery was probably necessary after SEMS insertion in metastatic patients (as a bridge to surgery) when a prolonged chemotherapy is considered with potential curative treatment of metastases. Regarding cost–benefit analysis, SEMS seems to be better than surgery in most of the studies [8, 9, 15]. In conjunction with shorter hospital stay and lower complications, cost reductions of 20 and 30 % have been reported in the palliative and bridge to surgery groups, respectively [16]. In the case of palliative treatment, risk factors for complication after stent insertion include proximal location of the stricture (right colon), extrinsic lesions, history of radiation and chemotherapy with bevacizumab [14, 17, 18].

14.2.2 SEMS as a "Bridge to Surgery"

SEMS as a "bridge to surgery" is used as a preoperative temporary step to relieve colonic obstruction before definitive "elective" one-stage surgical therapy 8–10 days later in patients with malignant colonic stenosis. Several studies have retrospectively compared SEMS and surgery used in combination to surgery alone and found that the combination of SEMS with surgery was associated with a lower need for stoma, shorter operative time, low morbidity rate, low intensive care stay and, at a lesser degree, a lower early mortality rate by comparison with surgery alone [8, 9].

One randomised controlled trial reported that SEMS as a "bridge to surgery" was associated with more occurrences of "one-step" surgery, less permanent stoma rate, low morbidity rate, less blood loss and less anastomotic fistulas or

wound infection [19]. Also, in a meta-analysis, SEMS as a "bridge to surgery" conveyed higher number of successful primary anastomosis and lower overall stoma rates, with no significant differences in complications and mortality rates [4]. This approach is now validated in the NICE (National Institute for Clinical Excellence) process [4, 20, 21]. Moreover, a recent meta-analysis showed that SEMS as a "bridge to surgery" was equivalent to emergency surgery in terms of overall survival, disease-free survival and recurrence [22].

To tone down some encouraging results, two randomised controlled trials have been terminated prematurely because of safety concerns due to colonic perforations and unexpected high morbidity rate [23, 24]. In the same time, concerns have been raised regarding oncological issues of SEMS. Of note, SEMS is associated with a high incidence of clinical and "silent" perforations, with an estimated incidence of 10–20 % [25, 26]. In this regard, clinical perforation of colon cancer is considered as a favouring factor for the development of peritoneal carcinomatosis after curative surgery for colon cancer [27]. Another putative risk comes from stent insertion itself and further expansion within the tumour. The problems resulting from stent insertion include tumour perforation, altered pathology and tumour cell dissemination [25, 28]. Indeed in a recent report, some authors have shown a lower overall and disease-free survival associated with shorter recurrence time in the group of patients who received stent placement by comparison with patients who had surgery [29]. Other authors observed that stent placement was associated with a significantly higher rate of local tumour recurrence compared to emergency resection ($P = 0.038$). However, none of these studies were randomised trials and therefore their results must be considered with caution.

14.2.3 External Malignant Colonic Stenosis

Colonic stenosis due to external compression by a tumour or peritoneal carcinomatosis usually results in failed SEMS placement. This is because such strictures are long and multiple, resulting in a failure rate of approximately 60 % [17]. Only strictures of the transverse colon due to gastric cancer compression have an acceptable rate of clinical success of approximately 80 % [30].

14.2.4 Benign Colonic Strictures

The use of SEMS in colonic obstruction due to a benign cause remains controversial and should be restricted to patients with tight, recurring strictures after repeated dilations or to patients who deny or who are not eligible to surgery [31–33]. The use of colonic stents for anastomotic, diverticular, radiation-induced and Crohn disease colonic strictures has been documented in retrospective studies and case reports [34]. The rate of technical success (i.e. successful stent placement) is between 90 and 100 %, but the clinical success rate is lower whatever the type of stent (uncovered, fully/partially covered stents). This is due to high morbidity rate along with a high rate of delayed complications [34]. Indeed stent migration has been reported in approximately 40 % of patients, especially in anastomotic strictures or when covered stents are used. The perforation rate in inflammatory stenosis is approximately 20 %, especially in diverticular diseases. Also, clinical success is low in radiation-induced stenosis because of marked parietal stiffness of the colon. Although several authors suggest avoidance of SEMS placement in diverticular or radiation-induced colonic strictures, its use in anastomotic strictures seems to be promising especially with biodegradable stents or covered stents that can be easily removed.

14.3 Results

Technical success of stent placement is defined by a successful insertion of the stent across the stricture. Technical success is obtained in 90 % of patients with colonic stenosis, whatever the causative lesion [8, 9]. Technical failure of SEMS placement is most commonly due to the inability to pass the guidewire across the stricture, especially in cases with tortuous angulated anatomy, poor colonic preparation, marked bowel peristalsis or marked strictures [9, 35, 36].

14.4 Complications of Colonic Stent Placement

Colonic stent placement is generally considered as a low risk procedure because of a mortality rate of approximately 1 % [37, 38].

Complications associated with colonic SEMS can be classified as early complications, including perforation, bleeding and misplacement, and late complications including mainly stent migration, reobstruction and erosion or fistulisation of the intestinal wall [36, 39]. Risk factors for complications are male gender, stent diameter ≤22 mm, complete colonic obstruction, operator experience and stricture dilation during SEMS insertion [14].

Self-limited haemorrhage occurs in less than 5 % of colonic stent placement and is generally a minor complication, most likely related to the tumour itself, and does not require a specific treatment [33, 36, 40].

Colonic perforation is the most serious complication and occurs in approximately 5 % of the procedures, with reported incidences ranging from 0 to 83 % [9, 37]. However, the mortality rate can reach up to 10 % [37]. In a systematic review, Khot et al. have reported 3 deaths in a total of 565 colonic stent placements; 2 of them were due to colonic perforation [37]. Colonic perforation is predominantly observed in patients who had balloon dilation of the colonic stenosis or incomplete initial stent deployment [37, 41, 42]. Risk factors for early perforation following stent placement are balloon dilation prior to stent insertion, which try to pass the stenosis with the endoscope or excessive manipulation of guidewires, especially in the presence of diverticular disease or colon wall ischaemia [42]. The type and size of the stent must be carefully selected to match stenosis and colonic features in order to avoid stent incarceration. Late perforations are generally associated with systemic chemotherapy and thus require surgery 3–6 months after stent insertion.

The migration rate of colonic stents is about 11 %, with reported incidences ranging from 0 to 50 % [9, 15]. Most of the stents migrate distally and are automatically expelled through the anus, while symptomatic stents may be removed endoscopically. Stent migration can be favoured by chemotherapy that is responsible for tumour shrinkage or can be observed in patients who had prior laser debulking or over balloon dilation that leads to secondary obstruction [36]. Others factors that predispose to stent migration include treatment of partial obstructions or extrinsic compressions, small stent diameter, colonic angulation, insufficient length to allow stent flaring, postoperative radiotherapy and benign lesions [33, 39, 41]. Stent migration occurs also three times more frequently with stents placed in the distal rectum compared to those placed in the left colon [43]. Use of non-covered or longer/larger diameter stents seems to reduce the risk of migration.

Stent obstruction is most frequently observed in patients who had palliative stent placement and occurs in about 10 % of these patients [38]. Tumour overgrowth is the most common cause of stent obstruction, whereas ingrowth through the stent lattice, mucosal prolapse, stent fracture and faecal impaction is less frequent [9, 37, 42]. In the case of stent obstruction due to cancer progression, laser/argon therapy, stent in stent, placement or surgery can be done [38]. In the case of stool impaction, medical or endoscopic desobstruction is mandatory. The risk of stool impaction can be limited using dedicated low-residue diet and use of osmotic laxative.

14.5 Imaging Features

Whereas X-ray imaging using enema with water-soluble contrast agent has been used in the past to assess the degree of luminal stenosis and the length of the stenosis, currently, multidetector-row computed tomography (MDCT) using water

enema is the favoured imaging technique for a comprehensive evaluation before colonic stent placement [44]. One advantage of MDCT is that it helps determine the cause of colonic obstruction. In this regard, obstruction can be due to intraluminal tumour process but also to extraluminal compression by pelvic neoplasm or peritoneal carcinomatosis. MDCT with water enema is also used to determine the site of the obstruction and the number of sites of obstruction. It is currently acknowledged that multiple sites of obstruction render the patient unsuitable for stent placement [42].

In patients with suspected complications following colonic stenting, MDCT is usually performed using oral water. The use of oral positive contrast material is restricted to patients with clinical suspicion of perforation or fistula.

Before stent placement, colon perforation must be excluded. This is best depicted using MDCT. After stent placement, X-ray image of the abdomen and pelvis is performed to ensure correct placement and optimal expansion. This is

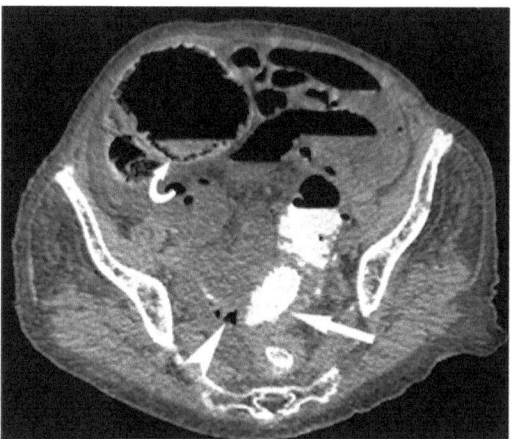

Fig. 14.1 A 98-year-old woman who had emergency colonic stent placement for acute left colonic obstruction. Axial MDCT image obtained after enema with water-soluble contrast agent showed metallic stent (*arrow*) in the sigmoid colon. The stent showed poor expansion. The extraintestinal gas bubble (*arrowhead*) indicated perforation. Because of incomplete expansion, persisting right colon dilatation was still present with parietal pneumatosis (*curved arrow*). The patient required emergency surgery

also helpful for further comparison should stent migration be suspected [42]. However, X-ray pelvic radiography may show initially incomplete stent expansion that subsequently becomes complete during the following days.

Following colonic stent placement in patients with major colonic dilatation, MDCT can reveal presence of marked colonic oedema, which is assumed to indicate colonic ischaemia [42].

Colonic perforation due to stent placement is confirmed by MDCT. MDCT usually shows pneumoperitoneum and pericolic fluid accumulation (Fig. 14.1) [42]. However, in some cases, extraluminal free air may be very limited so that its presence must be carefully searched for (Fig. 14.2). The use of multiplanar reconstructions is helpful to confirm extraintestinal gas bubbles. Infection of pericolic fluid collection can be managed percutaneously using drain placement.

Finally, MDCT is often performed in patients who had stent placement and symptoms suggestive of colonic obstruction. MDCT can reveal reobstruction, which is predominantly due to tumour overgrowth. However, stent migration, tumour ingrowth (Figs. 14.3 and 14.4) and faecal obstruction can be responsible for reobstruction. MDCT is helpful to confirm optimal stent deployment and exclude stent migration.

Conclusion

Except for emergencies, stent insertion has to be discussed during a multidisciplinary cancer conference in order to define its use in a comprehensive approach. Caution must be taken concerning oncologic outcomes of stent insertion in malignant strictures. Also, benign strictures are increasingly treated with stents even if a low efficacy and high morbidity rates reduce its use in such indications.

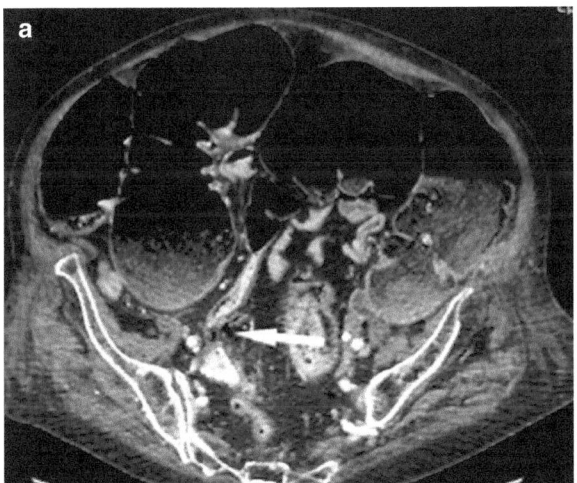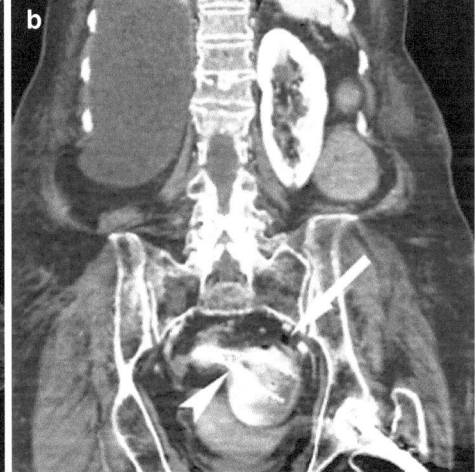

Fig. 14.2 An 83-year-old woman who had emergency colonic stent placement for acute left colonic obstruction and upstream colon dilatation. Axial MDCT image (**a**) obtained after enema with water-soluble contrast agent showed extraintestinal gas bubbles (*arrow*) indicating perforation. Because of incomplete expansion, marked right colon dilatation was still present. Coronal (**b**) MDCT image confirmed extraintestinal gas bubble (*arrow*) and incomplete expansion of metallic stent (*arrowhead*). The patient had emergency surgery

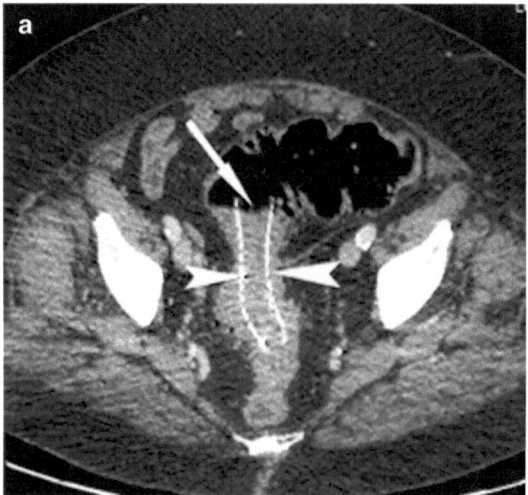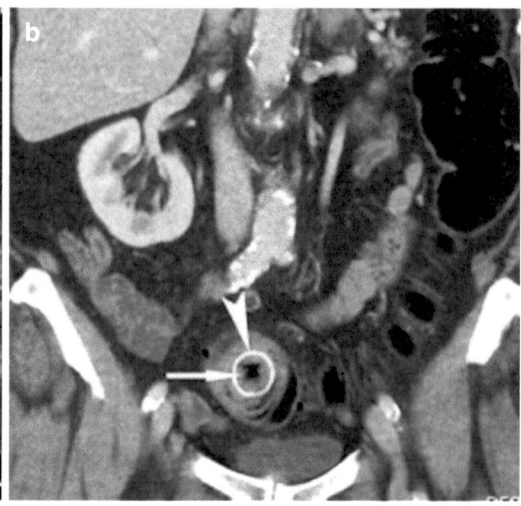

Fig. 14.3 An 83-year-old woman who had endoscopic metallic stent placement for adenocarcinoma of the sigmoid colon. Surgery was denied because of poor clinical status. Six months after stent placement axial (**a**) and coronal (**b**) MDCT images showed tumour ingrowth (*arrows*) within the stent lumen. The stent (*arrowhead*) showed normal deployment and no migration

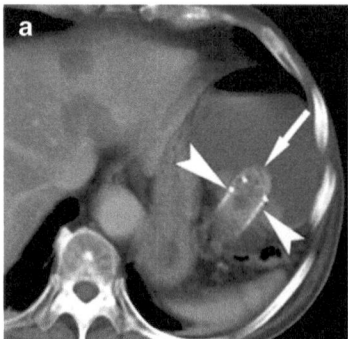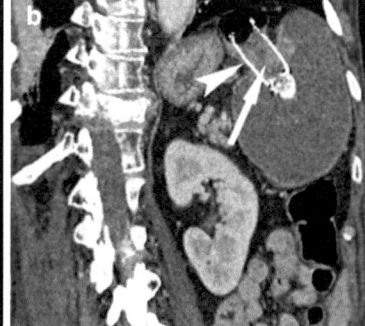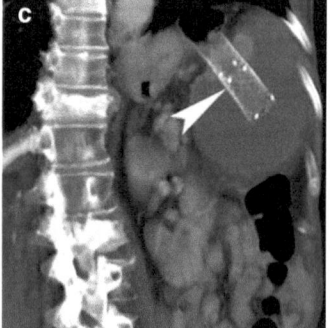

Fig. 14.4 A 66-year-old man who had endoscopic metallic stent placement for adenocarcinoma of the left colon. Four months after stent placement, the patient complained of abdominal distension and pain. Axial thick slab (**a**) and coronal (**b**) MDCT images showed tumour ingrowth (*arrow*) within the stent lumen. The stent (*arrowheads*) showed normal deployment and no migration. Coronal thick-slab (**c**) image confirmed correct position and optimal deployment of the stent (*arrowhead*)

References

1. Vibert E, Bretagnol F, Alves A, Pocard M, Valleur P, Panis Y (2007) Multivariate analysis of predictive factors for early postoperative death after colorectal surgery in patients with colorectal cancer and synchronous unresectable liver metastases. Dis Colon Rectum 50:1776–1782
2. Alves A, Panis Y, Mantion G, Slim K, Kwiatkowski F, Vicaut E (2007) The AFC score: validation of a 4-item predicting score of postoperative mortality after colorectal resection for cancer or diverticulitis: results of a prospective multicenter study in 1049 patients. Ann Surg 246:91–96
3. McArdle CS, Hole DJ (2004) Emergency presentation of colorectal cancer is associated with poor 5-year survival. Br J Surg 91:605–609
4. Tan CJ, Dasari BV, Gardiner K (2012) Systematic review and meta-analysis of randomized clinical trials of self-expanding metallic stents as a bridge to surgery versus emergency surgery for malignant left-sided large bowel obstruction. Br J Surg 99:469–476
5. Pearce NW, Scott SD, Karran SJ (1992) Timing and method of reversal of Hartmann's procedure. Br J Surg 79:839–841

6. Dohmoto M (1991) New method-endoscopic implantation of rectal stent in palliative treatment of malignant stenosis. Endosc Dig 3:1507–1512

7. Tejero E, Mainar A, Fernández L, Tobío R, De Gregorio MA (1994) New procedure for the treatment of colorectal neoplastic obstructions. Dis Colon Rectum 37:1158–1159

8. Tilney HS, Lovegrove RE, Purkayastha S, Sains PS, Weston- Petrides GK, Darzi AW et al (2007) Comparison of colonic stenting and open surgery for malignant large bowel obstruction. Surg Endosc 21:225–233

9. Watt AM, Faragher IG, Griffin TT, Rieger NA, Maddern GJ (2007) Self- expanding metallic stents for relieving malignant colorectal obstruction: a systematic review. Ann Surg 246:24–30

10. Karoui M, Charachon A, Delbaldo C, Loriau J, Laurent A, Sobhani I et al (2007) Stents for palliation of obstructive metastatic colon cancer: impact on management and chemotherapy administration. Arch Surg 142:619–623

11. Nagula S, Ishill N, Nash C, Markowitz AJ, Schattner MA, Temple L et al (2010) Quality of life and symptom control after stent placement or surgical palliation of malignant colorectal obstruction. J Am Coll Surg 210:45–53

12. Xinopoulos D, Dimitroulopoulos D, Theodosopoulos T, Tsamakidis K, Bitsakou G, Plataniotis G et al (2004) Stenting or stoma creation for patients with inoperable malignant colonic obstructions? Results of a study and cost-effectiveness analysis. Surg Endosc 18:421–426

13. Van Hooft JE, Fockens P, Marinelli AW, Timmer R, Van Berkel AM, Bossuyt PM et al (2008) Early closure of a multicenter randomized clinical trial of endoscopic stenting versus surgery for stage IV left-sided colorectal cancer. Endoscopy 40:184–191

14. Small AJ, Coelho-Prabhu N, Baron TH (2010) Endoscopic placement of self-expandable metal stents for malignant colonic obstruction: long-term outcomes and complication factors. Gastrointest Endosc 71:560–572

15. Sebastian S, Johnston S, Geoghegan T, Torreggiani W, Buckley M (2004) Pooled analysis of the efficacy and safety of self-expanding metal stenting in malignant colorectal obstruction. Am J Gastroenterol 99:2051–2057

16. Singh H, Latosinsky S, Spiegel BM, Targownik LE (2006) The cost- effectiveness of colonic stenting as a bridge to curative surgery in patients with acute left-sided malignant colonic obstruction: a Canadian perspective. Can J Gastroenterol 20:779–785

17. Keswani RN, Azar RR, Edmundowicz SA, Zhang Q, Ammar T, Banerjee B et al (2009) Stenting for malignant colonic obstruction: a comparison of efficacy and complications in colonic versus extracolonic malignancy. Gastrointest Endosc 69:675–680

18. Repici A, Adler DG, Gibbs CM, Malesci A, Preatoni P, Baron TH (2007) Stenting of the proximal colon in patients with malignant large bowel obstruction: techniques and outcomes. Gastrointest Endosc 66:940–944

19. Cheung HY, Chung CC, Tsang WW, Wong JC, Yau KK, Li MK (2009) Endolaparoscopic approach vs conventional open surgery in the treatment of obstructing left-sided colon cancer: a randomized controlled trial. Arch Surg 144:1127–1132

20. Van den Berg MW, Sloothaak DA, Dijkgraaf MG, van der Zaag ES, Bemelman WA, Tanis PJ et al (2014) Bridge to surgery stent placement versus emergency surgery for acute malignant colonic obstruction. Br J Surg 101:867–873

21. Choi JM, Lee C, Han YM, Lee M, Choi YH, Jang DK et al (2014) Long- term oncologic outcomes of endoscopic stenting as a bridge to surgery for malignant colonic obstruction: comparison with emergency surgery. Surg Endosc 28:2649–2655

22. Matsuda A, Miyashita M, Matsumoto S, Matsutani T, Sakurazawa N, Takahashi G et al (2015) Comparison of long-term outcomes of colonic stent as "bridge to surgery" and emergency surgery for malignant large bowel obstruction: a meta-analysis. Ann Surg Oncol 22:497–504

23. Van Hooft JE, Bemelman WA, Oldenburg B, Marinelli AW, Holzik MF, Grubben MJ et al (2011) Colonic stenting versus emergency surgery for acute left-sided malignant colonic obstruction: a multicentre randomised trial. Lancet Oncol 12:344–352

24. Pirlet IA, Slim K, Kwiatkowski F, Michot F, Millat BL (2011) Emergency preoperative stenting versus surgery for acute left-sided malignant colonic obstruction: a multicenter randomized controlled trial. Surg Endosc 25:1814–1821

25. Van Halsema EE, van Hooft JE, Small AJ, Baron TH, García- Cano J, Cheon JH et al (2014) Perforation in colorectal stenting: a meta-analysis and a search for risk factors. Gastrointest Endosc 79:970–982

26. Fryer E, Gorissen KJ, Wang LM, Guy R, Chetty R (2015) Spectrum of histopathological changes encountered in stented colorectal carcinomas. Histopathology 66:480–484

27. Honoré C, Goéré D, Souadka A, Dumont F, Elias D (2013) Definition of patients presenting a high risk of developing peritoneal carcinomatosis after curative surgery for colorectal cancer: a systematic review. Ann Surg Oncol 20:183–192

28. Maruthachalam K, Lash GE, Shenton BK, Horgan AF (2007) Tumour cell dissemination following endoscopic stent insertion. Br J Surg 94:1151–1154

29. Sabbagh C, Browet F, Diouf M, Cosse C, Brehant O, Bartoli E et al (2013) Is stenting as "a bridge to surgery" an oncologically safe strategy for the management of acute, left-sided, malignant, colonic obstruction? A comparative study with a propensity score analysis. Ann Surg 258:107–115

30. Shin SJ, Kim TI, Kim BC, Lee YC, Song SY, Kim WH (2008) Clinical application of self-expandable metallic stent for treatment of colorectal obstruction

caused by extrinsic invasive tumors. Dis Colon Rectum 51:578–583

31. Garcea G, Sutton CD, Lloyd TD, Jameson J, Scott A, Kelly MJ (2003) Management of benign rectal strictures: a review of present therapeutic procedures. Dis Colon Rectum 46:1451–1460

32. Paúl L, Pinto I, Gómez H, Fernández-Lobato R, Moyano E (2002) Metallic stents in the treatment of benign diseases of the colon: preliminary experience in 10 cases. Radiology 223:715–722

33. Suzuki N, Saunders BP, Thomas-Gibson S, Akle C, Marshall M, Halligan S (2004) Colorectal stenting for malignant and benign disease: outcomes in colorectal stenting. Dis Colon Rectum 47:1201–1207

34. Small AJ, Young-Fadok TM, Baron TH (2008) Expandable metal stent placement for benign colorectal obstruction: outcomes for 23 cases. Surg Endosc 22:454–462

35. Athreya S, Moss J, Urquhart G, Edwards R, Downie A, Poon FW (2006) Colorectal stenting for colonic obstruction: the indications, complications, effectiveness and outcome—5-year review. Eur J Radiol 60:91–94

36. Aitken DG, Horgan AF (2007) Endoluminal insertion of colonic stents. Surg Oncol 16:59–63

37. Khot UP, Lang AW, Murali K, Parker MC (2002) Systematic review of the efficacy and safety of colorectal stents. Br J Surg 89:1096–1102

38. Shim CS, Cho JY, Jung IS, Ryu CB, Hong SJ, Kim JO et al (2004) Through-the-scope double colonic stenting in the management of inoperable proximal malignant colonic obstruction: a pilot study. Endoscopy 36:426–431

39. Katsanos K, Sabharwal T, Adam A (2011) Stenting of the lower gastrointestinal tract: current status. Cardiovasc Intervent Radiol 34:462–473

40. Turégano-Fuentes F, Echenagusia-Belda A, Simó-Muerza G, Camuñez F, Muñoz-Jimenez F, Del Valle Hernandez E et al (1998) Transanal self-expanding metal stents as an alternative to palliative colostomy in selected patients with malignant obstruction of the left colon. Br J Surg 85:232–235

41. Baron TH, Dean PA, Yates MR, Canon C, Koehler RE (1998) Expandable metal stents for the treatment of colonic obstruction: techniques and outcomes. Gastrointest Endosc 47:277–286

42. Dharmadhikari R, Nice C (2008) Complications of colonic stenting: a pictorial review. Abdom Imaging 33:278–284

43. Alcantara M, Serra X, Bombardó J, Falcó J, Perandreu J, Ayguavives I et al (2007) Colorectal stenting as an effective therapy for preoperative and palliative treatment of large bowel obstruction: 9 years' experience. Tech Coloproctol 11:316–322

44. Ridereau-Zins C (2014) Imaging in colonic cancer. Diagn Interv Imag 95:475–483

Imaging Complications of Anorectal Endoscopic Procedures

15

Massimo Tonolini

15.1 Anorectal Iatrogenic Injuries: Imaging Techniques and Appearances

Nowadays, anoscopy and proctoscopy are commonly performed to investigate complaints and disorders pertaining to the anus and rectum. Furthermore, interventional endoscopic procedures may be performed to obtain tissue samples, to remove superficial lesions, to retrieve foreign bodies, to achieve haemostasis and to treat strictures. Although relatively uncommon compared to the large number of procedures performed, iatrogenic injuries such as haemorrhage, perforation, inflammation and infection may occur. High-risk situations include polypectomy, endoscopic mucosal resection (EMD), endoscopic submucosal dissection (ESD) and balloon dilatation [1, 2].

Patients with clinical suspicion of iatrogenic complications involving the anorectum require prompt dedicated imaging, due to the peculiar anatomic site and close proximity to the lower genitourinary tract. The rationale for early investigation involves (a) the increasing trend towards conservative treatment provided that injuries are promptly detected and categorised and (b) the possibility to adopt endoscopic treatments such as clip placement before further morbidity (particularly peritoneal contamination) occurs. In the vast majority of cases, multidetector CT with and without intravenous contrast medium (CM) is warranted and arguably the preferred technique to investigate suspected anorectal injuries prior to surgical consultation. However, ionising radiation exposure from CT represents a significant concern which should be taken into consideration particularly in children and young patients [1, 2]. Practically, the role of conventional abdominal radiographs is limited to the detection of pneumoperitoneum, signs of bowel obstruction, radio-opaque retained foreign bodies or surgical clips. Conversely, plain radiographs are insensitive for limited or extraperitoneal perforations [3, 4].

15.1.1 Rectal Perforation

Iatrogenic rectal perforation may occur during blind introduction of the endoscope, during the colonoscopic retroflexion manoeuvre or during stricture dilatation or biopsy; occasionally, perforation may be induced by anorectal manometry, particularly in patients with postsurgical anatomic changes [1, 5].

From the surgical viewpoint the key issue is the distinction between intraperitoneal and extraperitoneal rectal injuries. Perforations occurring at the serosalised anterior and lateral sidewalls of the upper two-thirds of the rectum are classified

M. Tonolini
Radiology Department, "Luigi Sacco" University Hospital, Via G.B. Grassi 74, Milan 20157, Italy
e-mail: mtonolini@sirm.org

© Springer International Publishing Switzerland 2016
M. Tonolini (ed.), *Imaging Complications of Gastrointestinal and Biliopancreatic Endoscopy Procedures*, DOI 10.1007/978-3-319-31211-8_15

as intraperitoneal and usually require surgical repair and faecal diversion. Conversely, lesions involving the distal one-third of the rectum circumferentially and the upper two-thirds of the rectum posteriorly are considered extraperitoneal and can be managed nonsurgically [6, 7].

Commonly observed CT findings after rectal interventional endoscopic procedures include increased "hazy" attenuation of the presacral or mesorectal fat (Fig. 15.1) corresponding to oedematous "fat stranding" and unspecific reversible rectal wall thickening (Fig. 15.2). Borrowing from experience with spontaneous perforations, CT is extremely sensitive for even small extraluminal gas collections from visceral perforation, which usually collect near the injury site, thus hinting at its location (Fig. 15.3). Air may remain within the subperitoneal space or track along the extraperitoneal and retroperitoneal fascial planes. Conversely, perforation of intraperitoneal rectal segments leads to the formation of peritoneal effusion and pneumoperitoneum (Fig. 15.3) [8, 9].

Whereas barium sulphate preparations are contraindicated when perforation is suspected, in selected patients retrograde administration of water-soluble iodinated CM before CT (Fig. 15.4) may be beneficial to confirm or exclude a concealed perforation. Borrowing from experience with traumatic lesions, this technique allows direct visualization of rectal perforations indicated by extraluminal CM leakage and differentiation between intra- and extra-peritoneal injuries, thereby providing correct injury diagnosis and presurgical classification [3, 7, 10, 11].

15.1.2 Rectal Bleeding

Early or delayed rectal haemorrhage is reported to occur after up to 1–2 % endoscopic procedures, most usually polypectomy, EMR or ESD, secondary to inadequate electrocautery or incomplete tissue shearing. Immediate bleeding detected during endoscopy may be controlled by cautery, epinephrine injection and placement of hemostatic clips. Conversely, when a patient presents with haematochezia after an endoscopic procedure, CT angiography with rapid

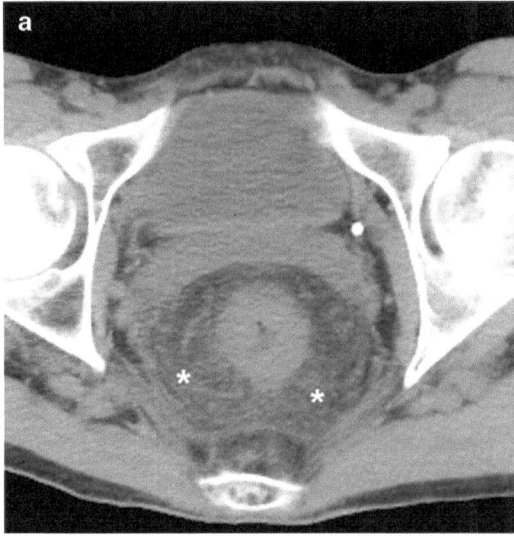
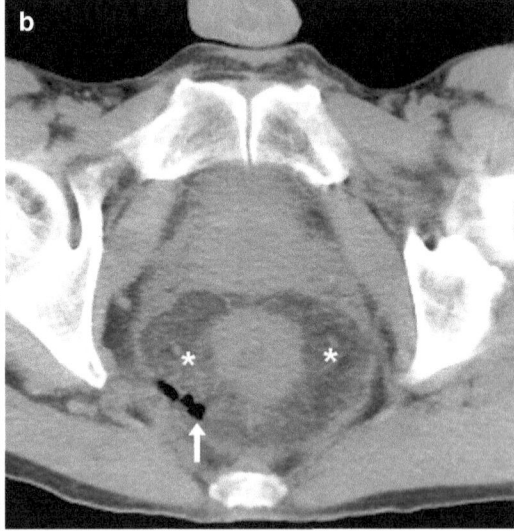
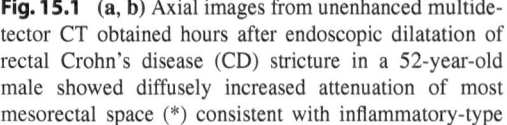

Fig. 15.1 (a, b) Axial images from unenhanced multidetector CT obtained hours after endoscopic dilatation of rectal Crohn's disease (CD) stricture in a 52-year-old male showed diffusely increased attenuation of most mesorectal space (*) consistent with inflammatory-type "fat stranding" plus a limited amount of extraluminal gas (*arrow*) abutting the right posterolateral aspect of the mesorectal fascia. The patient had an uneventful course after conservative treatment but later required elective surgical resection of the intractable stricture

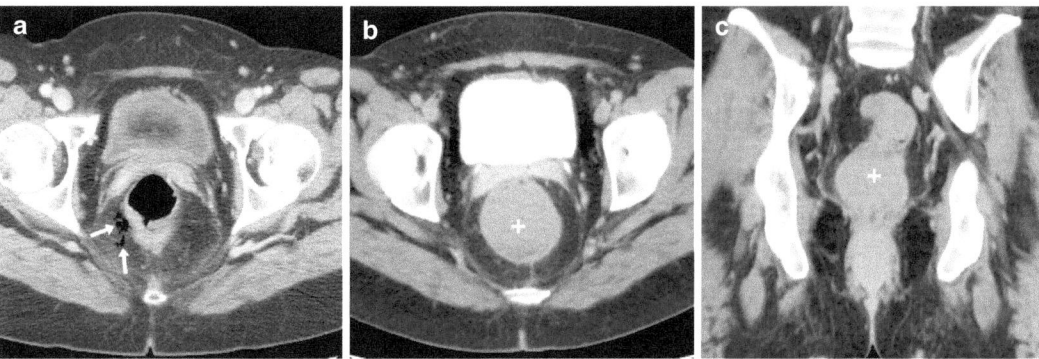

Fig. 15.2 Shortly after rectal endoscopic polypectomy, a 62-year-old female suffered from pelvic dull pain. Initial contrast-enhanced multidetector CT (**a**) showed minimal thickening of the posterior rectal wall and a limited collection of extraluminal air consistent with minimal perfora-tion. After conservative treatment, repeated unenhanced CT (**b**, **c**) with preliminary filling of the urinary bladder with iodinated contrast and of the rectosigmoid with tap water (+) demonstrated resolved rectal thickening and normalised mesorectal planes

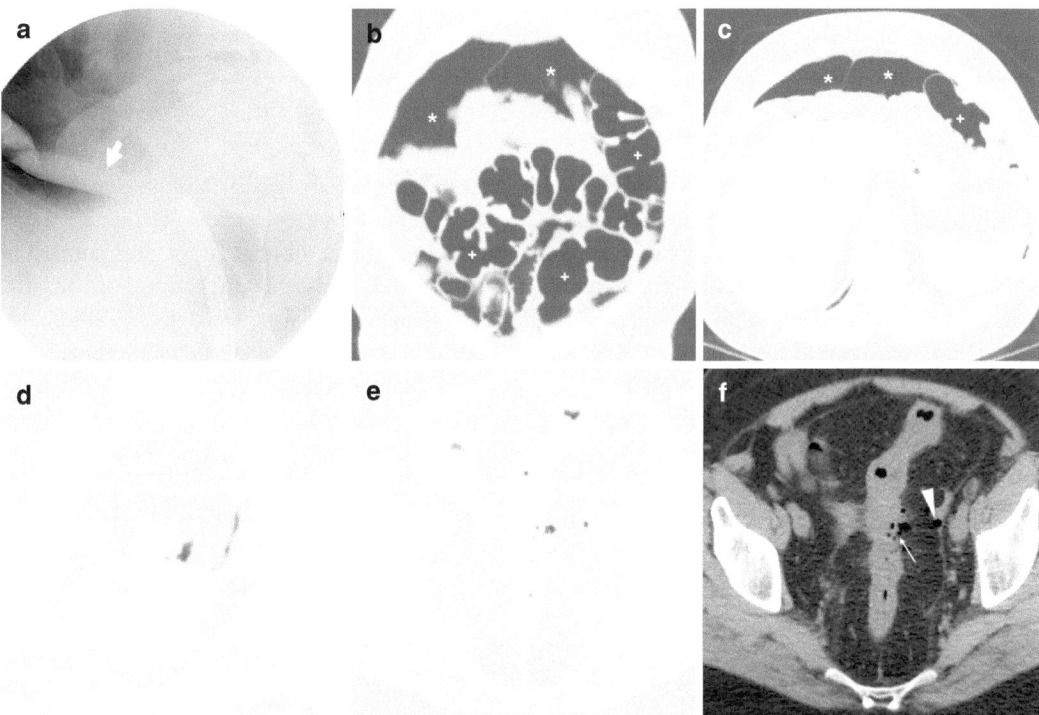

Fig. 15.3 A 53-year-old female was hospitalised to undergo endoscopic balloon dilatation (*short arrow* in **a**) of CD stricture of the rectosigmoid junction. Early post-procedural CT revealed the appearance of large, predomi-nantly supramesocolic intraperitoneal air (* in **b**, **c**). Note dilated large bowel after endoscopic insufflation (+). The site of perforation was identifiable at the rectosigmoid junction as a focal discontinuity (*thin arrows*) in the bowel wall, from which gas flowed out along the peritoneal serosa (*arrowheads*) (**d**–**f**). Follow-up imaging after conservative treatment (not shown) confirmed resolved pneumoperitoneum and excluded formation of abnormal fluid collections

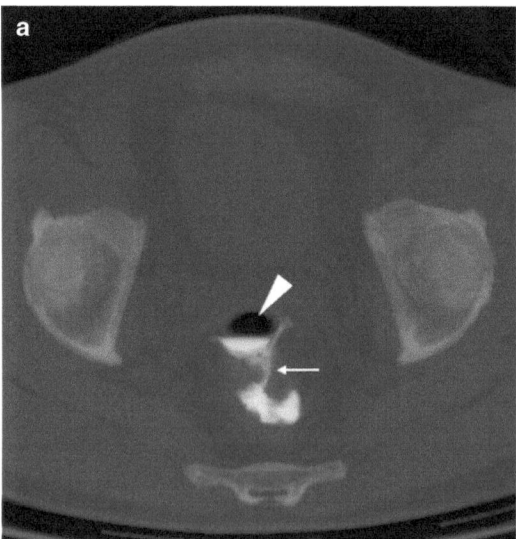 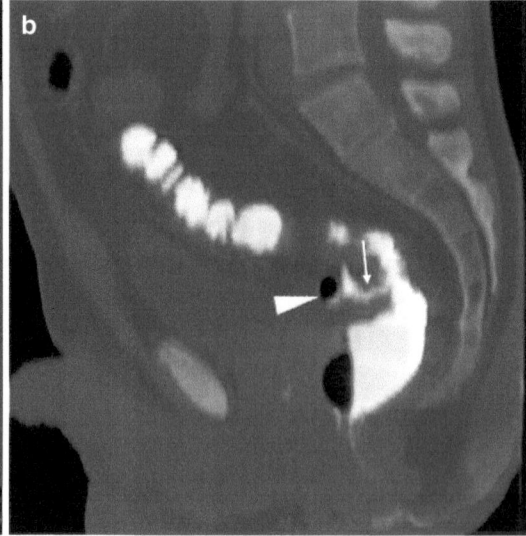

Fig. 15.4 Unenhanced CT obtained after administration of water-soluble contrast enema (sodium–meglumine diatrizoate, Gastrografin ®) through a thin, soft rectal tube in a 38-year-old male with rectal bleeding and pelvic and perineal pain after recreational rectal self-insertion of a hard-consistency, unsharp foreign object. Axial (**a**) and sagittal (**b**) images viewed at bone window settings showed well-distended rectum, an air–fluid collection (*arrowheads*) in the peritoneal cul-de-sac partially opacified through ventral extraluminal leak from the proximal rectum (*thin arrows*) and patent upstream sigmoid. Intraperitoneal rectal perforation was diagnosed and the patient underwent primary surgical repair (Adapted from Ref. [11])

(at least 3–4 ml/s) bolus injection of iodinated CM is warranted. When bleeding is suspected, the unnecessary oral or rectal administration of diluted CM should be obviated since it may mask haemorrhage. A preliminary unenhanced acquisition may reveal intraluminal dense fluid consistent with fresh blood or higher-attenuation clots hinting to the site of bleeding. Correlation with precontrast scans is necessary to differentiate haemorrhage from other high-density materials such as old enteral CM, pills or sutures. CM-enhanced acquisition, most usually including arterial and portal venous phases, depicts active bleeding as intraluminal CM extravasation with a variable configuration and attenuation generally exceeding 90–100 HU [8, 9, 12–15].

15.1.3 Iatrogenic Infections

Although magnetic resonance imaging (MRI) represents the best imaging technique to visualise perianal fistulas and abscesses, in acute settings, multidetector CT is more readily available and highly effective to investigate patients with clinical and laboratory features suggesting suspected anorectal sepsis. The use of MRI-like multiplanar reconstructions from volumetric multidetector CT acquisitions comprehensively depicts the relevant perianal and perineal structures (including the internal anal sphincter, the intersphincteric and anovaginal spaces and the external anal sphincter and levator ani muscles), thus allowing radiologists to provide surgeons a descriptive roadmap of the infectious process. The well-known CT appearance of abscesses includes variably shaped fluid collections with thickened enhancing walls, which may contain air and may be associated with surrounding inflammatory changes (see case presentation in paragraph 15.2). The intrinsic CT contrast resolution limits differentiation between soft tissue structures such as pelvic muscles, active inflammatory changes and fibrotic scar tissue. However, tubular fistulas can be identified when filled by air or fluid because of adequate contrast between their hypodense content and enhancing inflamed granulation tissue walls. Finally, an additional excretory-phase CT acquisition may be beneficial to assess possible associated urine leakage indicating injury to the lower urinary tract [14].

15.2 Case Presentation: Severe Perineal Infection Complicating Endoscopic Biopsy, Beware of Antibiotic Resistance!

A 61-year-old male suffered from high-grade fever, severe pain and tender hard-consistency perineal swelling without urinary symptoms, the day after anoscopy and biopsy of anal squamocellular carcinoma (Fig. 15.5). Laboratory assays revealed leukocytosis (20,000/mmc) and increased acute phase reactants (C-reactive protein 210 mg/L).

Urgent multidetector CT (Fig. 15.6) showed a post-biopsy fistula crossing the anorectal tumour and giving rise to a sizeable perineal abscess which extended along the anatomic site of the corpus spongiosum. Surgeons opted for incision and drainage of the perianal abscess. Pus cultures revealed antibiotic-resistant extended-spectrum beta-lactamase (ESBL)-producing *Escherichia coli*. Three days after surgery, with worsening perineal pain, scrotal swelling and septic fever, repeated CT (Fig. 15.7) showed persistent abscess with partial gaseous content,

dislocating the urethra but extrinsic to the spermatic fascia. Excretory-phase CT acquisition excluded urine leakage from iatrogenic lower urinary tract injury. Lack of clinical improvement after surgical drainage required creation of colostomy to allow fistula healing during planned chemoradiotherapy.

Following physical examination including digital rectal examination, proctologists commonly perform endoscopy and endoscopic-guided biopsy (AB) to diagnose abnormalities of the anorectal tract, particularly to differentiate precancerous (dysplastic) changes and invasive tumours from other non-malignant conditions. Similarly, urologists routinely perform transrectal ultrasound-guided prostate biopsy (TRUS-PB) to obtain tissue samples in patients with abnormal findings at digital examination or serum prostate-specific agent [16].

Routinely performed on outpatients using a standard empirical prophylaxis with ciprofloxacin, AB and TRUS-PB have been traditionally considered safe procedures. Limited complications including local bleeding and infection have been reported in less than 2 % of patients following TRUS-PB. However, in the current era of antibiotic resistance, rectal colonisation by fluoroquinolon-resistant bacteria poses an increasing concern for the development of post-biopsy complications. ESBL-producing organisms, mostly (83 %) represented by *Escherichia coli*, are present in the rectum in up to 8 % of

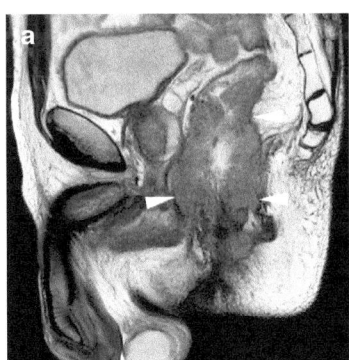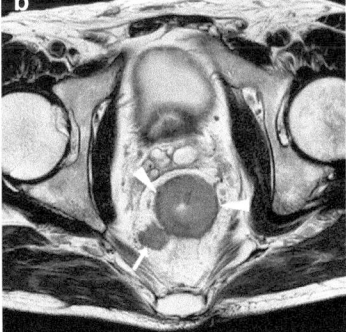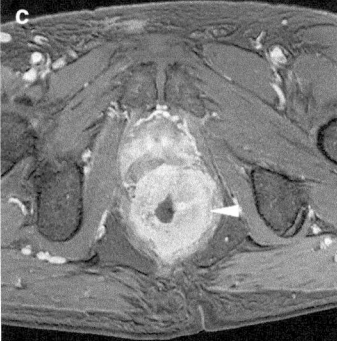

Fig. 15.5 Sagittal (**a**) and axial (**b**) T2-weighted MRI images show 9-cm long solid, circumferential mural thickening of the rectum (*arrowheads*) consistent with biopsy-proven squamocellular carcinoma, with a mesorectal adenopathy (*arrow* in **b**) and positive contrast enhancement on post-gadolinium fat-suppressed T1-weighted sequence (**c**)

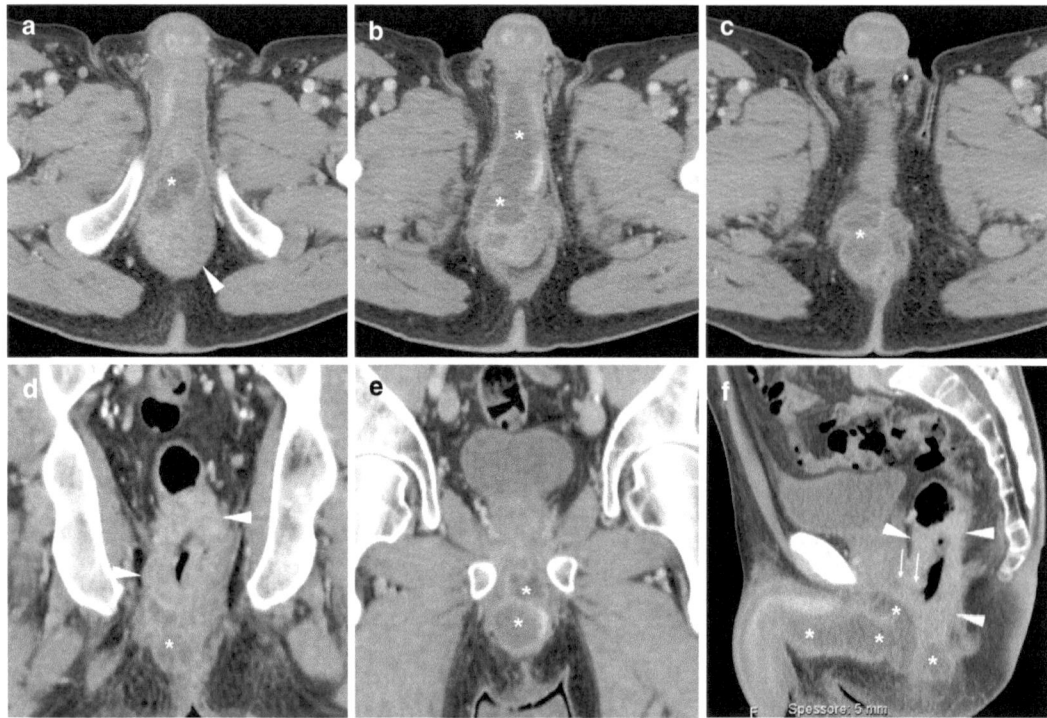

Fig. 15.6 Multiplanar contrast-enhanced images from post-biopsy multidetector CT of the pelvis. The known anorectal carcinoma (see Fig. 15.5) is clearly recognised as marked, homogeneously enhancing thickening (*arrowheads* in **d**, **f**). Additionally a hypoattenuating collection (*) with enhancing peripheral rim consistent with perineal abscess was seen abutting the ventral aspect of the distal anus (**a**, **b**, **c**, **e**) and extending along the anatomic site of the corpus spongiosum. Note ventral hypoattenuating track consistent with post-biopsy fistula (*thin arrows* in **f**) crossing through the tumour, giving rise to the perineal abscess

individuals. History of previous quinolone exposure represents a crucial risk factor for infection and subsequent hospitalisation following biopsy. Despite prophylaxis, documented rectal colonisation by resistant organisms is associated with a significantly increased risk of post-biopsy infection (6.6 % versus 1.6 %) and hospitalisation (4.4 % versus 0.95 %) [17–20]. Very recently, targeted antimicrobial prophylaxis and rectal cleansing by means of povidone–iodine enema are increasingly used and

seem effective to limit the rate of infectious complications (0.3 % versus 3.5 % without) after biopsy, by reducing the rectal bacterial load [19, 20].

As this case exemplifies, post-biopsy complaints (such as perineal pain or swelling, difficulty urinating, bleeding or discharge, fever and systemic signs of sepsis) and abnormal laboratory inflammatory markers should not be underestimated since they may herald a serious complication [17–20].

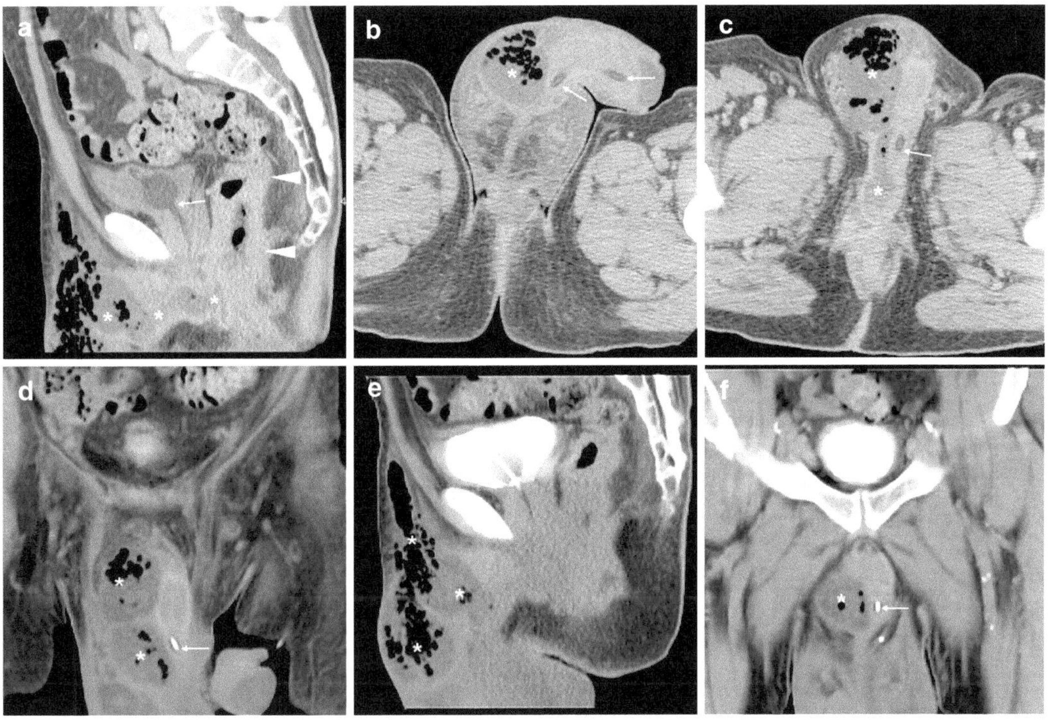

Fig. 15.7 Follow-up contrast-enhanced multidetector CT (**a–d**) after surgical drainage and catheterisation (*thin arrows*). Compared to Fig. 15.6, multiplanar images show persistent perineal abscess with partial gaseous content (*) extending ventrally from the anus, dislocating the ure- thra (*thin arrows*) but extrinsic to the ipsilateral spermatic fascia. Additionally, maximum intensity projection (MIP) reconstructions from excretory-phase acquisition (**e, f**) excluded extraluminal urine leak indicating injury to the lower urinary tract

References

1. Paspatis GA, Dumonceau JM, Barthet M et al (2014) Diagnosis and management of iatrogenic endoscopic perforations: European Society of Gastrointestinal Endoscopy (ESGE) position statement. Endoscopy 46:693–711
2. Sartelli M, Viale P, Catena F et al (2013) 2013 WSES guidelines for management of intra-abdominal infections. World J Emerg Surg 8:3
3. Hellinger MD (2002) Anal trauma and foreign bodies. Surg Clin N Am 82:1253–1260
4. Borofsky S, Taffel M, Khati N et al (2015) The emergency room diagnosis of gastrointestinal tract perforation: the role of CT. Emerg Radiol 22:315–327
5. Park JS, Kang SB, Kim DW et al (2007) Iatrogenic colorectal perforation induced by anorectal manometry: report of two cases after restorative proctectomy for distal rectal cancer. World J Gastroenterol 13:6112–6114
6. McGrath V, Fabian TC, Croce MA et al (1998) Rectal trauma: management based on anatomic distinctions. Am Surg 64:1136–1141
7. Weinberg JA, Fabian TC, Magnotti LJ et al (2006) Penetrating rectal trauma: management by anatomic distinction improves outcome. J Trauma 60:508–513; discussion 513–514
8. Saddala P, Ramanathan S, Tirumani SH et al (2015) Complications of minimally invasive procedures of the abdomen and pelvis: a comprehensive update on the clinical and imaging features. Emerg Radiol 22:283–294
9. Kim DH, Pickhardt PJ, Taylor AJ et al (2008) Imaging evaluation of complications at optical colonoscopy. Curr Probl Diagn Radiol 37:165–177
10. Bondia JM, Anderson SW, Rhea JT et al (2009) Imaging colorectal trauma using 64-MDCT technology. Emerg Radiol 16:433–440
11. Tonolini M (2013) Images in medicine: diagnosis and pre-surgical triage of transanal rectal injury using multidetector CT with water-soluble contrast enema. J Emerg Trauma Shock 6:213–215
12. Jaeckle T, Stuber G, Hoffmann MH et al (2008) Acute gastrointestinal bleeding: value of MDCT. Abdom Imaging 33:285–293
13. Horton KM, Jeffrey RB Jr, Federle MP et al (2009) Acute gastrointestinal bleeding: the potential role of

64 MDCT and 3D imaging in the diagnosis. Emerg Radiol 16:349–356

14. Khati NJ, Sondel Lewis N, Frazier AA et al (2015) CT of acute perianal abscesses and infected fistulae: a pictorial essay. Emerg Radiol 22:329–335

15. Wax BN, Katz DS, Badler RL et al (2006) Complications of abdominal and pelvic procedures: computed tomographic diagnosis. Curr Probl Diagn Radiol 35:171–187

16. Glynne-Jones R, Northover JM, Cervantes A (2010) Anal cancer: ESMO clinical practice guidelines for diagnosis, treatment and follow-up. Ann Oncol 21(Suppl 5):v87–v92

17. Taylor AK, Zembower TR, Nadler RB et al (2012) Targeted antimicrobial prophylaxis using rectal swab cultures in men undergoing transrectal ultrasound guided prostate biopsy is associated with reduced incidence of postoperative infectious complications and cost of care. J Urol 187:1275–1279

18. Liss MA, Taylor SA, Batura D et al (2014) Fluoroquinolone resistant rectal colonization predicts risk of infectious complications after transrectal prostate biopsy. J Urol 192:1673–1678

19. Gyorfi JR, Otteni C, Brown K et al (2014) Periprocedural povidone-iodine rectal preparation reduces microorganism counts and infectious complications following ultrasound-guided needle biopsy of the prostate. World J Urol 32:905–909

20. Hwang EC, Jung SI, Seo YH et al (2015) Risk factors for and prophylactic effect of povidone-iodine rectal cleansing on infectious complications after prostate biopsy: a retrospective cohort study. Int Urol Nephrol 47:595–601

Part V
Miscellanous Topics

Complications of Small Bowel Capsule Endoscopy

16

Massimo Tonolini

16.1 Capsule Endoscopy: Introduction and Indications

Available since 2001, capsule endoscopy (CE) has progressively emerged as an established, novel diagnostic tool that allows gastroenterologists to directly "see" the entire small bowel (SB) mucosa noninvasively. After being swallowed by the patient, the pill-like wireless videocapsule (Fig. 16.1) records over some hours of passage a digital image stream which is interpreted by the attending endoscopist. The majority (over 80%) of CE studies are completed with the capsule reaching the caecum within the recording time allowed by battery duration [1–3].

Although rather time consuming and without the ability to perform biopsy, currently CE represents the gold standard in evaluating obscure gastrointestinal bleeding, in which a potential cause is identified in approximately 70% of patients. Other indications include diagnosis and surveillance of hereditary polyposis syndromes and suspected SB tumours, nonsteroidal anti-inflammatory drug (NSAID)-induced injury and celiac disease [1–3].

Furthermore, CE may be useful in patients with suspected and established Crohn's disease

(CD) or indeterminate inflammatory bowel disease (IBD), with a complementary role to mural techniques such as CT-enterography (CT-E) and MR-enterography (MR-E). According to the guidelines from the European Crohn's and Colitis Organization (ECCO), CE is indicated in patients with high clinical suspicion of CD despite negative ileocolonoscopy and cross-sectional imaging. CE has higher diagnostic yield for superficial mucosal changes and proximal SB lesions compared to double-contrast SB studies, CT-E and MR-E and a high negative predictive value for CD. In patients with established CD, mural assessment with CT-E or MR-E is preferred over CE, which should be reserved for unexplained symptoms, obscure bleeding or iron deficiency [2–7].

16.2 Capsule Endoscopy: Safety Issues and Contraindications

Generally considered a safe procedure in the vast majority of patients, CE may occasionally (in less than 1% of examinations) have clinically significant complications, including bronchial capsule aspiration, interference with implantable cardiac devices and intestinal perforation. However, the commonest and most feared complication is videocapsule retention (VCR), associated with theoretical risk for SB obstruction. VCR is defined as the "presence of

M. Tonolini
Radiology Department, "Luigi Sacco" University
Hospital, Via G.B. Grassi 74, Milano 20157, Italy
e-mail: mtonolini@sirm.org

© Springer International Publishing Switzerland 2016
M. Tonolini (ed.), *Imaging Complications of Gastrointestinal and Biliopancreatic Endoscopy Procedures*, DOI 10.1007/978-3-319-31211-8_16

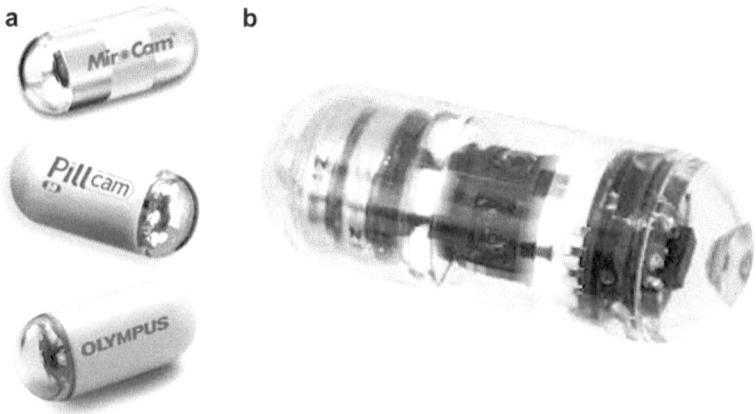

Fig. 16.1 Available from different manufacturers, wireless endoscopic videocapsules (**a**) measure approximately 2.5 cm in length and weigh less than 5 g. The internal structure of a videocapsule is partly perceptible (**b**, see radiographic image in Fig. 16.2b for comparison)

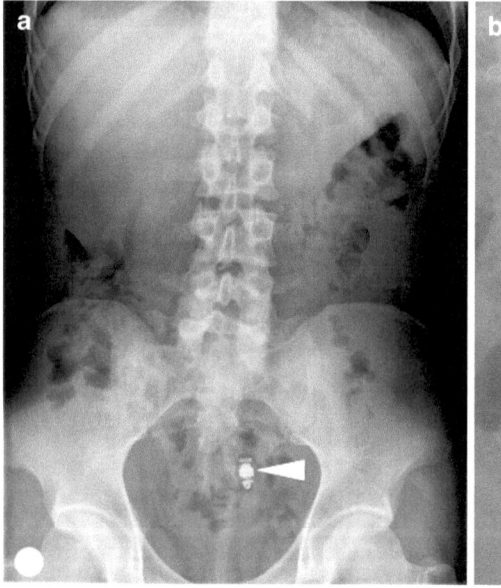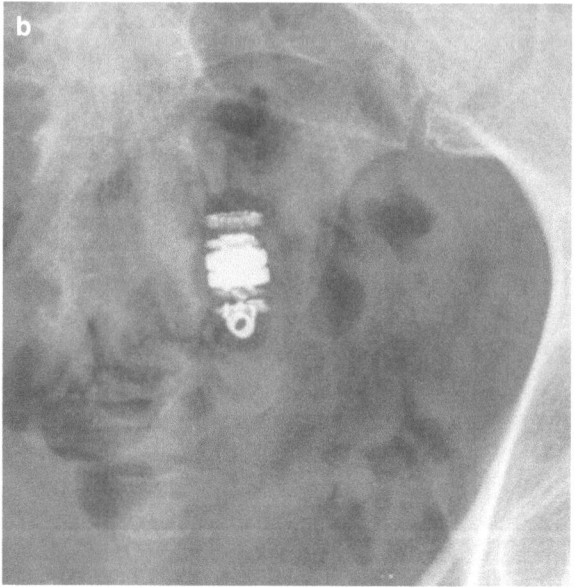

Fig. 16.2 On a supine plain abdominal radiograph, the endoscopic videocapsule (*arrowhead*) projects over the pelvic inlet (**a**) consistent with an ileal location. Detail radiographic view (**b**) allows to check for integrity of the retained endoscopic capsule (see Fig. 16.1b for comparison) and exclude detached radio-opaque fragments

the capsule in the digestive tract for at least 2 weeks after ingestion or when indefinite retention requires targeted medical, endoscopic or surgical treatment". Reported in 1.2–2.1 % of patients overall, VCR is favoured by inflammatory, neoplastic or postsurgical lumen narrowing reaching a 5–13 % incidence in patients with known CD [5, 8–13].

Commonly asymptomatic, VCR may last even for 2–3 years or alternatively cause partial or complete mechanical bowel obstruction within a month, occasionally SB perforation. Retained capsules are eventually evacuated in a highly variable proportion (13–71 %) of patients [3, 6, 8–13].

Due to its metallic internal parts, the endoscopic videocapsule is highly radio-opaque

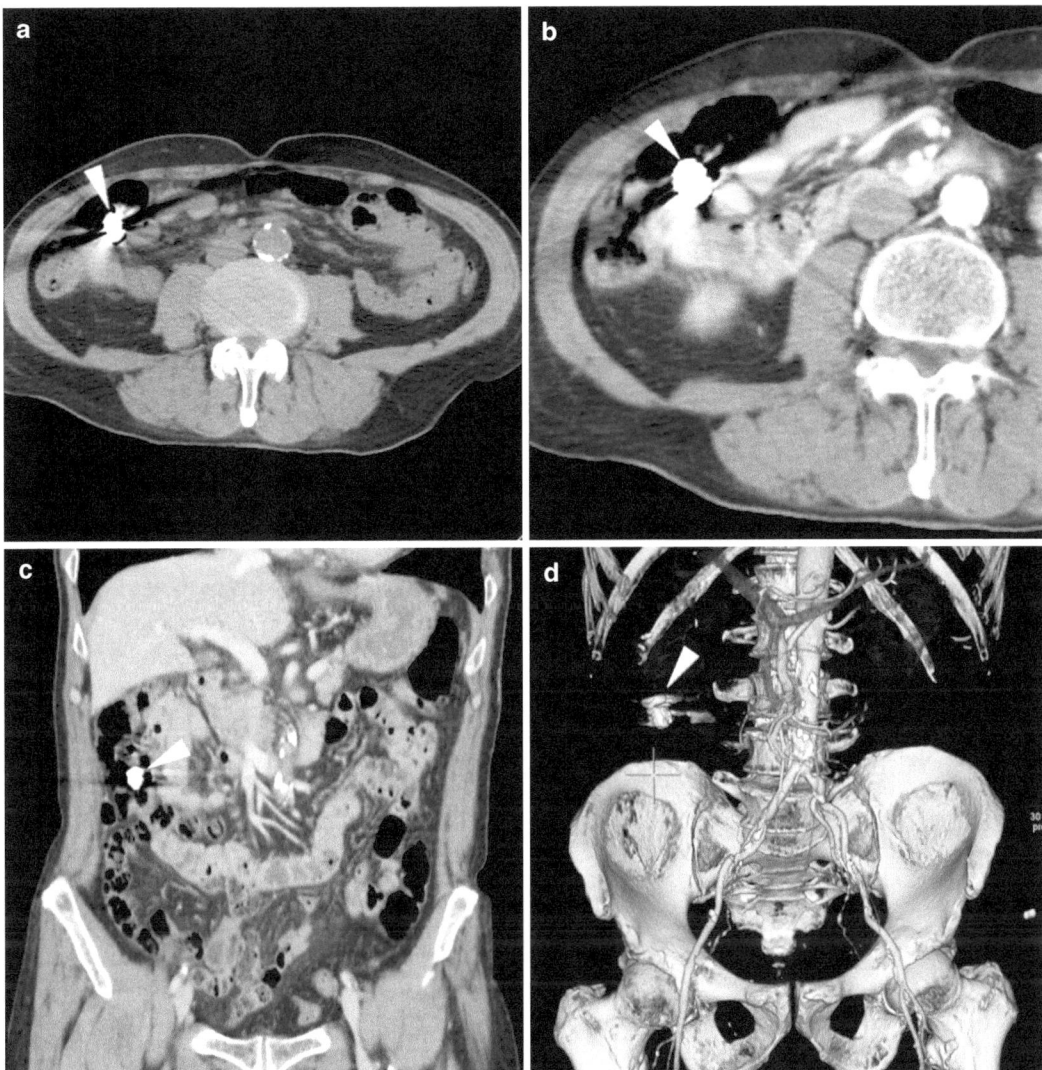

Fig. 16.3 Axial and coronal images from multidetector CT study requested from suspected acute bleeding during capsule endoscopy. Unenhanced acquisition (**a**) did not detect hyperattenuating intraluminal fluid consistent with fresh blood in the small bowel (SB) loops and colonic lumen. Repeated scanning after intravenous contrast medium (**b**, **c**) did not show contrast medium extravasa-tion indicating active arterial bleeding. Unfortunately, the CT study was significantly hampered by "streaky" beam-hardening artefacts caused from the metallic parts of the videocapsule (*arrowheads*) which appeared to be located in the ileum. Similarly, severe artefacts clearly alter the videocapsule's shape also in the volume-rendering three-dimensional image (**d**)

(Fig. 16.2) and therefore easily recognized on conventional radiographs (Fig. 16.2). As a result, bronchial videocapsule aspiration may also be diagnosed radiographically [1, 2].

Conversely, multidetector CT study of VCR may provide better anatomic delineation and clarify or exclude further complications such as bowel perforation, obstruction or acute bleeding. Unfortunately, CT images are significantly hampered by beam-hardening artefacts from the metallic structure of the videocapsule (Fig. 16.3). When failure of passage in stools occurs, serial radiographs (suggested on days 3, 7 and 14) allow to verify the intraabdominal location, to localize and monitor the videocapsule in the digestive tract, thus confirming diagnosis of VCR, and to detect signs of SB obstruction or perforation [12, 14, 15].

The choice between conservative, endoscopic and surgical management of VCR depends on the underlying cause and the capsule's position. Retained capsules requiring surgical removal are most commonly located proximally to ileal strictures from CD or NSAID enteritis, sometimes in the site of postoperative blind-ending loops, diverticula or obstructing tumours. Radiographic localisation of the retained capsule helps to confirm the diagnosis of VCR and to determine the retention site in the digestive tract and whether an upper, lower or complex (double-balloon enteroscopy) endoscopic approach is indicated. Surgery is performed in up to 29–87 % of VCR cases and is dictated by high-grade obstruction or signs of toxicity and necessary when endoscopic removal fails or is unfeasible [2, 3, 9–13]. Some authors advocate surgery for VCR to remove not only the capsule but also the causative stricture, thus relieving the patient's symptoms. On the other hand, VCR may lead to unnecessary surgery of lesions amenable to medical treatment such as active CD or medication-induced enteritis. After endoscopic or surgical removal of the retained videocapsule, prognosis of VCR is good unless in patients with underlying malignancy [5, 12, 16].

Considering the risk of VCR, contraindications for CE include bowel obstruction, known tumours, stricturing or extensive CD along with swallowing disorders and pregnancy. Unfortunately, a normal preprocedural radiographic study with SB follow-through or CT-E may under- or overestimate intestinal strictures and cannot effectively rule out the possibility of VCR. In recent years, the dissolving radio-opaque "patency test capsules" have been developed to confirm functional bowel patency. Therefore, their use is recommended to allow patients with obstructive symptoms, suspected or established CD to safely undergo CE [2–4, 6, 7, 9, 10].

16.3 Case Presentation: Endoscopic Videocapsule Retention in Crohn's Disease

In 2007, a 26-year-old male with medically treated SB CD since some years complained of low-grade obstructive symptoms. Prior to CE,

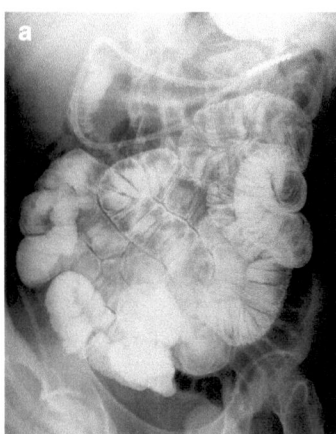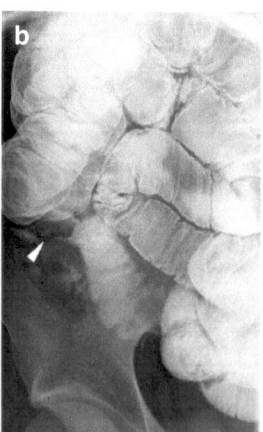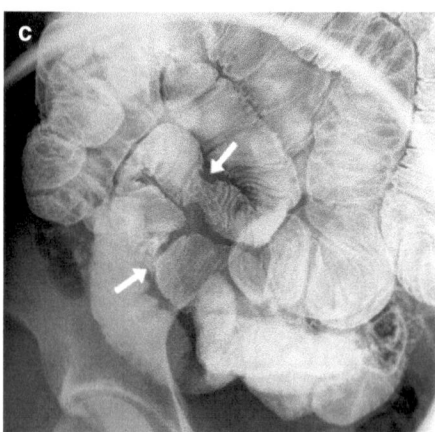

Fig. 16.4 A case of videocapsule retention (VCR) in a 26-year-old male. Prior to capsule endoscopy, double-contrast enteroclysis using duodenal intubation (**a**) showed a 6-cm stricture of the terminal ileum (*arrowhead* in **b**) in the characteristic site of known Crohn's disease (CD) plus two short poorly distended ileal segments (*arrows* in **c**) consistent with "skip" low-grade strictures

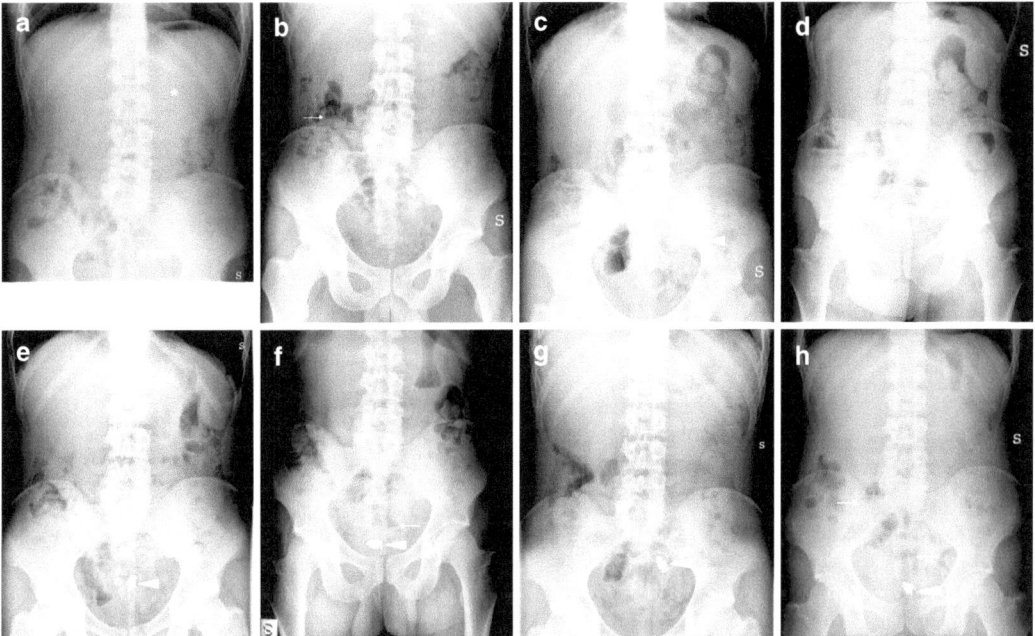

Fig. 16.5 Serial plain abdominal radiographs during VCR in CD. On day 3 after capsule ingestion, upright (**a**, **b**) films showed overdistended stomach (*) by ingested water. The radio-opaque endoscopic capsule (*arrowheads*) projected over the left pelvic inlet, consistent with location in the ileum. On day 7, repeated supine (**c**) and upright (**d**) radiographs showed unchanged position of the endoscopic capsule (*arrowheads*). On day 14, further supine (**e**) and upright (**f**) radiographs confirmed the pel-vic location of the endoscopic capsule (*arrowhead*), and still lodged in the ileum indicating VCR. Seven weeks after ingestion, before surgery with worsening abdominal discomfort supine (**g**) and upright (**h**) radiographs excluded pneumoperitoneum indicating bowel perforation, confirmed persistently retained endoscopic capsule (*arrowheads*). The progressive appearance of few air–fluid levels (*thin arrows* from **a–f**) was consistent with incomplete SB obstruction

with MR-enterography unavailable, the disease extent was assessed with double-contrast SB enteroclysis (Fig. 16.4). During reassessment for possible stricturoplasty or ileocaecal resection, gastroenterologists and surgeons requested CE. Within 3 days after ingestion, the videocapsule did not pass in stools. After failure of passage in stool, serial abdominal radiographs (day 3 to week 7 after ingestion, Fig. 16.5a–h) showed the radio-opaque endoscopic videocapsule projected over the left pelvis consistent with ileal location. According to clinical definition, diagnosis of VCR was confirmed radiographically on day 14. Meanwhile, the patient complained of intermittent abdominal pain and distension, with radiographic appearance (Fig. 16.5) of air–fluid levels consistent with incomplete bowel obstruction.

Seven weeks after ingestion, with worsening abdominal discomfort, repeated radiographs (Fig. 16.5g, h) excluded pneumoperitoneum and showed persistently retained videocapsule and ileal air–fluid levels.

Laparotomic surgery included enterotomy for removal of the retained videocapsule within a distal ileal loop, plus stricturoplasty of three ileal segments involved by circumferential CD strictures. Three years later, follow-up double-contrast SB enteroclysis (Fig. 16.6) showed good distension of most jejuno-ileal loops.

Fig. 16.6 Three years after episode of surgically treated VCR in CD, double-contrast SB enteroclysis showed good distension of most jejuno-ileal loops, with a residual short ileal segment (*arrows*) in the site of stricturoplasty

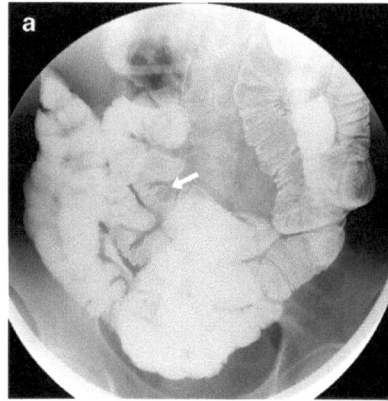
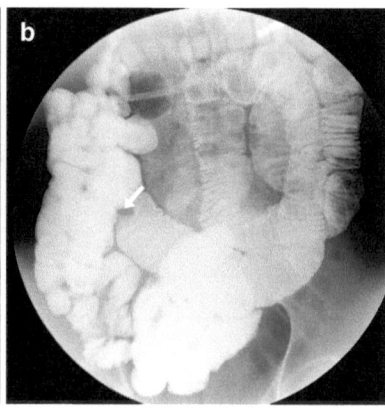

References

1. Rammohan A, Naidu RM (2011) Capsule endoscopy: new technology, old complication. J Surg Technol Case Rep 3:91–93
2. Rondonotti E, Soncini M, Girelli C et al (2010) Small bowel capsule endoscopy in clinical practice: a multicenter 7-year survey. Eur J Gastroenterol Hepatol 22:1380–1386
3. Van de Bruaene C, De Looze D, Hindryckx P (2015) Small bowel capsule endoscopy: where are we after almost 15 years of use? World J Gastrointest Endosc 7:13–36
4. Annese V, Daperno M, Rutter MD et al (2013) European evidence based consensus for endoscopy in inflammatory bowel disease. J Crohns Colitis 7:982–1018
5. Figueiredo P, Almeida N, Lopes S et al (2010) Small-bowel capsule endoscopy in patients with suspected Crohn's disease-diagnostic value and complications. Diagn Ther Endosc doi: 10.1155/2010/101285. Epub 2010 Aug 5
6. Kopylov U, Seidman EG (2014) Role of capsule endoscopy in inflammatory bowel disease. World J Gastroenterol 20:1155–1164
7. Van Assche G, Dignass A, Panes J et al (2010) The second European evidence-based consensus on the diagnosis and management of Crohn's disease: definitions and diagnosis. J Crohns Colitis 4:7–27
8. Bakhshi GD, Tayade MB, Jadhav KV et al (2014) Retention of an endoscopic capsule. J Minim Access Surg 10:163–165
9. Hoog CM, Bark LA, Arkani J et al (2012) Capsule retentions and incomplete capsule endoscopy examinations: an analysis of 2300 examinations. Gastroenterol Res Pract 2012:518718
10. Karagiannis S, Faiss S, Mavrogiannis C (2009) Capsule retention: a feared complication of wireless capsule endoscopy. Scand J Gastroenterol 44:1158–1165
11. Li F, Gurudu SR, De Petris G et al (2008) Retention of the capsule endoscope: a single-center experience of 1000 capsule endoscopy procedures. Gastrointest Endosc 68:174–180
12. Sachdev MS, Leighton JA, Fleischer DE et al (2007) A prospective study of the utility of abdominal radiographs after capsule endoscopy for the diagnosis of capsule retention. Gastrointest Endosc 66:894–900
13. Skovsen AP, Burcharth J, Burgdorf SK (2013) Capsule endoscopy: a cause of late small bowel obstruction and perforation. Case Rep Surg 2013:458108
14. Gayer G, Petrovich I, Jeffrey RB (2011) Foreign objects encountered in the abdominal cavity at CT. Radiographics 31:409–428
15. Shaish H, Gilet A, Gerard P (2015) "It's all foreign to me": how to decipher gastrointestinal intraluminal foreign bodies. Abdom Imaging, in press
16. Cheifetz AS, Lewis BS (2006) Capsule endoscopy retention: is it a complication? J Clin Gastroenterol 40:688–691

Interventional Radiology in the Treatment of Complications After Digestive and Biliopancreatic Endoscopy

17

Anna Maria Ierardi, Josè Urbano, Ejona Duka, Natalie Lucchina, and Gianpaolo Carrafiello

Iatrogenic complications are a major cause of morbidity and mortality. Advances in medicine have led to the development of sophisticated minimally invasive treatment techniques which have enabled to decrease the discomfort of iatrogenic complications.

Major adverse events related to diagnostic upper gastrointestinal (UGI) endoscopy are rare and include cardiopulmonary adverse events, infection, perforation and bleeding [1].

Procedures such as percutaneous drainage of fluid collections, percutaneous transhepatic biliary procedures, arterial embolisation and fistula embolisation are viable treatment options, with fewer complications compared with surgery, shorter hospital stay and faster recovery.

17.1 Percutaneous Drainage

Once an intra-abdominal collection is identified, in most cases it is possible to place a percutaneous drainage under image guidance.

The most common complications of endoscopic retrograde cholangiopancreatography (ERCP) and endoscopic ultrasonography-guided fine-needle aspiration (EUS-FNA) are acute pancreatitis and duodenal perforation. A pancreatic pseudocyst (PPC) is typically a complication of acute and chronic pancreatitis or pancreatic duct obstruction [2].

Several methods could be proposed to treat PPC. The recent trend in the management of symptomatic PPC has moved towards less invasive approaches such as endoscopic- and image-guided percutaneous catheter drainage (PCD). When possible, PCD is preferred because it permits monitoring, catheter manipulation and the analysis of cystic content. Earlier studies showed that conservative treatment in the hope of spontaneous resolution was not without risks. Several studies have warned against serious, life-threatening complications related to the conservative treatment of PPCs [3].

Complications related to PPC may be local (infection, haemorrhage and rupture) or may involve adjacent organs (stomach/duodenal stenosis and fistula, stenosis of common biliary duct, splenic rupture, arterial/venous erosion) [2]. In particular, PPC must be treated when

A.M. Ierardi (✉) • E. Duka • N. Lucchina
G. Carrafiello
Interventional Radiology Department, University of Insubria, Viale Borri 57, Varese 21100, Italy
e-mail: amierardi@yahoo.it; ejonaduka@hotmail.com; natalie.lucchina@hotmail.it; gcarraf@gmail.com

J. Urbano
Vascular and Interventional Radiology Department, Jiménez Díaz Foundation University Hospital, Av. Reyes Catolicos n° 2, Madrid 28040, Spain
e-mail: jurbano@fjd.es

© Springer International Publishing Switzerland 2016
M. Tonolini (ed.), *Imaging Complications of Gastrointestinal and Biliopancreatic Endoscopy Procedures*, DOI 10.1007/978-3-319-31211-8_17

symptomatic (abdominal distension, nausea and vomiting, pain, upper gastrointestinal bleeding) or when asymptomatic but >5 cm for more than 6 weeks and when thickness of cyst wall is more than 5 mm [2].

Image-guided percutaneous drainage of PPCs is a well-established and relatively inexpensive drainage method that involves either simple percutaneous aspiration or PCD. Single-step needle aspiration of PPCs is associated with a high recurrence rate (70 % or more) and cannot be considered the optimal treatment [4, 5].

The continuous vacuum drainage system is more effective because it continuously evacuates the cyst content and thereby avoids the lytic action of pancreatic enzymes that may lead to obliteration of the cyst cavity. This approach has achieved high initial drainage success rates (70–100 %) and reduced recurrence rates [4]. Patients with PPC-PD communication require a longer duration of drainage, as short-term drainage results in very high recurrence rates. However, some authors consider that the risk of septic complications is potentially increased with prolonged drainage periods [2].

Percutaneous techniques are usually performed under local anaesthesia and seem technically feasible in the most of patients. Transperitoneal, retroperitoneal, transhepatic, transgastric and transduodenal approaches are typically used.

When the collection is well visible using ultrasound (US), US-guided percutaneous drainage placement is generally the preferred choice, as US is widely available, easy to handle and allows for real-time monitoring of the drainage placement, being also free from ionizing radiation (Fig. 17.1a–d). When the collection is located deep in the abdomen and is not well seen at US, computed tomography (CT) generally offers good anatomical definition to guide the safe placement of a percutaneous drainage.

Depending on the operator's experience, drainage placement can be performed using the trocar or Seldinger technique. In the trocar technique, the drainage catheter containing a trocar needle is inserted directly into the collection. The trocar technique provides a fast deployment of the drainage that can be extremely helpful in critically ill or agitated patients. The Seldinger technique involves multiple steps: the collection is punctured with a small calibre needle, different calibre guidewires are inserted and the drainage is then advanced up to the collection over the guidewire. The Seldinger technique is especially useful when there is a small window to reach the collection, for example, when a retroperitoneal collection has to be drained through an anterior approach. The longer procedural time is the main disadvantage of this technique. The diameter of the draining tube should be bigger if the collections contain pus [6].

After complete evacuation of the cystic content, the catheter should be secured to the skin and connected to a pressure bag for continuous external drainage. Complications include catheter-related secondary infections (9 %), bleeding (1–2 %), inadvertent traversing of the pleural space or other viscera (1–2 %), catheter occlusion, cellulitis at the site of entry and sepsis [7]. Another limitation of PCD is the development of pancreatic-cutaneous fistulae [4, 8].

However, the resulting pancreatic-cutaneous fistula spontaneously resolves with time in 60–70 % of cases [4].

Even fluid collections that could arise from biliary or intestinal leak could also be managed with percutaneous drainage. Even acute diverticulitis after colonoscopy can hesitate in abscess development formation that may require percutaneous image-guided drainage [9, 10]. Same indications, considerations and techniques reported for PCD of PC may be considered in these cases [12].

17.2 Percutaneous Biliary Drainage

Possible iatrogenic complications that may arise after endoscopic procedures on the bile ducts and which can be treated with interventional radiology procedures are cholangitis and biliary leakage.

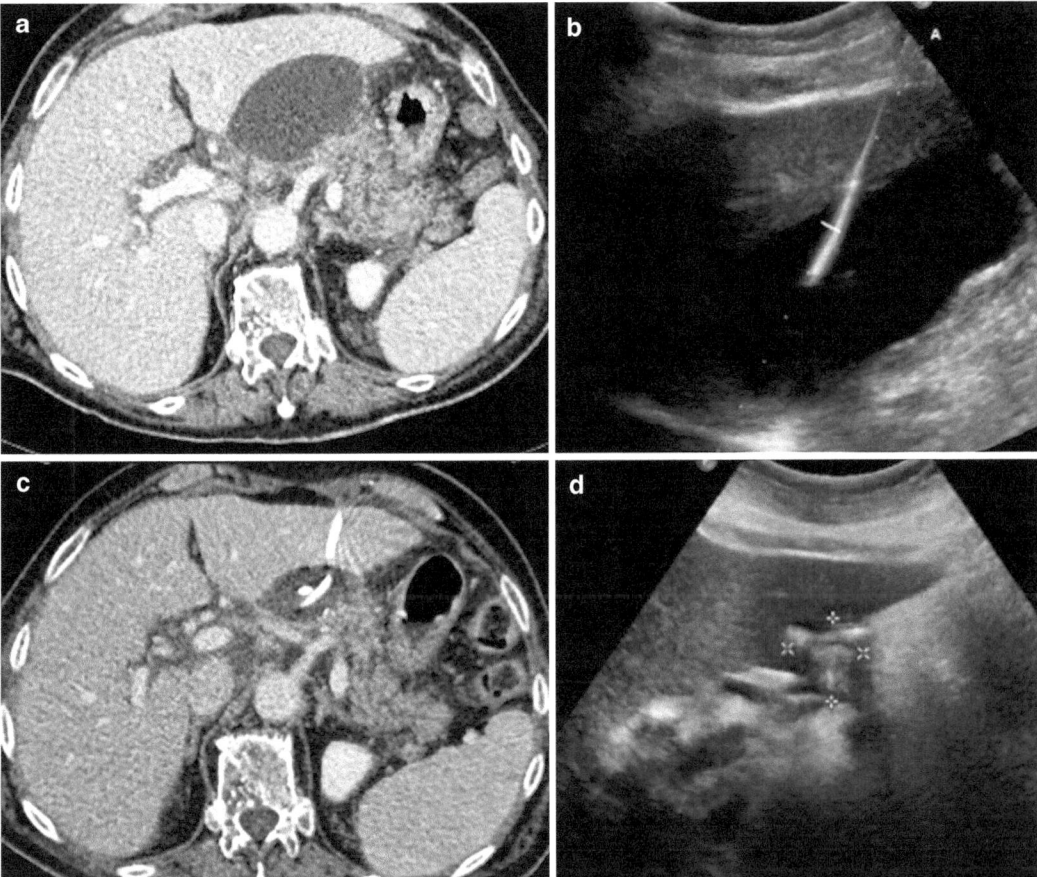

Fig. 17.1 (a–d) A 76-year-old woman after endoscopic retrograde cholangiopancreatography (ERCP) developed pancreatitis; a pseudocyst (PC) was observed during its evolution (a); a percutaneous drainage was deployed under ultrasound (US) guidance (b); CT scan performed after 15 days revealed shrinking of the PC (c); US performed after 28 days, before to remove drainage, confirmed further shrinking (d)

The first almost always occurs in the setting of a previously instrumented or manipulated biliary tree resulting from direct or enteric contamination of an obstructed system. Antibiotic therapy and "internal– external" drainage provides a minimally invasive treatment [7, 13].

In particular percutaneous drainage is indicated when medical therapy is ineffective or not enough. Excessive manipulation of catheters in the bile ducts should be avoided to reduce the risk of sepsis. In these patients, an external drain may be placed for 2–4 days to allow decompression and a course of antibiotic therapy to be administered before internal catheter placement is attempted [14].

Percutaneous drainage of a non-dilated biliary tree can be technically challenging (Fig. 17.2a, b).

The access to the biliary system is obtained by puncturing a peripheral bile duct under US and/or fluoroscopic guidance with conscious sedation. Peripheral access is preferred because the risk of bleeding and inadequate drainage rises with a central access. Classical teaching has been to approach the right hemiliver from the 11th intercostal space in the midaxillary line. A 22- or 21-gauge double-walled needle is advanced into the parenchyma of the liver. With the stylet removed, contrast may be gingerly injected while the needle is retracted until a bile duct is opacified. If the target duct is opacified, and the puncture is peripheral, it may be used for the drainage and the needle is exchanged for a coaxial system to upsize the system; a directional catheter is inserted and

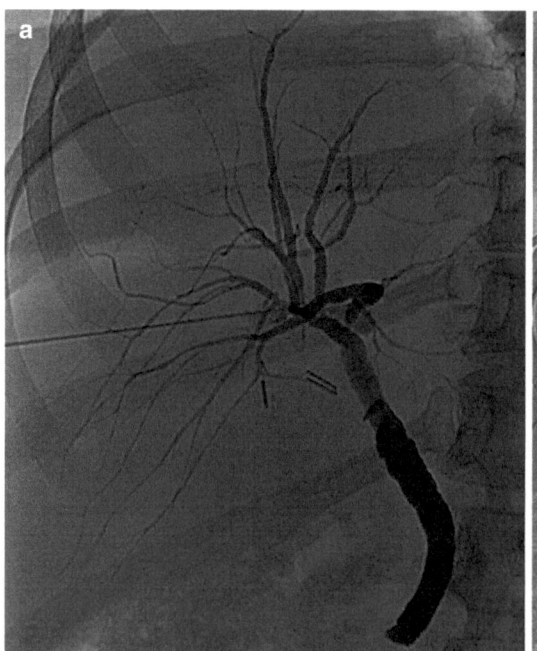 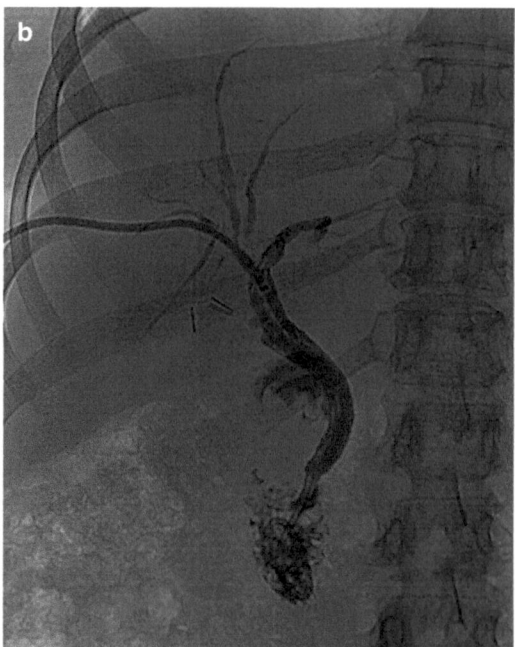

Fig. 17.2 (**a**, **b**) An endoscopic retrograde cholangiopancreatography (ERCP) to remove common bile duct stones was performed in a 56-year-old woman. The day after, the patient developed fever, leucocytosis and abdominal pain with increased transaminases. After 4 days of unsuccess- ful medical therapy, she was proposed for a percutaneous biliary drainage. The cholangiography revealed non-dilated intra-hepatic biliary ducts and mild dilatation of the common biliary duct related to the flogosis of the papilla (**a**); a biliary drainage was deployed (**b**)

advanced over a hydrophilic wire beyond the obstruction and into the small bowel. The catheter can then be exchanged over a stiffer wire for a multiside hole drainage catheter. This type of catheter is referred to as an "internal– external" catheter. A different and more recent technique is to use a covered stent that can close the bile leak and subsequently be retrieved percutaneously [11]. U-tube placement is a useful drainage tech- nique for the management of bile duct injuries requiring simultaneous biliary diversion and bili- ary drainage, such as common duct or hilar tran- section. A U-tube, which consists of a single straight drain with multiple side holes and two percutaneous exits, essentially serves the com- bined functions of a PTBD and a biloma drain [14]. A small rate of benign biliary strictures (BBS) is secondary to endoscopic sphincterot- omy, endoscopic injection sclerotherapy of duo- denal ulcer bleeding and even less due to post-cholangitis after ERCP [15].

Percutaneous approach is generally limited by the complication rates, discomfort due to long-standing indwelling catheters and high stricture recurrence rates. Still, the percutaneous approach can be useful in case of failure of ERCP for "rendezvous" techniques. ERCP for the treatment of BBS is preferred over surgery and the percutaneous approach due to its low invasiveness, because it is more patient friendly, safer and repeatable [15].

17.3 Angiographic Management of Bleeding and Pseudoaneurysm

Bleeding is another complication that can be encountered in digestive and biliopancreatic endos- copy. Its incidence has been variably reported in other studies, because of the difference in the defi- nition of bleeding. However, clinically significant bleedings have been reported to occur in 2–11 % of patients [16, 17].

Complication rates are manyfold higher for therapeutic procedures when compared to diagnostic ones. Transarterial embolisation (TAE) can be useful in case of haemorrhage which cannot be controlled endoscopically or in case of extraluminal bleeding. The major advantage of this method is that embolisation can be used to control bleeding sites observed on imaging [18].

17.3.1 Technique and Materials

Diagnostic angiography is most often performed only as a precursor to transarterial embolisation based on the knowledge of the vascular supply to the abnormal area. The initial artery catheterised is the one most suspected of bleeding based on previous imaging or endoscopy [7, 17].

A trans-femoral approach is usually used and involves placement of a 5F introducer sheath in the common femoral artery. A variety of introducers and selective catheters with a smaller calibre can be used to cannulate the artery that supplies bleeding. Once access is secured, arteriogram is performed to delineate the anatomy. Localisation of contrast extravasation is considered as a direct angiographic sign of active bleeding; other indirect angiographic signs that may be encountered are the visualisation of a pseudoaneurysm or an early venous drainage [19, 20]. Arteriography after superselective cannulation with a microcatheter may show extravasation that could have been missed during contrast injection in the main artery. Angiography can detect bleeding rates as low as approximately 0.5 ml/min and may be even more sensitive when using digital subtraction. Once the site of bleeding has been identified, several different techniques may be used to stop bleeding and achieve haemostasis. In case of terminal vascularisation, a proximal embolisation of the bleeding vessel may be enough to achieve the haemostasis, while in the presence of collaterals, it is crucial to embolise both the inflow and outflow vessels in order to avoid re-bleeding ("isolation technique") [7].

Many embolisation agents could be used in bleeding control: coils, vascular plugs, particulate material such as resorbable gelatin sponge and nonresorbable polyvinyl alcohol or trisacryl gelatin particles. Liquids such as N-butyl 2-cyanoacrylate glue or ethylene–vinyl alcohol copolymer are less popularly used. An advantage of coils is their ability to be picked up radiologically, and a size can be chosen to "fit" the required vessel. N-butyl 2-cyanoacrylate glue (NBCA) is a more recently developed liquid agent which has been tested successfully in several studies of lower GI bleeding. It is expensive and its use can be a technical challenge for those learning, but success rates seem to be high and ischaemic complications low. There is an additional advantage when compared with glue being easily visible fluoroscopically [21–24]. Recently, a liquid polyvinyl alcohol copolymer seems to have great potential in embolotherapy of acute arterial gastrointestinal bleeding [25].

Superselective arterial embolisation with a liquid polyvinyl alcohol copolymer in patients with acute gastrointestinal haemorrhage seems to be safe, in relation to its non-adhesiveness, progressive solidification and cohesiveness [26].

The choice of technique and embolic agents used anyway is conventionally dependent on the interventional radiologist's experience and preference, aetiology of bleeding and availability of the agent.

17.3.2 Management of Upper Gastrointestinal Bleeding (UGIB) After ERCP and Endoscopic Procedures and Pseudoaneurysm (PA) in Peripancreatic or Perihepatic Blood Vessels

UGIB after ERCP: Most ERCP-associated bleeding is intraluminal, although intraductal bleeding can occur and haematomas (hepatic, splenic and intra-abdominal) have been reported [27]. Haemorrhage is primarily a complication related to sphincterotomy rather than diagnostic ERCP

[28]. Haemorrhagic complications may be immediate or delayed, with recognition occurring up to 2 weeks after the procedure. The risk of severe haemorrhage (i.e. requiring >5 units of blood, surgery or angiography) is estimated to occur in fewer than 1 per 1000 sphincterotomies [29, 30]. Although sphincterotomy alone is a risk factor for haemorrhage, other factors identified in multivariate analysis include coagulopathy, the use of anticoagulants within 72 h of sphincterotomy, the presence of acute cholangitis or papillary stenosis, the use of precut sphincterotomy and low case volume of the endoscopist (i.e. one sphincterotomy per week or less) [16]. Observed bleeding during the initial examination is also predictive of delayed bleeding. Haemobilia is a rare cause of upper gastrointestinal bleeding (UGIB) that should be considered in the setting of recent hepatobiliary tree instrumentation, such as with endoscopic retrograde cholangiopancreatography. Bile duct and hepatic artery injuries are possible complications of this procedure, and patients can ultimately present with signs of UGIB. By skilled experienced hands, bleeding or haematoma associated with ERCP and involving the liver, spleen, intestinal wall or abdominal cavity turns out to be an extremely rare but potentially serious event which requires prompt recognition and treatment. Post-ERCP bleeding may either cease spontaneously or necessitate the use of endoscopic haemostatic techniques, such as epinephrine injection, balloon tamponade, electrocoagulation, argon plasma coagulation or hemoclip placement. Most often, bleeding originates from the edges of the sphincterotomy site; however, bleeding may also be consecutive to common bile duct (CBD) wall trauma. In this case, conventional endoscopic haemostatic techniques are inappropriate because they are only effective in treating bleeding originating from the duodenal papilla [31]. Most post-endoscopic sphincterotomy (post-ES) bleedings stop spontaneously, but significant bleeding may occur during the procedure or several days later. This type of bleeding is rarely encountered by interventional radiologists, unlike other nonvariceal upper gastrointestinal bleeding, because various haemostatic procedures are performed simultaneously or repeatedly during the endoscopic procedure. These endoscopic procedures or combined endoscopic therapies are considered to be the treatments of choice and have high success rates. However, in cases of endoscopic haemostasis failure caused by massive bleeding or technical failure, radiologic or surgical hemostasis may be required (Fig. 17.3a–f) [32–34].

The papillary artery originates from the communicating artery which connects the posterior superior pancreaticoduodenal artery (PSPDA) and the anterior superior pancreaticoduodenal artery (ASPDA), or directly from the posterior pancreaticoduodenal artery as a vasa recta type. According to previous reports, since the duodenum has a rich vascular network, rebleeding after embolisation is common when the embolisation has been performed incompletely or coagulopathy has existed [35, 36]. On the other hand, embolisation may cause ischaemic complications of the duodenum when the gastroduodenal artery is embolised or the patient has had surgically altered anatomy. Therefore, selective embolisation of bleeding branch for post-ES bleeding is required to reduce rebleeding or ischaemic complication related to embolisation [17, 35, 36]. The pancreaticoduodenal artery is a short vascular arcade between the celiac trunk and the SMA, and flow in this vascular segment is highly susceptible to pressure-gradient changes. Embolising under the principle of proximal and distal embolisation of the bleeding vessel is especially important during the embolisation of vessels with a direct collateral channel like the pancreaticoduodenal artery. The aim is to embolise the bleeding branch as selectively as possible to avoid duodenal ischaemia. Rebleeding from the same branch which was previously embolised can occur. In this case, a second embolisation can be performed. Different materials can be used to embolise like microcoils, NBCA (n-butyl cyanoacrylate) or Gelfoam particles [17].

UGIB and endoscopic procedures: Clinically significant bleeding is a rare adverse event of diagnostic UGI endoscopy [1]. Mallory-Weiss tears occur in less than 0.5 % of diagnostic UGI endoscopic procedures and usually are not associated with significant bleeding [37]. Bleeding

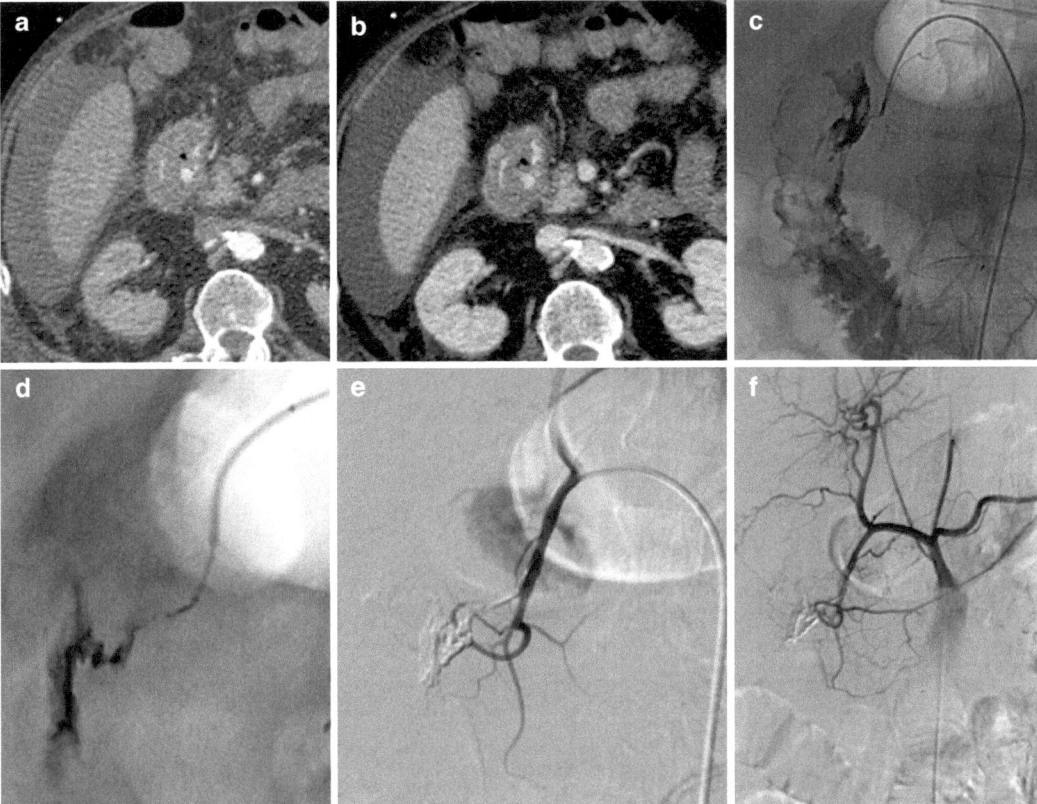

Fig. 17.3 (**a–f**) Massive UGIB due to a peptic ulcer in a 48-year-old man. After therapeutic gastroscopy, the bleeding persists and the patient was unstable. A CT was requested to rule out underlying problems (**a**, **b**). An urgent arteriography (**c**) was performed and embolisation which was done with ethylene–vinyl alcohol copolymer was performed (**d**). Final selective (**e**) and non-selective (**f**) angiography revealed complete embolisation

may be more likely in individuals with thrombo-cytopenia and/or coagulopathy. The minimum threshold platelet count for the performance of diagnostic UGI endoscopy has not been estab-lished [1]. Diagnostic endoscopy may induce bleeding from iatrogenic Mallory-Weiss tears and endoscopic biopsies. Bleeding from endo-scopic biopsies is rarely clinically significant. Therapeutic procedures, such as sclerotherapy or gastroduodenal polypectomy, have much higher bleeding complication rates. For example, bleed-ing complications from gastroduodenal polypec-tomies have been reported to occur in 0.2–8 %. Bleeding from polypectomy may be immediate as a result of inadequate coagulation or delayed for several days because of ulceration at the pol-ypectomy site. Upper gastrointestinal endoscopy rarely causes mesenteric vascular shearing and intraperitoneal bleeding from stretch and torque of the intestine [38]. The risk of inducing haem-orrhage is decreased by a meticulous endoscopic technique.

Haemorrhage from endoscopy may be imme-diate or delayed. Bleeding from endoscopy is classified as immediate when observed during (or appreciated within 1 h after) endoscopy or as delayed when first noted (>1 h) after endoscopy. Delayed bleeding is classified as early when observed within 24 h after endoscopy or as late when observed more than 24 h after endoscopy. Bleeding is classified as minor when haemody-namically insignificant, when not requiring transfusion of packed erythrocytes and when accompanied by a haematocrit decline of less than 4 %. Bleeding is classified as significant (moderate) when haemodynamically significant, when requiring transfusion of 1 unit of packed erythrocytes or when accompanied by a haematocrit decline greater than 4 %. Bleeding is classified as major when requiring transfusion of more than 1 unit of packed erythrocytes, when requiring surgery or angiographic intervention or when resulting in medical complications, such as myocardial infarction or acute tubular necrosis. Immediate haemorrhage should be immediately treated by endoscopic haemostatic therapy, including injection therapy, thermocoagulation or electrocoagulation. Delayed haemorrhage generally requires repeat endoscopy for diagnosis and therapy, using the same haemostatic techniques [38]. Diagnostic angiography for UGIB is centred on the anatomy of the celiac artery and the SMA. Blind or empiric is defined as embolisation without angiographic proof of extravasation and is typically guided by endoscopic information regarding the location of the bleeding vessel. Coils and gelatin sponge are then often used in such a situation [19, 36].

Pseudoaneurysm (PA) in peripancreatic or perihepatic blood vessels as a complication of pancreatic pseudocysts or in the setting of recent hepatobiliary tree instrumentation, respectively, may be responsible for UGIB. Recently, transarterial embolisation has generated considerable interest as the first-line therapeutic method for PAs (Fig. 17.4a–d). The success rate is high, ranging from 62 to 100 % in visceral PAs and the morbidity and mortality rates are low [19, 39]. Most investigators agree that coils are the most appropriate embolic material [36, 39]. However, the traditional technique for PA embolisation includes isolating the lesion by deploying coils in the parent artery, covering both sides of the PA neck to prevent back bleeding via collaterals (sandwich technique). Embolisation of PAs using a combination of gelatin sponge and coils, NBCA and coils, coils alone or NBCA has also been described [39, 40]. The main drawback of these techniques is the compromised patency of the parent vessel with potential ischaemic complications. Modification of the embolisation technique can help to preserve the patency of parent artery while achieving complete embolisation. Superselective arterial embolisation is achieved by three-dimensional coil packing of the PA sac using controlled, detachable microcoils placed in a concentric fashion.

17.3.3 Management of Lower Gastrointestinal Bleeding (LGIB)

Colonoscopic polypectomy causes bleeding much more frequently than diagnostic colonscopy. The bleeding can be intraluminal or extraluminal. Intraluminal haemorrhage after optical colonscopy is well documented and is the most frequent complication. It can occur in 1–2 % of therapeutic colonscopies. This may occur from inadequate coagulation after transection of a pedunculated polyp, but large sessile polyps (>1 cm) have the greatest risk for acute haemorrhage, which may be attributed to inadequate heat seal of the blood supply after tissue transaction [41]. Intraluminal haemorrhage is usually evident and can be treated using endoscopy by resnaring techniques or by injecting epinephrine at the bleeding site. Endoscopic hemoclips may also be used. Extraluminal haemorrhage is unusual and may occur as a result of peri-intestinal blood vessel injury during polyp coagulation. It may manifest as free bleeding into the peritoneal space or as bleeding into the retroperitoneal space when it involves the retroperitoneal portions of the ascending and descending colon. Such instances of haemorrhage can result from mechanisms of excessive force and possible weakness of the colonic wall. This is an uncommon complication for which a high clinical suspicion is also necessary. TAE can be useful in case of haemorrhage which cannot be controlled endoscopically or in case of extraluminal bleeding (Fig. 17.5a–c).

Diagnostic angiography for lower gastrointestinal bleeding (LGIB) is centred on the anatomy of the SMA and IMA [42]. If bleeding appears to originate in the proximal colon, the SMA is initially evaluated. If bleeding appears to originate in the distal colon, the IMA is selected [42]. When a bleeding site is identified, the aim is "superselective embolisation", i.e. of a target vessel as close as possible to the site of

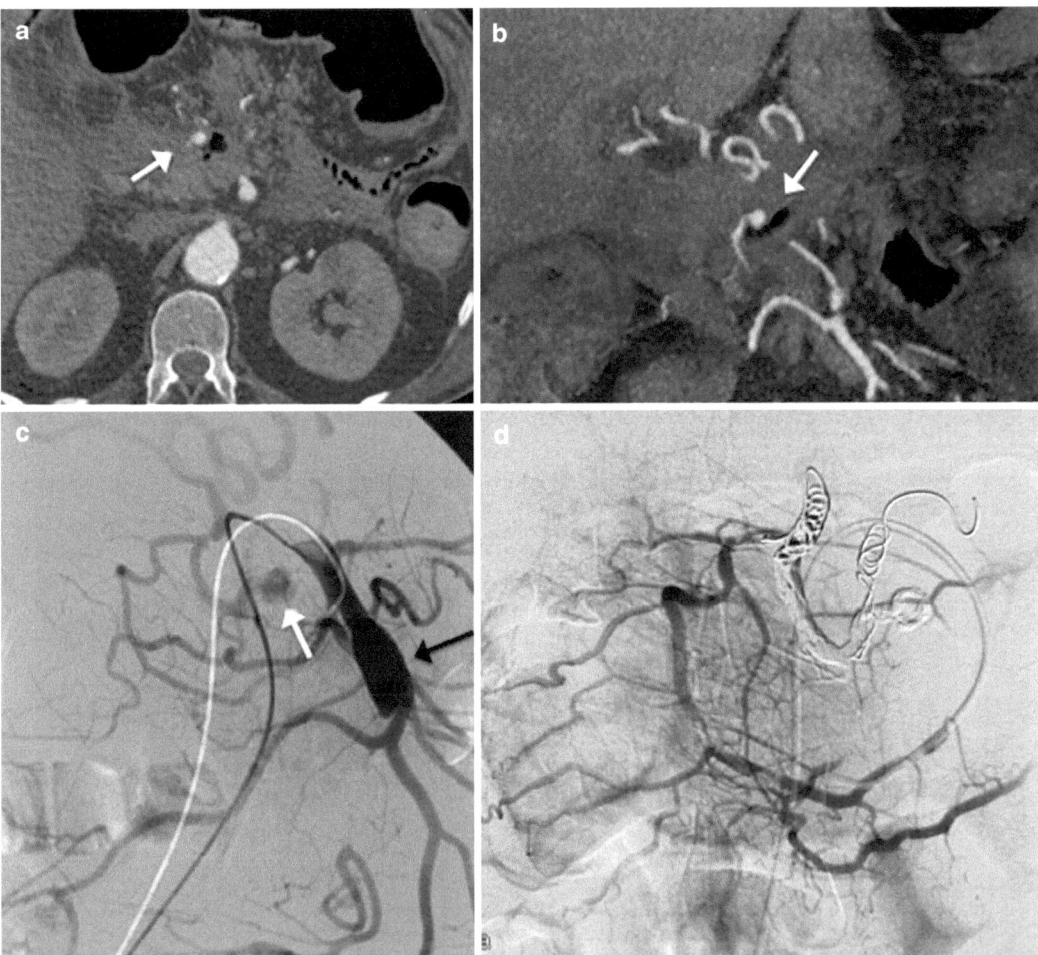

Fig. 17.4 (**a–d**) Post-pancreatitis saccular pseudoaneurysm (PSA) in the pancreaticoduodenal arcade: CT (**a**, **b**, *arrow*) finding. Angiography confirmed the PSA (**c**, *white arrow*); also a fusiform aneurysm of the superior mesenteric artery was detected (*black arrow*). Final angiogram performed after embolisation with coils showed complete embolisation (**d**)

bleeding (Fig. 17.6a–e). This is particularly important because occlusion of a distal supply should only be of vessels supplying a small segment of bowel to minimise the risk of bowel ischaemia [43]. Embolisation to treat LGIB has been performed with gelatin sponges, particles, coils and microcoils and, more recently, glue [44]. There are no guidelines for the choice of embolic material used, and the final decision is specific to each case. The most commonly used embolic material is 0.018-in. pushable microcoils. The efficacy of embolisation depends on a combination of bleeding site occlusion, the patient's clot-forming ability and local vasospasm. The main concern with embolic agents is rebleeding and the risk of secondary bowel ischaemia. The efficacy of microcoils, gelatin sponges and particles is dependent on a normal coagulation status, and the rate of clinical failure after embolisation is higher when the patient has coagulopathy. Glue has a high haemostatic effect with a low recurrent bleeding rate, but vascular glue penetration can be difficult to control and requires considerable experience [45]. Ethylene–vinyl alcohol copolymer (Onyx Liquid Embolic System; ev3 Neurovascular, Irvine, California)

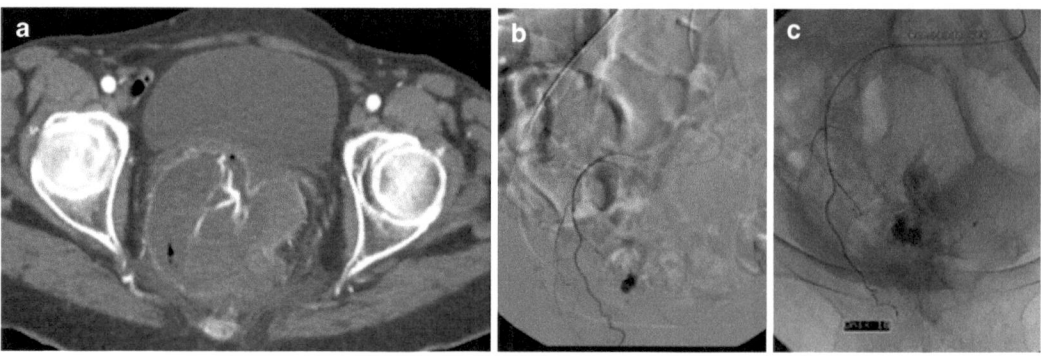

Fig. 17.5 (**a–c**) Massive rectal bleeding after polypectomy in an old man: CT scan showed active bleeding (**a**); an urgent embolisation (**b**) and selective embolisation with polyvinyl alcohol copolymer (**c**) were performed

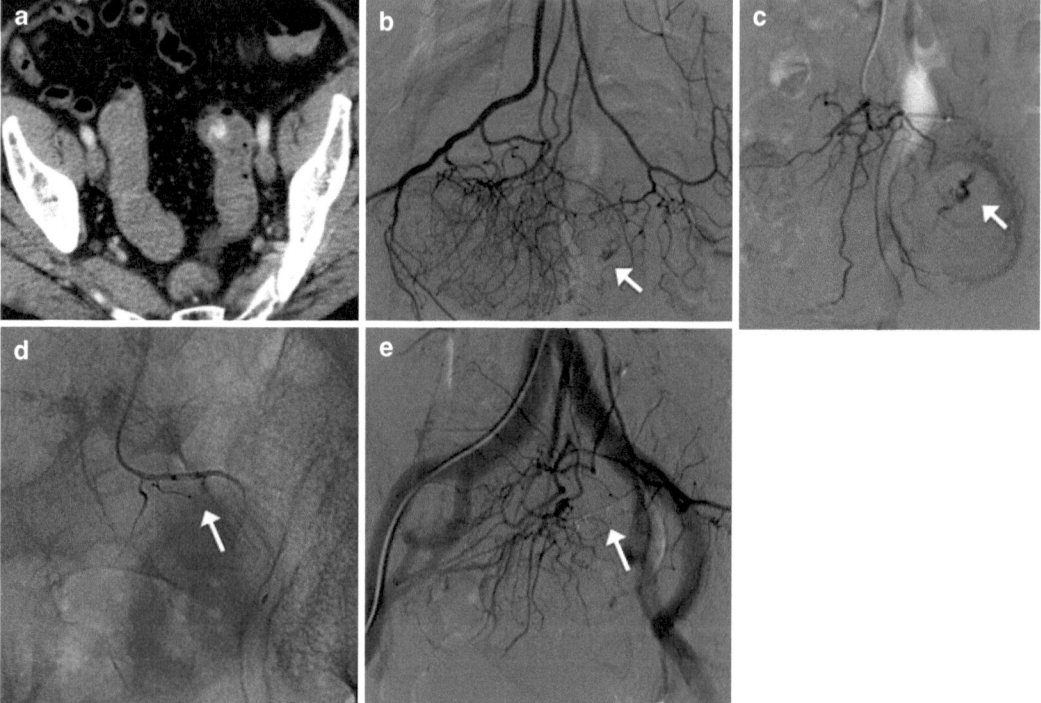

Fig. 17.6 (**a–e**) An endoscopic sigmoidal polypectomy was performed in a 69-year-old woman. Three days later, a massive LGIB was observed: bleeding site was diagnosed with CT (**a**); angiography of the inferior mesenteric artery (IMA) was performed (**b**); selective (**c**) branches of the IMA were catheterised, and superselective embolisation with polyvinyl alcohol copolymer (**d**, *arrow*) was performed; final non-selective angiogram confirmed complete embolisation (**e**)

is a liquid embolic agent that has some theoretical advantages owing to its controlled delivery injection, nonadhesive nature, high radiopacity and high haemostasis effect [46].

Moreover, onyx seems to be particularly useful in tortuous or rigid vessels, where it is occasionally impossible to deploy microcoils as selectively as would be desirable [46]. Furthermore, modern tools available in high-flow interventional radiology centres permit to identify and to reach the bleeding site faster than when only the two-dimensional angiography is applied. On the basis of the data reported by Iwazawa and Carrafiello, the use of angiographic CBCT and automatic vessel detection software during embolisation of arterial bleedings can improve operator confidence with embolisation techniques in emergency settings, reduce overall procedural time and total contrast media administration and ultimately have an impact on treatment outcome [47, 48].

17.3.4 Splenic Injury

An unusual but under-recognised and serious complication of optical colonoscopy is splenic laceration or rupture. The mechanism by which laceration occurs may be direct trauma leading to partial capsular avulsion as a result of colonoscopic manoeuvres. Protracted direct compression on the spleen by the colonoscope may be more likely to develop in patients with an acutely angled splenic flexure. Stretching of the colon during optical colonoscopy with consequent excessive traction or torsion on the phrenicocolic ligament is another likely precipitating cause. Splenic injuries also may be facilitated by adhesions from prior surgery, previous pancreatitis or inflammatory bowel disease. This complication is also seen more often in women and where the colonoscopic procedure is reported to have been technically difficult. All of these factors can contribute to splenic injury, leading to subcapsular haematoma development or capsular rupture with subsequent free intraperitoneal haemorrhage. A high clinical suspicion is required for the prompt diagnosis of this rare but serious and occasionally fatal complication. In case of active bleeding identified at CT examination, percutaneous trans-arterial embolisation has a role in the treatment of these patients (Fig. 17.7a–c) [49–51].

If arterial extravasation was seen on celiac arteriography, selective splenic artery catheterisation is attempted for embolisation by using stainless steel coils, gelatine particles or a combination of both. Splenic artery embolisation could be distal (selective), proximal (splenic artery) or combined [52]. As a rule, proximal SAE is indicated in hilar lesions, distant or selective SAE for limited vascular injuries and combined SAE for

multiple vascular injuries. By decreasing the blood flow and intrasplenic pressure, haemostasis could be obtained; the viability of the remaining spleen is ensured by collateral blood flow.

17.3.5 Post-endoscopic Ultrasound and Fine-Needle Aspiration (EUS-FNA) Bleeding

Overall, haemorrhagic complications from EUS-FNA appear to be infrequent and largely self-limited. A small amount of luminal bleeding is often present endoscopically at FNA puncture sites, but generally is without clinical sequelae. Extraluminal bleeding is rare, as endosonographers can avoid visible vessels detected by colour flow Doppler [53].

17.3.6 Post-percutaneous Endoscopic Gastrostomy (PEG) Bleeding

Haemorrhage is an uncommon complication after PEG, with a reported incidence of 0.2–2.5 % [54]. The most common cause of bleeding is erosion or ulceration of the gastric wall at the stoma. The ulceration is ascribed to pressure necrosis at the gastric stoma from excess bumper traction or mucosal abrasion from bumper friction. Another source of bleeding is cutaneous bleeding that can occur from trauma to a large vessel in the abdominal wall during trans-abdominal puncture. Cirrhotics are at increased risk for this bleeding because of formation of large, high-pressure veins on the abdominal skin from portosystemic shunting and their frequent mild coagulopathy. Oesophageal trauma during passage of the guidewire or PEG passage through tight benign or malignant oesophageal strictures may cause mucosal shearing and bleeding [38]. The onset of UGIB following percutaneous endoscopic gastrostomy tube placement may be delayed. Transcatheter embolisation is a highly effective technique for treatment. In view of the multiple sources of arterial supply to the stomach, including the left gastric, right gastric, short gastric and

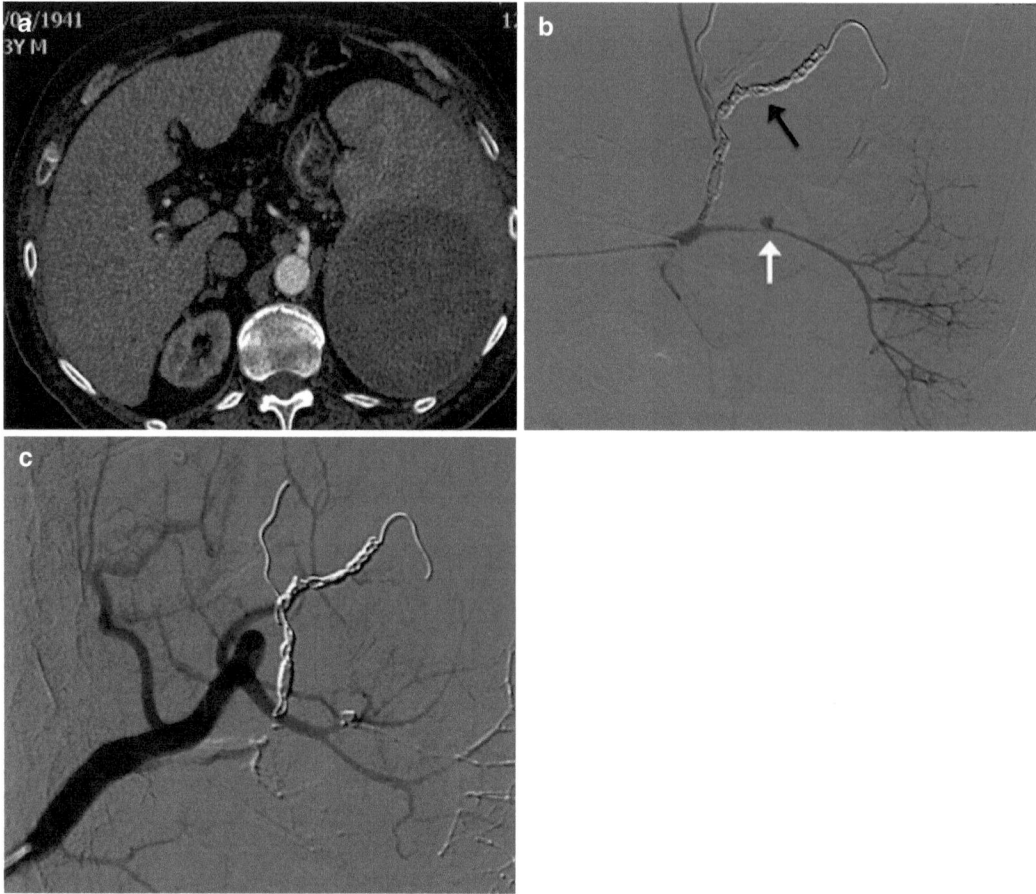

Fig. 17.7 (**a–c**) Subcapsular splenic haematoma in a 73-year-old man with left flank pain and anemisation were observed 8 h after diagnostic coloscopy (**a**); nonselective embolisation (**b**, *black arrow*) with coils and selective embolisation of a pseudoaneurysm with polyvinyl alcohol copolymer (**b**, *white arrow*) was performed; final angiogram (**c**) showed complete embolisation of the area of the haematoma

gastroduodenal artery and the right and left gastroepiploic arteries, gastric ischaemia usually does not represent a problem [55]. Singh et al. retrospectively evaluated 1541 PEG patients and found directly attributed to PEG bleeding in six cases (0.4 %) [56]. In literature only few cases are reported of bleeding after PEG managed with transarterial embolisation [55–57]. Techniques and materials for embolisation have already been explained in the previous paragraphs.

Conclusions

Interventional radiology plays an increasing, crucial role in the multidisciplinary management of complications after digestive and biliopancreatic endoscopy with the known advantages of a minimally invasive therapy in particular in critical patients, with correlated reduction of recovery time and avoiding surgery morbidity.

The Interventional radiology procedures described may be considered consolidated, safe and effective techniques.

References

1. ASGE Standards of Practice Committee, Ben-Menachem T, Decker GA, Early DS, Evans J, Fanelli RD, Fisher DA, Fisher L, Fukami N, Hwang JH, Ikenberry SO, Jain R, Jue TL, Khan KM, Krinsky ML, Malpas PM, Maple JT, Sharaf RN, Dominitz JA, Cash BD (2012) Adverse events of upper GI endoscopy. Gastrointest Endosc 76:707–718

2. Zerem E, Hauser G, Loga-Zec S et al (2015) Minimally invasive treatment of pancreatic pseudocysts. World J Gastroenterol 21(22):6850–6860
3. Cheruvu CV, Clarke MG, Prentice M et al (2003) Conservative treatment as an option in the management of pancreatic pseudocyst. Ann R Coll Surg Engl 85:313–316
4. Bhattacharya D, Ammori BJ (2003) Minimally invasive approaches to the management of pancreatic pseudocysts: review of the literature. Surg Laparosc Endosc Percutan Tech 13:141–148
5. Zerem E, Imamović G, Omerović S et al (2010) Percutaneous treatment for symptomatic pancreatic pseudocysts: long-term results in a single center. Eur J Intern Med 21:393–397
6. ASGE Standards of Practice Committee, Fisher DA, Maple JT, Ben-Menachem T, Cash BD, Decker GA, Early DS, Evans JA, Fanelli RD, Fukami N, Hwang JH, Jain R, Jue TL, Khan KM, Malpas PM, Sharaf RN, Shergill AK, Dominitz JA (2011) Complications of colonoscopy. Gastrointest Endosc 74:745–752
7. Mauri G, Mattiuz C, Sconfienza LM, Pedicini V, Poretti D, Melchiorre F, Rossi U, Lutman FR, Montorsi M (2015) Role of interventional radiology in the management of complications after pancreatic surgery: a pictorial review. Insights Imaging 6:231–239
8. Pitchumoni CS, Agarwal N (1999) Pancreatic pseudocysts. When and how should drainage be performed? Gastroenterol Clin North Am 28:615–639
9. Loperfido S, Angelini G, Benedetti G et al (1998) Major early complications from diagnostic and therapeutic ERCP: a prospective multicenter study. Gastrointest Endosc 48:1–10
10. Jones WB, Blackwell J, McKinley B, Trocha S (2014) What is the risk of diagnostic endoscopic retrograde cholangiopancreatography before cholecystectomy? Am Surg 80:746–751
11. Covey AM, Brown KT (2008) Percutaneous transhepatic biliary drainage. Tech Vasc Interv Radiol 11(1):14–20
12. Lorenz JM, Al-Refaie WB, Cash BD et al (2015) ACR appropriateness criteria radiologic management of infected fluid collections. J Am Coll Radiol 12(8):791–799
13. Burke DR, Lewis CA, Cardella JF et al (2003) Quality improvement guidelines for percutaneous transhepatic cholangiography and biliary drainage. J Vasc Interv Radiol 14(9 Pt 2):S243–S246
14. Thompson CM, Saad NE, Quazi RR et al (2013) Management of iatrogenic bile duct injuries: role of the interventional radiologist. RadioGraphics 33:117–134
15. Costamagna G, Boškoski I (2013) Current treatment of benign biliary strictures. Ann Gastroenterol 26(1):37–40
16. Freeman ML, Neslon DB, Sherman S et al (1996) Complications of endoscopic biliary sphincterotomy. N Engl J Med 335:909–918
17. So YH, Choi YH, Chung JW, Jae HJ, Song SY, Park JH (2012) Selective embolization for post-endoscopic sphincterotomy bleeding: technical aspects and clinical efficacy. Korean J Radiol 13:73–81
18. Tonolini M, Pagani A, Bianco R (2015) Cross-sectional imaging of common and unusual complications after endoscopic retrograde cholangiopancreatography. Insights Imaging 6:323–338
19. Loffroy RF, Abualsaud BA, Lin MD, Rao PP (2011) Recent advances in endovascular techniques for management of acute nonvariceal upper gastrointestinal bleeding. World J Gastrointest Surg 3:89–100
20. Miller M, Smith TP (2005) Angiographic diagnosis and endovascular management of nonvariceal gastrointestinal hemorrhage. Gastroenterol Clin North Am 34:735–752
21. Moss AJ, Tuffaha H, Malik A (2016) Lower GI bleeding: a review of current management, controversies and advances. Int J Colorectal Dis 31(2):175–188
22. Ramaswamy RS, Choi HW, Mouser HC, Narsinh KH, McCammack KC, Treesit T, Kinney TB (2014) Role of interventional radiology in the management of acute gastrointestinal bleeding. World J Radiol 6(4):82–92
23. Lubarsky M, Ray C, Funaki B (2010) Embolization agents-which one should be used when? Part 2: small-vessel embolization. Semin Interv Radiol 27(1):99–104
24. Yata S, Ihaya T, Kaminou T, Ohuchi Y, Hashimoto M, Umekita Y, Ogawa T (2013) Transcatheter arterial embolization of acute arterial bleeding in the upper and lower gastrointestinal tract with N-butyl-2-cyanoacrylate. J Vasc Interv Radiol 24(3):422–431
25. Lenhart M, Paetzel C, Sackmann M et al (2010) Superselective arterial embolisation with a liquid polyvinyl alcohol copolymer in patients with acute gastrointestinal haemorrhage. Eur Radiol 20(8):1994–1999
26. Kolber MK, Shukla PA, Kumar A et al (2015) Ethylene vinyl alcohol copolymer (onyx) embolization for acute hemorrhage: a systematic review of peripheral applications. J Vasc Interv Radiol 26(6):809–815
27. ASGE Standards of Practice Committee, Anderson MA, Fisher L, Jain R, Evans JA, Appalaneni V, Ben-Menachem T, Cash BD, Decker GA, Early DS, Fanelli RD, Fisher DA, Fukami N, Hwang JH, Ikenberry SO, Jue TL, Khan KM, Krinsky ML, Malpas PM, Maple JT, Sharaf RN, Shergill AK, Dominitz JA (2012) Complications of ERCP. Gastrointest Endosc 75(3):467–473
28. Andriulli A, Loperfido S, Napolitano G et al (2007) Incidence rates of post-ERCP complications: a systematic survey of prospective studies. Am J Gastroenterol 102:1781–1788
29. Freeman ML (2003) Adverse outcomes of endoscopic retrograde cholangiopancreatography: avoidance and management. Gastrointest Endos Clin N Am 13:775–798, xi
30. Ferreira LE, Baron TH (2007) Post-sphincterotomy bleeding: who, what, when, and how. Am J Gastroenterol 102:2850–2858
31. Valats JC, Funakoshi N, Bauret P et al (2013) Covered self-expandable biliary stents for the treatment of bleeding after ERCP. Gastrointest Endosc 78(1):183–187

32. Muhldorfer SM, Kekos G, Hahn EG et al (1992) Complications of therapeutic gastrointestinal endoscopy. Endoscopy 24:276–283

33. Kim HJ, Kim MH, Kim DI et al (1999) Endoscopic hemostasis in sphincterotomy-induced hemorrhage: its efficacy and safety. Endoscopy 31:431–436

34. Sherman S, Hawes RH, Nisi R et al (1992) Endoscopic sphincterotomy induced hemorrhage: treatment with multipolar electrocoagulation. Gastrointest Endosc 38:123–126

35. Poultsides GA, Kim CJ, Orlando R 3rd, Peros G, Hallisey MJ, Vignati PV (2008) Angiographic embolization for gastroduodenal hemorrhage: safety, efficacy, and predictors of outcome. Arch Surg 143:457–461

36. Loffroy R, Guiu B, Cercueil JP, Lepage C, Latournerie M, Hillon P et al (2008) Refractory bleeding from gastroduodenal ulcers: arterial embolization in high-operative-risk patients. J Clin Gastroenterol 42:361–367

37. Montalvo RD, Lee M (1996) Retrospective analysis of iatrogenic Mallory-Weiss tears occurring during upper gastrointestinal endoscopy. Hepatogastroenterology 43:174–177

38. Cappell MS, Abdullah M (2000) Management of gastrointestinal bleeding induced by gastrointestinal endoscopy. Gastroenterol Clin North Am 29:125–167

39. Lau KY, Wong TP, Wong WW, Chan JK, Kan WK, Chan YF, Lee AS (2005) Transcatheter embolisation of visceral pseudoaneurysms – technical difficulties and modification of embolisation technique. Eur J Vasc Endovasc Surg 30:133–136

40. Tokuda T, Tanigawa N, Shomura Y, Kariya S, Kojima H, Komemushi A, Shiraishi T, Sawada S (2009) Transcatheter embolization for peripheral pseudoaneurysms with n-butyl cyanoacrylate. Minim Invasive Ther Allied Technol 18:361–365

41. MacRae FA, Tank KG, Williams CB (1983) Toward safer colonoscopy: a report on the complications of 5000 diagnostic or therapeutic colonoscopies. Gut 24:37–383

42. Walker TG, Salazar GM, Waltman AC (2012) Angiographic evaluation and management of acute gastrointestinal hemorrhage. World J Gastroenterol 18:1191–1201

43. Funaki B, Kostelic JK, Lorenz J, Ha TV, Yip DL, Rosenblum JD, Leef JA, Straus C, Zaleski GX (2001) Superselective microcoil embolization of colonic hemorrhage. AJR Am J Roentgenol 177(4):829–836

44. Hur S, Jae HJ, Lee M, Kim HC, Chung JW (2014) Safety and efficacy of transcatheter arterial embolization for lower gastrointestinal bleeding: a single-center experience with 112 patients. J Vasc Interv Radiol 25:10–19

45. Navuluri R, Kang L, Patel J, Van Ha T (2012) Acute lower gastrointestinal bleeding. Semin Intervent Radiol 29:178–186

46. Urbano J, Manuel Cabrera J, Franco A et al (2014) Selective arterial embolization with ethylene-vinyl alcohol copolymer for control of massive lower gastrointestinal bleeding: feasibility and initial experience. J Vasc Interv Radiol 25:839–846

47. Iwazawa J, Ohueo S, Hashimoto N, Mitani T (2014) Feasibility of using vessel-detection software for the endovascular treatment of visceral arterial bleeding. Diagn Interv Radiol 20:160–163

48. Carrafiello G, Ierardi AM, Duka E et al (2015) Usefulness of cone-beam computed tomography and automatic vessel detection software in emergency transarterial embolization. Cardiovasc Intervent Radiol. doi:10.1007/s00270-015-1213-1

49. Daly B, Lu M, Pickhardt PJ, Menias CO, Abbas MA, Katz DS (2014) Complications of optical colonoscopy: CT findings. Radiol Clin North Am 52:1087–1099

50. Fishback SJ, Pickhardt PJ, Bhalla S et al (2011) Delayed presentation of splenic rupture following optical colonoscopy: clinical and CT findings. Emerg Radiol 18:539–544

51. Holzer K, Thalhammer A, Bechstein WO (2004) Splenic trauma: a rare complication during optical colonoscopy. J Gastroenterol 42:509–512

52. Sclafani SJ, Shaftan GW, Scalea TM et al (1995) Nonoperative salvage of computed tomography diagnosed splenic injuries: utilization of angiography for triage and embolization for hemostasis. J Trauma 39(5):818–825

53. Ho S (2008) Risks of endoscopic ultrasound and endoscopic ultrasound-guided fine-needle aspiration. Tech Gastrointest Endosc 10:22–24

54. Chung RS, Schertzer M (1990) Pathogenesis of complications of percutaneous gastrostomy. Am Surg 56:134–137

55. Lewis MB, Lewis JH, Marshall H et al (1999) Massive hemorrhage complicating percutaneous endoscopic gastrostomy: treatment by means of transcatheter embolization of the right and left gastroepiploic arteries. J Vasc Interv Radiol 10:319–323

56. Singh D, Laya AS, Vaidya OU, Ahmed SA, Bonham AJ, Clarkston WK (2012) Risk of bleeding after percutaneous endoscopic gastrostomy (PEG). Dig Dis Sci 57:973–980

57. Shigoka H, Maetani I, Saito M (2013) Pseudoaneurysm developed after percutaneous endoscopic gastrostomy: a report of two cases. Eur J Gastroenterol Hepatol 25:1484–1487

Index

© Springer International Publishing Switzerland 2016
M. Tonolini (ed.), *Imaging Complications of Gastrointestinal and Biliopancreatic Endoscopy
Procedures*, DOI 10.1007/978-3-319-31211-8